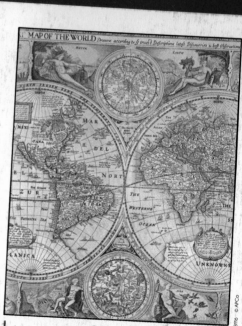

Regional Anesthesia

An Atlas of Anatomy and Techniques

Regional Anesthesia

An Atlas of Anatomy and Techniques

Marc B. Hahn, D.O.

*Director of the Pain Management
and Palliative Care Center
The Milton S. Hershey Medical Center;
Associate Professor, Department of Anesthesia
The Pennsylvania State University College of Medicine
Hershey, Pennsylvania*

Patrick M. McQuillan, M.D.

*Assistant Professor, Department of Anesthesia
The Pennsylvania State University College of Medicine
Hershey, Pennsylvania*

George J. Sheplock, M.D.

*Assistant Professor, Department of Anesthesia
Indiana University School of Medicine;
Staff Anesthesiologist, Riley Hospital for Children
Indianapolis, Indiana;
Center Associate, Center for Excellence in Education
Indiana University
Bloomington, Indiana*

■

with 304 illustrations

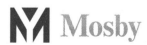

St. Louis Baltimore Boston Carlsbad Chicago Naples New York Philadelphia Portland
London Madrid Mexico City Singapore Sydney Tokyo Toronto Wiesbaden

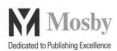

Mosby
Dedicated to Publishing Excellence

A Times Mirror
Company

Editor-in-Chief: Susan M. Gay
Senior Editor: Laurel Craven
Developmental Editor: Sandra Clark Brown
Project Manager: Dana Peick
Production Editor: Cindy Deichmann
Manufacturing Supervisor: Betty Richmond
Book Designer: Amy Buxton
Electronic Production Coordinator: Chris Robinson

The processes and development of x-ray images and other computer-enhanced images were based on previous original work by George J. Sheplock, M.D.

Printed in the United States of America

Composition by Mosby Electronic Production
Illustration preparation by Black Dot
Printing/binding by Von Hoffman Press
Mosby–Year Book, Inc.
11830 Westline Industrial Drive
St. Louis, MO 63146

Library of Congress Cataloging-in-Publication Data
Regional anesthesia : an atlas of anatomy and techniques / [edited by]
    Marc B. Hahn, Patrick M. McQuillan, George J. Sheplock.
        p. cm.
    Includes index.
    ISBN 0-8151-4121-1 (hardcover)
    1. Conduction anesthesia—Atlases. I. Hahn, Marc B.
II. McQuillan, Patrick M. III. Sheplock, George J.
    [DNLM: 1. Anesthesia, Local—methods—atlases. 2. Anatomy,
Regional—atlases. WO 517 R336 1995]
RD84.R4223 1995
617.9'64—dc20
DNLM/DLC
for Library of Congress   95-31275
                                                              CIP

96 97 98 99 00 / 9 8 7 6 5 4 3 2

CONTRIBUTORS

Marshall D. Bedder, M.D.
Director, Advanced Pain Management
  Group
Providence St. Vincent Hospital and
  Medical Center
Portland, Oregon

Jon W. Blank, M.D.
Staff Anesthesiologist
Raleigh Anesthesia Associates
Carolina Pain Consultants
Raleigh, North Carolina

Lynn M. Broadman, M.D.
Professor of Anaesthesia and Pediatrics
Director, Pain Management Center
West Virginia University
Morgantown, West Virginia

Kenneth Drasner, M.D.
Associate Professor
Department of Anesthesia
University of California—San Francisco
San Francisco, California

Marc B. Hahn, D.O.
Director of the Pain Management and
  Palliative Care Center
The Milton S. Hershey Medical Center;
Associate Professor
Department of Anesthesia
The Pennsylvania State University
  College of Medicine
Hershey, Pennsylvania

Robert C. Hamilton, M.B., B.Ch.,
  F.R.C.P.C.
Clinical Professor
Department of Anaesthesia
The University of Calgary;
Senior Anaesthesiologist
Gimbel Eye Centre
Calgary, Alberta, Canada

Quinn Hogan, M.D.
Associate Professor of Anesthesiology
Medical College of Wisconsin;
Director, Pain Management Center
Milwaukee County Medical Complex
Milwaukee, Wisconsin

Cynthia H. Kahn, M.D.
Director, Clinical Pain Research
Department of Anesthesia
Beth Israel Hospital
Boston, Massachusetts

John C. Keifer, M.D.
Associate Professor
Department of Anesthesia
The Pennsylvania State University
  College of Medicine
Hershey, Pennsylvania

Patrick M. McQuillan, M.D.
Assistant Professor
Department of Anesthesia
The Pennsylvania State University
  College of Medicine
The Milton S. Hershey Medical Center
Hershey, Pennsylvania

Jeffrey S. Morrow, M.D.
Staff Anesthesiologist
Hartford Hospital
Hartford, Connecticut

Michael F. Mulroy, M.D.
Staff Anesthesiologist
Department of Anesthesiology
Virginia Mason Clinic
Seattle, Washington

Umeshraya T. Pai, M.D.
Clinical Professor of Anesthesiology
Associate Professor of Anatomy
Department of Anesthesiology
The University of Cincinnati
  Medical Center
Cincinnati, Ohio

Winston C.V. Parris, M.D., F.A.C.P.M.
Professor of Anesthesiology
Director, Vanderbilt Pain Control Center
Vanderbilt University Medical Center
Nashville, Tennessee

Richard B. Patt, M.D.
Associate Professor of Anesthesiology
  and Neuro-Oncology
Deputy Chief, Pain and Symptom
  Management Section
University of Texas
M.D. Anderson Cancer Center
Houston, Texas

Ricardo Plancarte, M.D.
Chairman, Anesthesiology
Critical Care and Pain Management
Instituto Nacional de Cancerologia
Mexico City, Mexico

P. Prithvi Raj, M.D.
Professor of Clinical Anesthesiology
Academic Director of Pain Medicine
UCLA School of Medicine
Los Angeles, California

Linda Jo Rice, M.D.
Director of Anesthesia Research
Hartford Hospital
The Connecticut Children's Medical Center
Hartford, Connecticut

John C. Rowlingson, M.D.
Professor of Anesthesiology
Director, Pain Management Center
University of Virginia
  Health Science Center
Charlottesville, Virginia

George J. Sheplock, M.D.
Assistant Professor
Department of Anesthesia
Indiana University School of Medicine;
Staff Anesthesiologist
Riley Hospital for Children
Indianapolis, Indiana;
Center Associate
Center for Excellence in Education
Indiana University
Bloomington, Indiana

Richard Sheppard, M.D.
Director, Orthopaedic Anesthesia
Staff Anesthesiologist
Hartford Hospital
Hartford, Connecticut

John M. Stamatos, M.D.
Co-Director, Pain Management Services
St. Vincent's Hospital and Medical Center;
Assistant Professor of Anesthesiology
New York Medical College
New York, New York

Gale E. Thompson, M.D.
Department of Anesthesiology
Virginia Mason Clinic
Seattle, Washington

Steven D. Waldman, M.D., M.B.A.
Director, Pain Consortium of Greater
  Kansas City;
Clinical Professor of Anesthesiology
University of Missouri at Kansas City
  School of Medicine
Kansas City, Missouri

Carol A. Warfield, M.D.
Director of Pain Management
Beth Israel Hospital
Boston, Massachusetts

Mark J. Williams, M.D.
Staff Anesthesiologist
Longview Regional Hospital
Longview, Texas

To my wife, Robin, *and my children,* Bradley *and* Erin,
*for without their support and understanding I could not have completed
this project. And to my father,* Charles, *and the memory of my mother,*
Barbara, *for their unconditional love and guidance.*
Marc B. Hahn

To Randi, *my wife, and* Stephen, *my son, for their patience,
encouragement, and understanding during the preparation of this book.
To* Helen, *my mother, for the lifelong loving devotion encouraging
greater efforts, and to the memory of my father.*
Patrick M. McQuillan

To my wife, Lynne, *and daughter,* Kara; *this project would not have
been possible without your encouragement, support, and love.
And to my parents,* George *and* Delores, *for their love and guidance.*
George J. Sheplock

The ability to succinctly convey the anatomic location of nerves is the foundation for effectively teaching regional anesthesia. The purpose of this text is to offer the clinician a three-dimensional understanding of human anatomy as it pertains to regional anesthesia. With this approach, the relationship of nerves and other deep structures to the surface anatomy becomes easily recognizable. This knowledge allows the clinician to fully understand proper needle placement for successful neural blockade, while at the same time minimizing complications. This synthesis of anatomic specimens, descriptions of techniques, and computer-enhanced images offers the reader a complete guide for the safe and successful performance of regional anesthesia.

The principal intent of this text is to convey the cognizance of anatomy and technique. However, indications, side effects, and complications are also discussed.

Techniques, illustrated in this text, are demonstrated without the use of surgical drapes or discoloring skin disinfectants to avoid obscuring important topographic landmarks. In practice, all techniques should be performed in an aseptic manner using thorough skin preparation and surgical drapes, with specific attention paid to the practice of universal precautions.

Anatomy is the study of the structure of the body and the relationship of its constituent parts to each other. An understanding of the nomenclature describing anatomic positioning is paramount for complete understanding of anatomic relationships for regional anesthetic techniques. All descriptions of the human body are based on the assumption that the patient is standing in the anatomic position (Fig. 1). In this position the patient is erect, arms by the sides, with the face and palms of the hands directed forward.

To understand the orientation of the anatomic specimen, it is fundamental to recognize the plane from which the specimen was taken, as well as the surface orientation and direction.

Planes are described as:

Median sagittal:	Vertical plane passing through the center of the body between the eyes, dividing the body into equal right and left halves.
Paramedian or parasagittal:	Plane situated to one or the other side of the median plane and parallel to it.
Coronal:	Vertical planes at right angles to the median plane.
Transverse:	Horizontal plane at right angles to both the median and coronal planes.

Surface orientations and directions are described as:

Anterior or ventral:	The front of the body.
Posterior or dorsal:	The back of the body.
Superficial and deep:	Indicates relative distances of structures from the surface of the body.
Palmar and dorsal:	Used in place of anterior and posterior, respectively, when describing the hand.
Plantar and dorsal:	Used in place of lower and upper, respectively, when describing the foot.
Superior or cephalad:	Denotes levels directed toward the upper end of the body.
Inferior or caudad:	Denotes levels directed toward the lower end of the body.
Proximal and distal:	Indicates relative distances from the origin of a limb, with proximal being the closer.
Medial:	Indicates a structure nearer to the median sagittal plane than another structure.
Ipsilateral:	Refers to structures on the same sides of the body.
Contralateral:	Refers to structures on opposite sides of the body.
Prone:	Lying with the anterior or ventral surface down.
Supine:	Lying with the posterior or dorsal surface down.

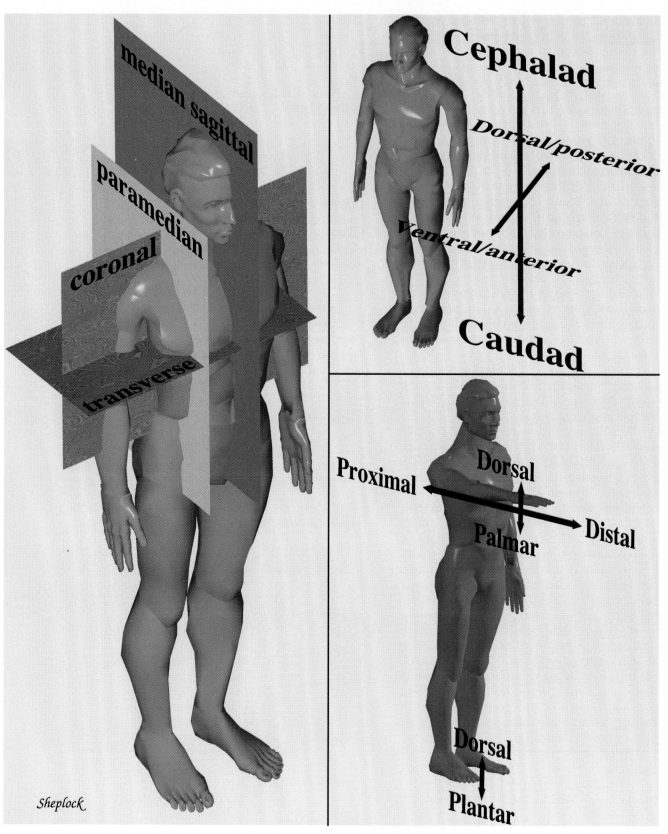

Fig. 1 *Nomenclature for anatomic positioning.*

When performing regional anesthetic techniques, it is also important to understand the descriptive terms used to relate movement (Fig. 2). Movement takes place at joints, the site where two or more bones come together.

Directions of motion are described as:

Flexion: Movement that takes place in a sagittal plane. It is usually an anterior movement that causes a bending at the joint.

Extension: Movement involving straightening a joint, which usually takes place in a posterior direction.

Lateral flexion: Movement of the trunk in the coronal plane.

Abduction: Movement, usually of a limb, in the coronal plane away from the midline of the body.

Adduction: Movement, usually of a limb, in the coronal plane towards the midline of the body.

Rotation: Movement of a part of the body around its long axis.

Pronation: Medial rotation, usually of an arm, resulting in an anterior surface facing posteriorly.

Supination: Lateral rotation, usually of an arm, from the pronated position, resulting in the anterior surface facing anteriorly.

Inversion: Movement of the foot resulting in the sole facing in the medial direction.

Eversion: Movement of the foot resulting in the sole facing in the lateral direction.

An understanding of the segmental nerve supply to the skin, subcutaneous tissues, and bone is crucial in the rendering of regional anesthesia. Dermatome mapping of the skin describes which nerve roots or peripheral nerves need to be anesthetized for various diagnostic, therapeutic, or operative procedures (Fig. 3).

A thorough understanding of anatomic relationships no doubt leads to successful regional anesthetic techniques. In addition, this knowledge leads to an awareness of the etiology of various side effects, as well as the avoidance of complications.

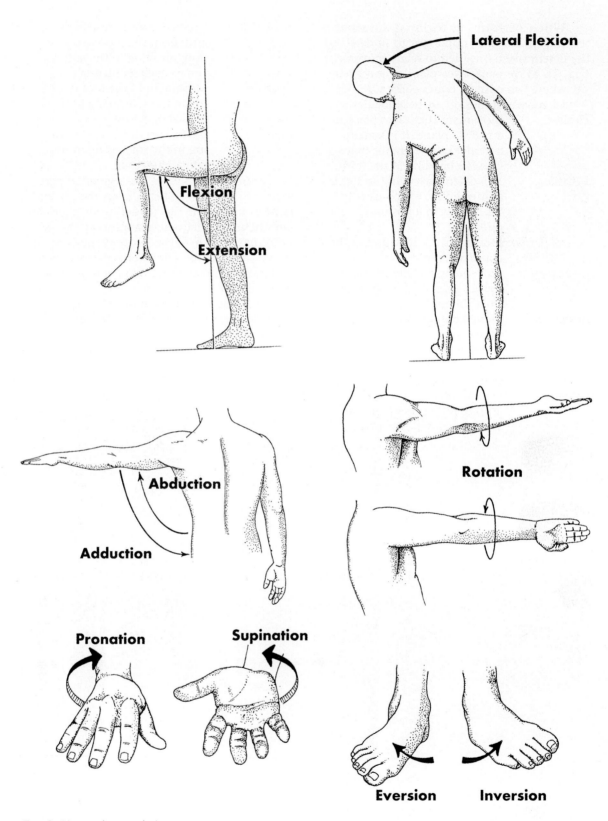

Fig. 2 *Nomenclature relating to movement.*

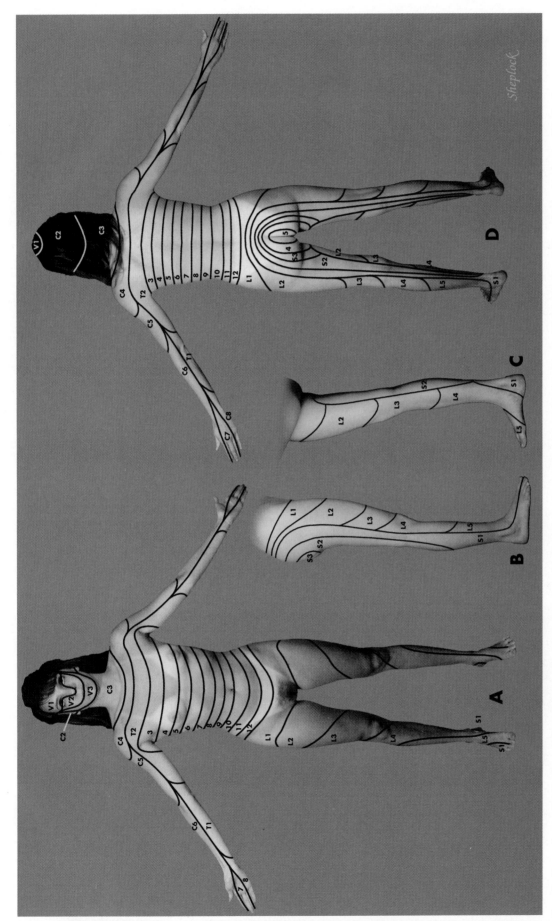

Fig. 3 *Dermatome distribution of the various nerve roots.* Developed by John J. Bonica, M.D., D.Sc., D.Med.Sc.(Hon.), F.F.A.R.C.S.(Hon.). As published in Bonica JJ (editor): *The management of pain*, ed 2, Philadelphia, 1990, Lea and Febiger.

ACKNOWLEDGMENTS

For their contributions to the preparation of this book, the editors wish to express our deepest thanks to:

Harold Carron, M.D. *(1916-1991), Professor Emeritus of Anesthesiology, The University of Virginia, Charlottesville, Virginia, and Georgetown University, Washington, D.C., for his relentless dedication to the advancement of regional anesthetic techniques for both operative anesthesia and the management of pain, as well as for his caring, support, and commitment to my professional and personal development, without which I would never have undertaken this project.* **MBH**

Geoff Greenwood *of Times Mirror International Publishers, Ltd. and R.M.H. McMinn, R.T. Hutchings, J. Pegington and P.H. Abrahams for their gracious use of illustrations from* Color Atlas of Human Anatomy, *third edition, 1993.*

Lynn Broadman, M.D. *Professor and Vice Chairman, Department of Anesthesiology, West Virginia University, Morgantown, West Virginia, for his unfailing commitment to the research, practice, and teaching of regional anesthesia, as well as for his years of personal encouragement and guidance in the development of this project.*

Sheila M. Muldoon, M.D. *Professor and Chairperson, Department of Anesthesiology, The Uniformed Services University of the Health Sciences, Bethesda, Maryland, for the years of support and encouragement.*

Julien F. Biebuyck, M.B., *D.Phil., Eric A. Walker Professor and Chairman, Department of Anesthesia, The Pennsylvania State University, M.S. Hershey Medical Center, Hershey, Pennsylvania, for his unfailing support and gracious commitment of departmental resources to enable this book to come to fruition.*

Robert K. Stoelting, M.D, *Professor and Chairman, Department of Anesthesia, Indiana University School of Medicine, Indianapolis, Indiana, for his lifelong commitment to education in anesthesia and his valued support during this project.*

Umeshraya T. Pai, M.D. *Clinical Professor of Anesthesiology and Associate Professor of Anatomy, Department of Anesthesiology, The University of Cincinnati Medical Center, Cincinnati, Ohio, for his invaluable assistance in the identification of all anatomic structures described in this text.*

Ronald S. Wade *in his positions as Director, Maryland State Anatomy Board and Director, Anatomic Services Division, The University of Maryland School of Medicine, Baltimore, Maryland, for his assistance in the procurement, through the Anatomic Gift Program, and preparation of anatomic specimens.*

George S. Holborow *Anatomical Curator, Anatomic Teaching Laboratory, The Uniformed Services University of the Health Sciences, Bethesda, Maryland, for his assistance in the preparation of anatomic specimens.*

Yvette Legrande *Plastination Technician, The Armed Forces Institute of Pathology, Washington, DC., for her meticulous preparation and plastination of anatomic specimens.*

John Biondi *Senior Medical Photographer, Department of Educational Resources, Division of Medical Photography, The Pennsylvania State University, M.S. Hershey Medical Center, for his patience and skill in preparing anatomic specimen and model photographic layouts.*

Susan M. Gay *Editor-in-Chief, and Sandra Clark Brown, Developmental Editor, for their enthusiastic support and guidance in the preparation of this book.*

Lisa Rothermel *Departmental Secretary, Department of Anesthesia, The Pennsylvania State University, Hershey, Pennsylvania, for her editorial assistance in preparing this manuscript.*

Melanie Berrier *and* **Brian Slater** *of Fashion Mystique Modeling, Harrisburg, Pennsylvania.*

James J. Richter, M.D., *Ph.D., Director, Department of Anesthesiology, Hartford Hospital, Hartford, Connecticut, and his staff, for their support during the beginning of this project.*

The Men and Women of the United States Army, Navy, Air Force, and Marine Corps.

Marc B. Hahn
Patrick M. McQuillan
George J. Sheplock

Illustrator's PREFACE

Perhaps the greatest impact of the recent advancements in personal computing technology is in empowering educators to create new and exciting educational resources. These educational resources can range from computer-enhanced images and multimedia presentations to interactive hypermedia software and virtual reality. These advancements are resulting in monumental changes in the manner in which information is processed and presented. Furthermore, these new computer-enhanced educational resources have the potential to make learning more efficient and enjoyable.

Performing regional anesthesia successfully requires an accurate vision and understanding of the anatomy underlying the surface landmarks. The study and depiction of anatomy has evolved over time from the spoken word and sketches to high-fidelity drawings and high-resolution photographs. Today the latest advancements in personal computing and digital imaging technology are enabling educators to take this evolutionary process another step forward. The digital cadaver images and computer-enhanced illustrations in this atlas were created to develop a more accurate understanding of the important *in vivo* anatomic relationships.

In order to illustrate the anatomy underlying the surface landmarks, cadaver and live model photographs were digitized and processed using the latest imaging techniques. This process resulted in digital images that reveal the underlying anatomy along with surface landmark features. In addition, some of the images contain realistic-appearing needles and pointers to demonstrate the proper placement of the needle. To both enhance the illusion of "x-ray vision" and limit the distortion of the anatomy, only the major structures are labeled. Hopefully, these computer-generated images will aid in developing a clearer understanding and vision of the anatomy that will lead to a more successful regional anesthetic technique.

I would like to acknowledge some of the very many people who have made it possible for me to develop the computer-enhanced images in this atlas:

To Howard L. Zauder, M.D., who fostered my initial interest in academics, for all his support and guidance.

To Gary Philips, for developing my initial interests in computer programming, and especially for all his dedicated efforts in motivating students to learn and enjoy mathematics.

To Enrico M. Camporesi, M.D., P. Sebastian Thomas, M.D., John I. Gerson, M.D., and Win Rice, Ph.D., for assisting and guiding me in my initial interests in computer-based instructional technologies.

To Lac Tran, Lt. Col. Jay S. Ellis, M.D., and the anesthesia staff and residents of Wilford Hall Medical Center, USAF, for their support and commitment to exploring and utilizing these new learning technologies.

To Apple Computer, Inc., especially to Jim Pile, Bert Creighton, and Ron Amenta, for all their assistance, resources, and guidance.

To Robert K. Stoelting, M.D., Gopal Krishna, M.D., Stephen F. Dierdorf, M.D., and the anesthesia staff at Riley Hospital for Children for their unending support and guidance.

George J. Sheplock

"Imagination is more important than knowledge..."
A. Einstein

CONTENTS

Regional Anesthesia

An Atlas of Anatomy and Techniques

Pharmacology

Part 1

CHAPTER 1

Pharmacology for Regional Anesthetic Techniques

■

Mark J. Williams

■

Introduction The placement of local anesthetics at various sites along the neural axis to produce anesthesia or analgesia is classified as *regional anesthesia*. The application of these techniques is used for surgical anesthesia and postoperative analgesia and as acute or chronic pain management modalities.

Local anesthetics can be used in combination or with other adjuvant medications to potentiate speed of onset and duration of action or to increase the intensity of anesthesia or analgesia. It is important to know the pharmacology of these medications to select the appropriate drug for a specific therapeutic task. Chemical structure determines metabolism and elimination of these drugs from the body. Local anesthetics exist in two chemical forms, amino esters and amino amides (see Fig. 1-1). Amino esters are ester derivatives of para-aminobenzoic acid and are metabolized by plasma cholinesterase. The metabolic byproduct is para-aminobenzoic acid, a known allergen, so allergic reactions are not uncommon. On the other hand, amino amides are compound with amide linkages and are metabolized for the most part by the liver. Their potentials for allergic reactions are extremely small.

Local anesthetics can also be classified, on the basis of their clinical properties, into three basic categories:

1. Low potency/short duration: procaine, 2-chloroprocaine;
2. Intermediate potency/intermediate duration: lidocaine, mepivacaine, prilocaine;
3. High potency/long duration: bupivacaine, tetracaine, etidocaine.

The difference in clinical activities among the local anesthetics can be explained by their inherent physicochemical properties.

PHYSICAL AND CHEMICAL PROPERTIES

Lipid solubility, protein binding, and pK_a of the local anesthetic agents are important factors that directly influence potency, onset of action, and duration of action (see Table 1-1). In addition, some local anesthetics exist as chemical isomers (chiral forms) and may further create differences in their inherent activity and toxicity.

Lipid Solubility

The potency of a local anesthetic is influenced in a nonlinear manner by its lipid solubility. The more lipid-soluble a local anesthetic is, the more potent the local anesthetic

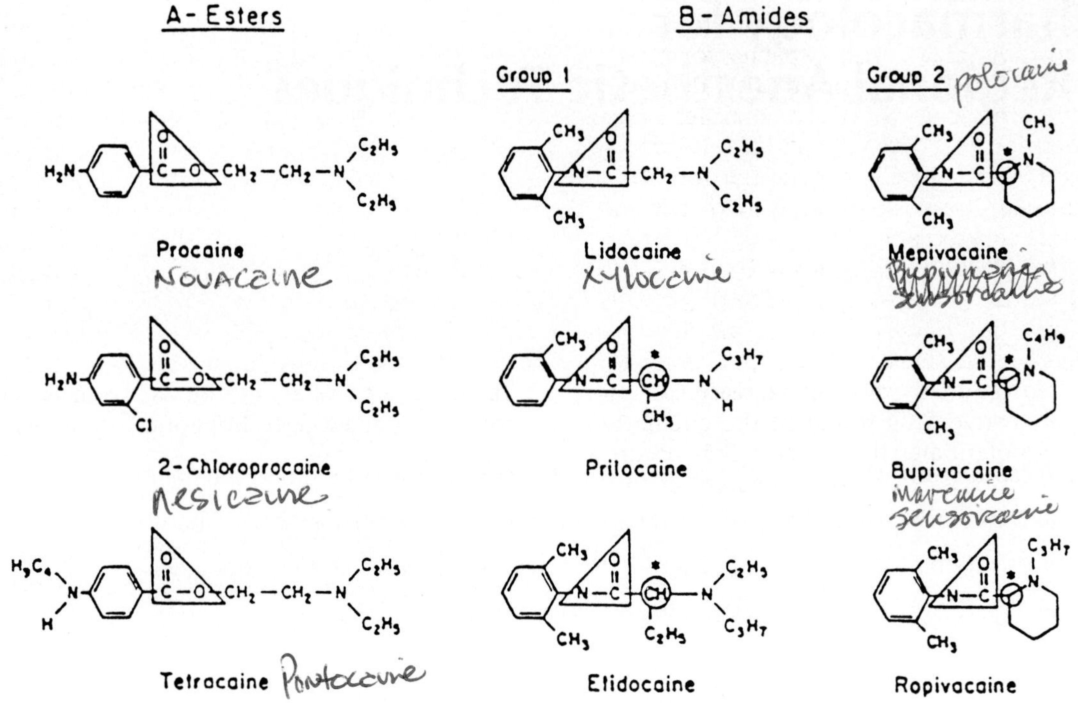

A- Esters   **B - Amides**

Group 1   Group 2 *polocaine*

Procaine
Novacaine

Lidocaine
Xylocaine

Mepivacaine

2-Chloroprocaine
Nesicaine

Prilocaine

Bupivacaine
marcaine
sensorcaine

Tetracaine *Pontocaine*

Etidocaine

Ropivacaine

FIG. 1-1 *Local anesthetic structures with the ester and amide link shown within the superimposed triangle. When present, the asymmetric carbon is circled, shaded, and marked with an *. (From DiFazio CA, Woods AM: Pharmacology of local anesthetics. In Raj PP, editor: Practical management of pain, ed. 2, St. Louis, 1992, Mosby.)*

Table 1-1   Physical properties and equipotent concentrations of local anesthetics

	PROCAINE	LIDOCAINE	MEPIVACAINE	BUPIVACAINE	ETIDOCAINE	ROPIVACAINE
Molecular weight	236	234	246	288	276	274
pK_a	8.9	7.7	7.6	8.1	7.7	8.0
Lipid solubility	1	4	1	30	140	2.8
Partition coefficient	0.02	2.9	0.8	28	141	9
Protein binding	5	65	75	95	95	90-95
Equipotent concentration		2.0	1.5	0.5	1.0	0.75

From DiFazio CA, Woods AM: Pharmacology of local anesthetics. In Raj PP, editor: Practical management of pain, ed. 2, St. Louis, 1992, Mosby.

effect. The major determinant of the lipid solubility is the aromatic group (benzene ring) found on the local anesthetic molecule. The measurement of solubility is performed by studying the base form's solubility in organic solvents. However, experimental evaluations of solubility differ from clinical effect in that local anesthetics clinical potency increases to a point and then levels off. This leveling off occurs at a lipid partition coefficient of about four. The plateauing of clinical potency is surmised to be related to the surrounding fat and blood vessels adjacent to the nerve. These may act as a depot and pull local anesthetic away, thereby decreasing the total amount of drug available to the nerve.

Protein Binding

Local anesthetics bind to both plasma proteins and tissue proteins. Local anesthetics with a high protein-binding capacity will stay on the protein receptor for a longer time, producing an increased duration of effect. Also, when these molecules are bound to the plasma proteins, they are not pharmacologically active; this affects their activity, toxicity, and metabolism. The two main binding plasma proteins are albumin and α_1-acid glycoprotein. Alpha$_1$-acid glycoprotein is described as having a high affinity and low capacity for binding with the local anesthetics, whereas albumin has a lower affinity and higher capacity. In other words, albumin, which has less affinity, will bind larger amounts of local anesthetics long after the α_1-acid glycoprotein capacity to bind has been maximized. This capacity for binding local anesthetics is concentration-dependent, decreasing in a curvilinear manner as concentration increases. The clinical importance of this fact is that the potential for toxicity increases disproportionately with increased plasma concentrations.

Protein binding is also influenced by the pH of the plasma. The percentage of the bound drug decreases as the pH decreases. Therefore, in acidotic states, for a given total concentration there is an increased fraction of free active drug found in the circulation, which potentiates the toxicity. This occurs at the receptor proteins in the sodium channels as well, and may decrease duration of the local anesthetic effect.

Ionization

The amino acid group on the local anesthetic molecule determines the ionization of the molecule and, thus, the hydrophilic activity. This amino group is capable of accepting a hydrogen ion (H+), and in so doing converts the unionized base form of the drug into the cationic form of the drug. The proportions of these forms present in solution determined by the pK_a is defined as the pH at which 50% of the local anesthetic will remain in the uncharged (basic) form and 50% will exist in the charged (cationic) form. This relationship between the pH and the pK_a and the concentrations of the cation and the base forms is described by the Henderson-Hasselbach equation:

$$pK_a = pH + \log(\text{cation/base})$$

The pK_a is important in determining the speed of onset of the local anesthetic. It is believed that the unionized form is responsible for diffusion across the nerve membrane, whereas the ionized form produces blockade of the sodium ion movement through the sodium channel by binding to the receptor proteins. Hence both uncharged and charged forms are important for local anesthetic neural blockade. For local anesthetics the pK_a falls within a narrow range, 7.6 to 8.9; thus these drugs at equilibrium exist predominantly in the cationic form at normal pH. Even still agents with a pK_a closest to the body's pH will have the fastest onset of action, because a major portion will exist in the uncharged forms.

Chiral Forms

The identification of stereo isomers for some of the local anesthetics like bupivacaine, mepivacaine, etidocaine, prilocaine, and ropivacaine have led to further evaluations into potential differences in potency, toxicity and duration between them. For stereo isomers to exist, an asymmetric carbon atom must be present in the molecule. The nomenclature used to describe these isomers has changed in recent years, and now terms like "D" and "L" have been replaced by "R" and "S" respectively. Details for these differences are noted in Table 1-2, but as a rule the "S" form is less toxic and has a longer duration of anesthesia.

MECHANISMS OF LOCAL ANESTHETIC FUNCTION

A good way to explain the mechanism of local anesthetic action is to relate anesthetic activity to the transmission of the nerve impulse. Stimulation of the nerve results in a propagated impulse that passes along the course of the nerve. This electric signal results from a propagation of ionic currents. These currents are created by a transient fluctuation in the ion concentrations across a lipoprotein membrane. The main ionic species are Na+, which is concentrated mostly extracellularly, and K+, which is concentrated mostly intracellularly. These gradients are maintained by an ion-translocating, Na+K+ adenosine triphosphate (ATP) pump mechanism within the nerve cell. The resulting resting electrical potential across the membrane is about -90 mV, with the exterior being positive. This is in large part due to a difference in the membrane's permeability for K+ over that for Na+. In other words, the ionic leakage down the concentration gradient occurs more for the K+ than for the NA+ ions at the resting potential.

Table 1-2 Anesthetic duration and toxicity of local anesthetic isomers

Drug	Duration	Toxicity
Etidocaine	S = R	S = R
Mepivacaine	S > R	S = R
Bupivacaine	S > R	S < R
Ropivacaine	S > R	S < R

From DiFazio CA, Woods AM: Pharmacology of local anesthetics. In Raj PP, editor: Practical management of pain, *ed 2, St. Louis, 1992, Mosby.*

As the nerve impulse spreads, partial depolarization exceeds the threshold potential and triggers depolarization via a major increase in the permeability to Na^+. With the influx of Na^+, the membrane potential transiently becomes negative relative to the inside, and depolarization is electrically conducted to the adjacent areas of the membrane. At the same time, K^+ ion outflow commences. This outflow occurs later and at a slow rate than that for Na^+, and peaks after the Na^+ influx has subsided. In the late phase of depolarization, the membrane becomes again less permeable to Na^+, and, as the ATP ion pump exchanges ions, the membrane returns to its resting potential. This sequence of events occurs successively as the impulse spreads down the nerve. At present, investigators postulate that the action potential causes conformational changes in the nerve membrane lipoproteins; these changes result in the actual opening of the Na^+ channel gates, which consist of two proteins designated as the "m" and "h" gate proteins. These channels, because of their size and charges, are specific for the Na^+ ion.

Local anesthetics act on the membrane by interfering with its ability to undergo the specific changes that result in the altered permeability to Na^+. Thus local anesthetics increase the threshold for electrical excitation in the nerve, slow the propagation of the impulse, reduce the rate of rise of the action potential, and eventually block the conduction. Several theories have been postulated over the years as to the exact mechanism of local anesthetics.

The most popular theories at present are the combination of the receptor and the membrane expansion theories (see Fig. 1-2). The membrane expansion theory states that local anesthetic in its uncharged base form dissolves in the nerve membrane, causing an expansion of the membrane. This produces conformational changes between the proteins and their association with the membrane lipids and results in the partial collapse of these ionic channels, thus impeding the passage of Na^+ ions. The receptor theories basically state that the local anesthetic bind to receptors at the cell membrane and prevent the opening of channels or pores for the passage of ions.

Local anesthetics are believed to diffuse through the lipid bilayer structure of the cell membrane in their lipid-soluble, uncharged base form. They then equilibrate in the axoplasm of the nerve into the charged (cationic) and uncharged form in accordance with the drug's pK_a and the pH of the axoplasm. The cationic form then enters the Na^+ channel from the intracellular side, binds to the anionic site within the Na^+ channel, and physically or ionically blocks the movement of the Na^+ ions. Therefore the local anesthetic prevents the action potential from developing in the nerve by inhibition of the movement of Na^+ into the cell. The resulting effect is a nondepolarization block, similar to the action of curare at the neuromuscular junction.

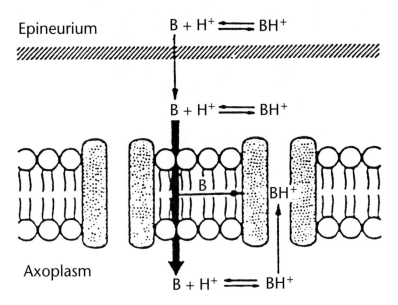

Fig. 1-2 *Local anesthetic access to the sodium channel. The uncharged molecule diffuses most easily across lipid barriers and interacts with the channel through the axolemma interior. The charged species formed in the axoplasm gains access to a specific receptor via the sodium channel pore.* (From Carpenter RL, Mackey DC: Local anesthetics. In Barash PG, Cullen BF, Stoelting RK, editors: *Clinical anesthesia*, Philadelphia, 1989, JB Lippincott.)

NERVE FIBER SIZE

The varying effect on nerve conduction is termed "differential blockade." Although each local anesthetic has its own inherent hydrophilic or hydrophobic properties that produce this effect, other factors also explain this phenomenon. Nerve-fiber diameter and myelinization play an important role in the physical function and modality of the nerve. They also affect the sensitivity of the nerve fiber to local anesthetic blockade. Nerve fibers are categorized into three major anatomic classes (see Table 1-3). Myelinated somatic nerves are called "A fibers," myelinated preganglionic autonomic nerves are called "B-fibers," and nonmyelinated axons are called "C fibers." The A fibers are further divided into four other groups according to decreasing size: alpha, beta, gamma, and delta.

In general, the thicker the nerve, the greater the amount of local anesthetic required to block the conduction. B fibers, preganglionic autonomic fibers, are an exception to the rule because, although they are myelinated, they are more easily blocked than other fiber groups. This fact explains why one sees the sympathetic blockade with epidural or subarachnoid blocks extending several segments beyond the cutaneous block.

Another factor is the geographic arrangement of the nerve fibers within a peripheral nerve (see Fig. 1-3). Simply stated, the nerve fibers that are located in the outer layers of the nerve bundles will be exposed to and blocked by the effects of the local anesthetic before more internal ones are affected.

Next is the concept of conduction safety. The distance between the nodes of Ranvier increases as the size of the myelinated nerve fibers increases. Conduction safety proposes that a requirement of at least three nodes of Ranvier must be exposed to local anesthetic before conduction can be halted. Therefore the variation in the distances between the nodes of Ranvier plays a major role in the

Table 1-3 Classification of nerve fibers

CONDUCTION/ BIOPHYSICAL CLASSIFICATION	ANATOMIC LOCATION	MYELIN	DIAMETER (μ)	RATE (MS⁻¹)	Function
A fibers					
A alpha A beta	Afferent to and efferent from muscles and joints	Yes	6-22	30-85	Motor and proprioception
A gamma	Efferent to muscle spindles	Yes	3-6	15-35	Muscle tone
A delta	Sensory roots and afferent peripheral nerves	Yes	1-4	5-25	Pain Temperature Touch
B fibers	Preganglionic sympathetic	Yes	<3	3-15	Vasomotor Visceromotor Sudomotor Pilomotor
C fibers sC	Postganglionic sympathetic	No	0.3-1.3	0.7-1.3	Vasomotor Visceromotor Sudomotor Pilomotor
drC	Sensory roots and afferent peripheral nerves	No	0.4-1.2	0.1-2.0	Pain Temperature Touch

From Carpenter RL, Mackey DC: Local anesthetics. In Barash PG, Cullen BF, Stoelting RK, editors: Clinical anesthesia, *Philadelphia, 1989, JB Lippincott.*

variability of blockade (see Fig. 1-4). In addition, the degree of impulse activity, the effects of CO_2 tension, pH, the local ion gradients, the degree of myelination on the nerve, and the concentration of a given local anesthetic drug all appear to contribute to this known clinical phenomena. The importance of the differential block of nerve conduction plays a major role in the proper use of these medications and adds to the armamentarium of those proficient in regional anesthesia.

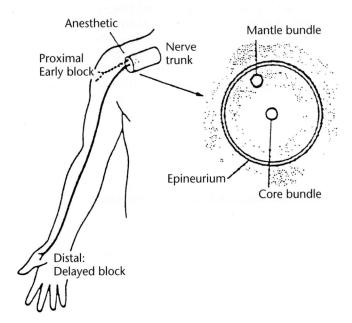

FIG. 1-3 *Representation of the somatotropic arrangement of fibers in the trunks of the brachial plexus. Nerve fibers in the mantle (or peripheral) bundles innervate the proximal arm, and fibers in the core (or central) bundles innervate the distal arm. The concentration gradient that develops during initial diffusion of local anesthetic into the nerve trunk causes onset of anesthesia to proceed from proximal to distal. (From Carpenter RL, Mackey DC: Local anesthetics. In Barash PG, Cullen BF, Stoelting RK, editors: Clinical anesthesia, Philadelphia, 1989, JB Lippincott.)*

FIG. 1-4 *Differential blockade of myelinated nerve fibers of differing diameters. Intermodal distance is proportional to axon diameter, and conduction blockade occurs when at least three adjacent nodes of a nerve fiber are exposed to blocking concentrations of the local anesthetic agent. Thus equivalent spread of local anesthetic may produce conduction blockade of a thin axon, but not the adjacent thick axon. (Modified from Franz DN, Perry RS: Mechanisms of differential block among single myelinated and nonmyelinated axons by procains, J Physiol (Lond) 236:193, 1974.)*

EXTERNAL FACTORS THAT AFFECT BLOCKADE
Volume and Concentration

The total milligrams of the agents ultimately will dictate the onset, quality, and duration of the block, so that with increasing doses of local anesthetic one can make the onset faster and the duration longer (see Table 1-4). Using the same volume, rapid onset and better quality and duration of the block are observed with varying concentrations of local anesthetics. On the other hand, it has been shown epidurally that, when the concentration is varied and the volume is adjusted in order to maintain the same milligram dosage, no difference is noted in the onset, duration, and quality of the block; however, the spread of the block may be higher when using the larger volume. It must be noted that the potential for increased serum levels and toxicity is also seen with increased dosages.

Addition of Vasoconstrictor Agents

The addition of epinephrine, norepinephrine, and phenylephrine is frequently used with different local anesthetics to hasten onset and improve the quality and duration of the analgesia (see Table 1-5). These drugs reverse the known intrinsic vasodilatation effects found among most of the local anesthetics. Vasoconstriction caused by these chemicals will reduce the absorption of the local anesthetics; hence more agent is available for the neural blockade.

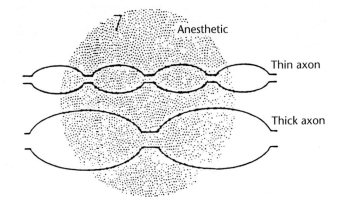

Site of the Injection

The proximity to the nervous tissues and the anatomic structures located at the site of injection can influence onset, duration, and peak serum levels. An example is seen with the subarachnoid route of administration, which is associated with a faster onset than epidural placements.

The potential for decreased duration of effect and increased serum levels of local anesthetics is noted to be related to amount of blood flow at the site of injection. In decreasing order the potential for these effects is seen with intercostal, caudal, epidural, brachial plexus, and sciatic or femoral nerves.

Bicarbonation and Carbonation of Local Anesthetics

The addition of bicarbonate to local anesthetics is associated with faster onset and spread of the block. Local anesthetics are often supplied at low pH to prolong the shelf life. The addition of bicarbonate will increase the pH of these solutions and ultimately the percentage of the uncharged form that is important for diffusion through the nerve membrane.

The mixing of CO_2 (700 mmHg) with local anesthetic will also shorten the onset time, but by a different mechanism. The CO_2 diffuses rapidly across the axonal membrane and thus decreases the intracellular pH. This will increase the concentration of the charged form of the local anesthetic, which is important for receptor binding and neural blockade.

Temperature

Warming local anesthetic has been observed to reduce the onset of epidural blockade because the elevation of the temperature decreases the pK_a of the drug.

Pregnancy

The requirements for local anesthetic in parturient women have been observed to be decreased compared to their nonpregnant counterparts. Onset has been shown to be

Table 1-4 Effects of dose and epinephrine on local anesthetic properties

	INCREASED DOSE (CONCENTRATION OR VOLUME)	ADDITION OF EPINEPHRINE
Onset time	↓	↓ (Minimal effect for etidocaine)
Degree of motor blockade	↑	↑
Degree of sensory blockade	↑	↑
Duration of blockade	↑	↑
Area of blockade	↑	↑
Peak plasma concentration	↑	↓

From Covino BG: Clinical pharmacology of local anesthetic agents. In Cousins MJ, Bridenbaugh PO, editors: Neural blockade in clinical anesthesia and management of pain, Philadelphia, 1988, JB Lippincott.

Table 1-5 Comparative onset times and analgesic durations of various local anesthetic agents and effects of epinephrine (5 μg/ml) on duration and peak plasma levels (C_{max})

ANESTHETIC TECHNIQUE	ANESTHETIC AGENT	USUAL CONCENTRATION (%)	AVERAGE ONSET TIME (MIN ± SE)	AVERAGE ANALGESIC DURATION (MIN ± SE)	ADDITION OF EPI % CHANGE DURATION	C_{MAX}
Brachial plexus block (40-50 ml)	Lidocaine	1.0	14 ± 4	195 ± 26	+50	−20 - 30
	Mepivacaine	1.0	15 ± 6	245 ± 27	−	−20 - 30
	Bupivacaine	0.25-0.5	10-25	572	−	−10 - 20
	Etidocaine	0.5	9	572	−	−10 - 20
Epidural anesthesia (20-30 ml)	Lidocaine	2.0	15	100 ±20	+50	−20 - 30
	Mepivacaine	2.0	15	115 ± 15	+50	−20 - 30
	Bupivacaine	0.5	17	195 ± 30	+0 - 30	−10 - 20
	Etidocaine	1.0	11	170 ± 57	+0 - 30	−10 - 20
Local infiltration	Lidocaine	0.5		75 (35-340)	+200	−50
	Mepivacaine	0.5		108 (15-240)	+120	−
	Bupivacaine	0.25		200 ± 33	+115	−

From Carpenter RL, Mackey DC: Local anesthetics. In Barosh PG, Cullen BF, Stoelting RK, editors: Clinical anesthesia, Philadelphia, 1989, JB Lippincott.

faster with the use of epidural and spinal anesthesia or peripheral nerve blocks. Progesterone is suspected as a factor in this reported effect.

Combination of Local Anesthetics

Combination of local anesthetics has been done to hasten the onset of action, as well as to improve the quality of block. However, this may not always be the case. For example, the addition of 2-chloroprocaine with bupivacaine improves the onset and quality of the sensory block, but the combination has been shown to shorten the duration of bupivacaine. The cause may be related to the possible interference by 2-chloroprocaine or its metabolites with the binding of bupivacaine to the receptors.

LOCAL ANESTHETICS

Esters

Cocaine is a rather complex alkaloid originally obtained from the Peruvian coca plant. Cocaine is used solely for topical anesthesia. Because of its unique vasoconstrictive action, which is related to its abilities to inhibit the reuptake of norepinephrine, it is especially useful during procedures on the oral and nasal cavities. Addiction and high toxicity are the main drawbacks to its use. The metabolism is by two pathways of hydrolysis, but 20% is still excreted in the urine unchanged.

Procaine (Novocain) is one of the first synthetic para-aminobenzoic acid esters. Its use has declined because of its low potency, slow onset, short duration of action, and the advent of the more lipid-soluble amide-linked anesthetics. Although the potential for systemic side effects is low, the agent can cause allergic reactions. Currently it is mainly used for local infiltration anesthesia and in differential spinal blocks for chronic patients' evaluations.

2-Chloroprocaine (Nesacaine) is an analog of procaine. It is hydrolyzed four times faster then procaine in human plasma, thus it is less toxic than procaine. Its rapid onset, brief duration, and low systemic toxicity have made it popular, especially in obstetrics, because it can be metabolized by the fetal enzyme system. It is not used intrathecally secondary to reports of neurotoxicity. However, this has been associated with the low pH and buffers used in the solution mixture. It is also proven to be valuable for peripheral nerve blocks.

Tetracaine (Pontocaine, Amethocaine, Pantocaine) is also an analog of procaine with radically different local anesthetic properties. It is ten times more potent and toxic but about four times slower to hydrolyze than procaine. The main benefit is its long duration of action, which can be further potentiated with the use of vasoconstrictors. Because of its poor diffusion qualities, it is not a good agent for peripheral nerve blockade except in combination with other fast-onset local anesthetics. Also, its potential for systemic side effects is increased with the larger dosages required for these types of nerve blocks. Tetracaine does possess excellent topical anesthetic properties, and it was used in the past to topically anesthetize the oral mucosa; however, rapid absorption with aerosol mixtures led to some reports of fatalities. Its elimination is believed to be through excretion by the biliary tree.

Benzocaine is an ethyl ester of para-aminobenzoic acid that lacks the hydrophilic amine tail. In addition, the pK_a of benzocaine is well below physiologic range, which means it exists almost entirely as the unionized base form. These differences make it nearly insoluble in water and limit its use solely to topical application because it causes irritation on injection.

Amino Amides

Lidocaine (Xylocaine, Lignocaine) remains the most versatile and commonly used local anesthetic because of its inherent potency, rapid onset, and moderate duration of action. It is used in infiltration; peripheral nerve block; and epidural, spinal, and topical anesthesia. Given intravenously (IV) it acts as a systemic analgesic for blunting the response to intubation in the operating room and in the treatment of certain chronic pain syndromes secondary to its direct effects on the CNS. Generally, the duration of lidocaine is 1 to 3 h for various regional anesthetic procedures; however, the addition of epinephrine to the dosage will increase its onset, extend the duration, and at the same time decrease its toxicity by limiting peak levels in the serum. Lidocaine is metabolized in the liver and, although the metabolites are excreted by the biliary tree, they are reabsorbed by the circulation only to be excreted in the urine. Only a small portion of lidocaine is excreted in the urine unchanged.

Bupivacaine (Marcaine, Sensorcaine) is a butyl derivative of a ringed piperidine carboxylic acid amide. It is used in infiltration, peripheral nerve block, and epidural and spinal anesthesia, but not for topical anesthesia. Bupivacaine's duration is two to three times longer then lidocaine's, but so is its toxicity. It is this severe toxic profile that prevents its use for IV regional or systemic anesthesia. Because it offers excellent differential blockade between different nerve fibers, it has gained popularity for use in obstetric, acute postoperative, and chronic pain anesthetic techniques. Its longest duration of action occurs when it is used for peripheral nerve blockade; it has been reported to last up to hours or even longer. The addition of epinephrine does influence its vascular absorption and its effect on target sites. Other facts of interest are that, as an intrathecal agent, it has a better satisfactory anesthetic effect than tetracaine and reportedly less potential for hypotensive side effects. Also, the degree of motor blockade is greater when isobaric solutions of bupivacaine are used, as opposed to hyperbaric formulations.

Etidocaine (Duranest) is a longer-acting derivative of lidocaine that has been found to be four times more potent and toxic than lidocaine. It is characterized by a very rapid onset, prolonged duration, and profound sensory and motor blockade. It is formulated for infiltration, peripheral nerve block, and epidural uses. It differs from bupivacaine in that it produces a more profound motor block than sensory block, which makes it primarily useful for surgical procedures that require muscle relaxation, but limits use for obstetric and postoperative analgesia.

Mepivacaine (Carbocaine) is a methyl derivative of a ringed piperidine rather than an alkylamino compound. Its duration is slightly longer than lidocaine. It is known to have some vasoconstrictive activity, but the addition of epinephrine affects its duration, onset, and potential for toxicity just as with lidocaine. Mepivacaine is used in infiltration, peripheral nerve, and epidural anesthesia in the United States, but it is not effective as a topical agent. Also, metabolism is markedly decreased in the fetus and the newborn with its use so it is infrequently used to obstetric anesthesia. Although it is eliminated by the same mechanism as lidocaine, metabolites are also excreted by the salivary glands and gastric mucosa.

Prilocaine (Citanest, Propitocaine) is a secondary amine analog of lidocaine. It is as potent as lidocaine, but it is the least toxic of all the amino amide local anesthetics, due to the fact that levels in the blood are cleared quickly secondary to rapid uptake by the tissues. It has a rapid onset, a moderate duration, and profound depth of conduction blockade. Prilocaine is used in infiltration, peripheral nerve blocks, and epidural anesthesia. No specific formulas for topical or spinal use are available because of its short duration of action. During metabolism it is biotransformed to an amino-phenol end product. This compound can oxidize hemoglobin to methemoglobin, which can result in cyanosis; thus the total dose needs to be limited to 600 mg. Also, its use in obstetric anesthesia and IV analgesic techniques has been abandoned. The metabolism of prilocaine is via lung, liver, and kidney.

Ropivacaine is a propyl derivative of an n-alkyl piperidine amide. Ropivacaine is a chiral drug, but in its production the racemic mixture exists almost as a pure solution of one isomer. It is believed that this isomer possesses the most therapeutic qualities and the safest cardiac profile. In fact, one of the main advantages of ropivacaine over bupivacaine is its reduced cardiotoxic potential. The physicochemical properties of ropivacaine are similar to those of bupivacaine except that it is less lipid-soluble (Table 1-5). This may explain why, although ropivacaine and bupivacaine have equipotent effects on C-fiber action potentials, ropivacaine is less potent in blocking A-fiber activity. In other words, when compared with bupivacaine, the sensory anesthetic profiles of the two drugs are similar in onset, depth, and duration, but the depth and duration of the motor block are less with ropivacaine. It is felt that ropivacaine may possess an even greater potential for a differential sensory motor blockade compared to bupivacaine. However, this differential blocking effect has been shown to be overcome by increasing the concentration of the ropivacaine. This would make ropivacaine superior to bupivacaine and an extremely useful agent for obstetric anesthesia and postoperative epidural analgesia. Ropivacaine has been found to be an effective local anesthetic agent for infiltration, epidural, spinal, and brachial plexus anesthesia. Also, the addition of epinephrine has not been shown to alter the onset or duration of its action significantly because of its own inherent vasoconstrictive activity. For a summary of the local anesthetics clinical profile, see Table 1-6.

TOXICITY OF LOCAL ANESTHETICS

Allergic reactions to local anesthetics are known to occur mainly with the amino ester-linkage local anesthetics. This has been documented especially with procaine, but crossover hypersensitivity has been seen with the other ester amide-linkage drugs as well. It is believed to happen because of a cross-sensitivity with para-aminobenzoic acid. True allergic reactions to amino amide local anesthetics are extremely rare and are usually related not to the drug but to the preservative methylparaben. Paraben esters have excellent bacteriostatic and fungistatic properties, and are widely used in multidose vials. In the past, skin testing of those suspected of possible allergic reactions to local anesthetics was felt to be the best way to identify these patients. However, this may not be scientifically reliable because only a small amount of drug is used; a conjugation of the drug may be needed with a carrier molecule before allergic reactions can occur. Also, the possibility of a severe anaphylactic reaction could put the patient's life at risk.

Local Tissue Toxicity

Tissue toxicity is rare when proper technique and concentrations of local anesthetics are used. However, serious neurotoxicity may result from intraneural injections, needle trauma, injections of large concentrations or volumes, chemical contamination, and neural ischemia produced by local neural compression or systemic hypotension. Examples of this are the neurologic deficits reported with the use of 2-chloroprocaine in epidural anesthesia. Although the 2-chloroprocaine itself did not appear to have neurotoxic effects at a clinical level, the preservative sodium bisulfite and the low pH of the solution were felt to be the culprit, which resulted in the reformulation of this local anesthetic.

Recent reports of neurotoxicity with the administration of local anesthetics through small-gauged subarachnoid catheters exist. At present, the proposed theory is that use of these catheters results in a maldistribution of local anesthetic. This in turn leads to localized areas of the cauda equina being continuously exposed to high concentrations of local anesthetics, which results in direct local anesthetic neurotoxicity. Therefore a ban on the use of these smaller catheters is in place until further investigation.

Table 1-6 Clinical profile of local anesthetic agents

Agent	Concentration (%)	Clinical use	Onset	Usual Duration (H)	Recommended Maximum Single Dose (MG)	Comments	pH of Plain Solutions
Amides							
Lidocaine	0.5-1.0	Infiltration	Fast	1.0-2.0	300	Most versatile agent	6.5
	0.25-0.5	IV regional			500 + epinephrine		
	1.0-1.5	Peripheral nerve blocks	Fast	1.0-3.0	500 + epinephrine		
	1.5-2.0	Epidural	Fast	1.0-2.0	500 + epinephrine		
	4	Topical	Moderate	0.5-1.0	500 + epinephrine		
	5	Spinal	Fast	0.5-1.5	100		
Prilocaine	0.5-1.0	Infiltration	Fast	1.0-2.0	600	Least toxic agent Methemoglobinemia occurs usually above 600 mg	4.5
	0.25-0.5	IV regional			600		
	1.5-2.0	Peripheral nerve blocks	Fast	1.5-3.0	600		
	2.0-3.0	Epidural	Fast	1.0-3.0			

table continues on next page

Agent	Concentration (%)	Clinical Use	Onset	Usual Duration (H)	Recommended Maximum Single Dose (MG)	Comments	pH of Plain Solutions
Mepivacaine	0.5-1.0	Infiltration	Fast	1.5-3.0	400 500 + epinephrine	Duration of plain solutions longer than lidocaine without epinephrine	4.5
	1.0-1.5	Peripheral nerve blocks	Fast	2.0-3.0			
	1.5-2.0	Epidural	Fast	1.5-3.0		Useful when epinephrine is contraindicated	
	4.0	Spinal	Fast	1.0-1.5	100		
Bupivacaine	0.25	Infiltration	Fast	2.0-4.0	175 225 + epinephrine	Lower concentrations provide differential sensory/motor block.	4.5-6
	0.25-0.5	Peripheral nerve blocks	Slow	4.0-12.0	225 + epinephrine	Ventricular arrhythmias and sudden	
	0.25-0.5	Obstetric epidural	Moderate	2.0-4.0	225 + epinephrine	cardiovascular collapse reported	
	0.5-0.75	Surgical epidural	Moderate	2.0-5.0	225 + epinephrine	following rapid IV injection	
	0.5-0.75	Spinal	Fast	2.0-4.0	20		
Etidocaine	0.5	Infiltration	Fast	2.0-4.0	300 400 + epinephrine	Profound motor block useful for surgical anesthesia but not for obstetric analgesia	4.5
	0.5-1.0	Peripheral	Fast	3.0-12.0	400 + epinephrine		
	1.0-1.5	Surgical epidural	Fast	2.0-4.0	400 + epinephrine		
Dibucaine	0.25-0.5 hyperbaric	Spinal	Fast	2.0-4.0	10	Recommended only for spinal and topical use	
	0.00067 hypobaric	Spinal	Fast	2.0-4.0	10		
	1.0	Topical	Slow	30-60	50		
Esters							
Procaine	1.0	Infiltration	Fast	30-60	1000	Used mainly for infiltration and differential spinal blocks.	5-6.5
	1.0-2.0	Peripheral nerve blocks	Slow	30-60	1000		
	2.0	Epidural	Slow	30-60	1000	Allergic potential after repeated use	
	10.0	Spinal	Moderate	30-60	200		
Chloroprocaine	1.0	Infiltration	Fast	30-60	800 1000 + epinephrine	Lowest systemic toxicity of all local anesthetics	2.7-4
	2.0	Peripheral nerve block	Fast	30-60	1000 + epinephrine	Intrathecal injection may be associated with sensory/motor deficits	
	2.0-3.0	Epidural	Fast	30-60	1000 + epinephrine		
Tetracaine	1.0	Spinal	Fast	2.0-4.0	20	Use is primarily limited to spinal and topical anesthesia	
	2.0	Topical	Slow	30-60	20		4.5-6.5
Cocaine	4.0-10.0	Topical	Slow	30-60	150	Topical use only. Addictive, causes vasoconstriction. CNS toxicity marked excitation ("fight or flight" response). May cause cardiac arrhythmias owing to sympathetic stimulation.	
Benzocaine	Up to 20	Topical	Slow	30-60	200	Useful only for topical anesthesia.	

Modified from Covino BG: Clinical pharmacology of local anesthetic agents. In Cousins MJ, Bridenbaugh PO, editors: Neural blockade in clinical anesthesia and management of pain, *Philadelphia, ed 2, 1988, JB Lippincott.*

Systemic Toxicity

The systemic effects of local anesthetic—ranging from therapeutic to toxic—can best be described as a continuum that is dependent on blood level concentrations. Systemic toxicity most frequently arises from one of two causes: (1) accidental vascular injections, or (2) administration of an excessive dose (see Table 1-7). The main toxic effects occur in the CNS and cardiovascular systems, but the cardiovascular system is four to seven times more resistant to these effects; in other words, seizures will occur with lower concentrations than are required to produce cardiovascular collapse.

CNS TOXICITY

The continuum of symptoms related to CNS toxicity appears to be not only related to concentration but also to the rate at which it presents itself to the nervous system.

For example, small amounts of local anesthetic can induce side effects, even seizures, if their application to the CNS is instantaneous, as with inadvertent intraarterial injections. On the other hand, high blood concentrations can be tolerated without signs of systemic toxicity if they are applied over long periods of time with continuous perineural and epidural infusions. The progression of CNS toxic symptoms results from selective depression of inhibitory fibers or centers in the CNS that results in excessive excitatory input. Early signs of toxicity differ between the ester and amide-linkage local anesthetics.

The former generally produce stimulant and euphoric symptoms, whereas the latter tend to produce sedation and amnesia. Beyond this all the local anesthetics produce similar toxic symptoms. Commonly reported symptoms in association with rising blood levels are headache, lightheadedness, numbness and tingling of the perioral area or distal extremities, tinnitus, drowsiness, a flushed or chilled sensation, and blurred vision or difficulty focusing the eyes. Objectively, signs of obtundation, confusion, slurred speech, nystagmus, and muscle tremors or twitches can be observed. It is important to recognize these signs, as they can foreshadow an impending seizure. The seizures appear to arise from subcortical levels in the brain, mainly the amygdala and the hippocampus, and then subsequently spread, producing a generalized grand mal seizure.

Other factors affect the CNS toxicity of local anesthetics. Increases in PCO_2 may possibly have an effect by increasing cerebral blood flow and therefore increasing delivery to the CNS, as well as enhancing excitatory effects on the brain tissue. Similarly, a decrease in pH may increase the concentration of the active cationic form in the brain cells. It also has been shown that cimetidine can increase the toxicity of local anesthetics by slowing their elimination.

Likewise, the toxic effects of local anesthetics can be decreased by the effects of barbiturates, benzodiazepines, and inhalation anesthetics by raising the seizure threshold of the CNS.

Table 1-7   Comparable safe doses of local anesthetics (mg/kg)*

| | | AREAS INJECTED | | |
| | | CENTRAL BLOCKS‡ | | INTERCOSTAL BLOCKS§ with |
DRUGS	PERIPHERAL BLOCKS‡	PLAIN	WITH EPINEPHRINE 1:200,000	EPINEPHRINE 1:200,000
2-Chloroprocaine	–	20	25	–
Procaine	–	14	18	–
Lidocaine	20	7	9	6
Mepivacaine	20	7	9	6
Bupivacaine	5	2	2	2
Tetracaine	–	2	2	–

*Estimated to produce peak plasma levels that are less than half the plasma levels at which seizures could occur
‡Areas of low vascularity, i.e., axillary blocks using local anesthetic solutions containing 1:200,000 epinephrine
§Areas of high vascularity, i.e., intercostal blocks using local anesthetic solutions containing 1:200,000 epinephrine
From DiFazio CA, Woods AM: Pharmacology of local anesthetics. In Raj PP, editor: Practical management of pain, ed. 2, St. Louis, 1992, Mosby.

Cardiovascular System Toxicity

Although the cardiovascular system is more resistant to the toxic effects of local anesthetics, CVS toxicity can be severe and difficult, if not impossible, to treat. Decreases in myocardial contractility, rates of cardiac electrical impulse conduction, and effects on smooth muscle contractual functions are dose-dependent. Cardiac arrhythmias and hypertension develop as dosages increase. At one time the potency of the local anesthetics was thought to be directly related to their cardiac toxicity. However, it is now known that bupivacaine and etidocaine have a more profound effect on the electrophysiology of the heart. Bupivacaine is approximately 70 times more potent than lidocaine in blocking cardiac conduction, yet it is only four times more potent in blocking the conduction of nerves. This is felt to be due to the slower dissociation of bupivacaine from the cardiac Na^+ channels than that of lidocaine. This lack of complete dissociation leads to a progressive number of blocked Na^+ channels during diastole, which leads to subsequent cardiac depression and failure. Also, there is an indirect contribution to the cardiac toxicity by the local anesthetic's suppressive effects on the CNS. In addition, local anesthetics have both a direct and an indirect (via the autonomic system) effect on the vascular smooth muscle tone, resulting in either vasoconstriction and/or vasodilatation in different vascular beds, which is related to different levels of dosages. Cardiovascular toxicity is increased by hypoxia, acidosis, pregnancy, and hyperkalemia.

Table 1-8   Differential diagnosis of local anesthetic reactions

ETIOLOGY	MAJOR CLINICAL FEATURES	COMMENTS
Local anesthetic toxicity		
Intravascular injection	Immediate convulsion and/or cardiac toxicity	Injection into vertebral or carotid artery may cause convulsion after administration of small dose
Relative overdose	Onset in 5 to 10 min. of irribility, progressing to convulsions	
Reaction to vasoconstrictor	Tachycardia, hypertension, headache, apprehension	May vary with vasopressor used
Vasovagal reaction	Rapid onset Bradycardia Hypotension Pallor, faintness	Rapidly reversible with elevation of legs
Allergy		
Immediate	Anaphylaxis ($\downarrow$ BP, bronchospasm, edema)	Allergy to amides extremely rare
Delayed	Urticaria	Cross-allergy possible, for example, with preservatives in local anesthetics and food
High spinal or epidural block	Gradual onset Bradycardia* Hypotension Possible respiratory arrest	May lose consciousness with total spinal block and onset of cardio-respiratory effects more rapid than with high epidural or with subdural block
Concurrent medical episode (e.g., asthma attack, myocardial infarct)	May mimic local anesthetic reaction	Medical history important

*Sympathetic block above T4 adds cardioaccelerator nerve blockade to the vasodilatation seen with blockade below T4; total spinal block may have rapid onset.
From Covino BG: Clinical pharmacology of local anesthetic agents. In Cousins MJ, Bridenbaugh PO, editors: Clinical anesthesia and management of pain, Philadelphia, 1988, JB Lippincott.

PROCEDURAL USE OF LOCAL ANESTHETICS

Before the application of neural blockade, the patient's present physical condition should be assessed and a complete history taken to assure the appropriateness for the patient's procedure. It is important to ascertain if the patient has had any past reactions to local anesthetics. Patients scheduled for nerve blocks should refrain from eating at least 4 h before the procedure because vomiting may occur either as a psychogenic response or secondary to a systemic reaction. Ambulatory patients need transportation home provided and should not be permitted to drive home. Consent should be obtained only after full disclosure of the purposes of the blockade, the procedural steps, and effect and duration of the medications, and discussion of possible side effects and complications. Intravenous access should be assured and monitoring of the vital signs is mandatory. Not only will sedation with a benzodiazepine allay apprehension, but it will also protect the patient from possible systemic reaction by increasing the level for CNS seizure threshold. One should calculate in advance the appropriate amount of the drug needed and assure toxic dose potentials are avoided. This is done by understanding the anatomic considerations, as well as knowing the optimal site for injection so that the desired effects can be attained with the least amount of local anesthetic solution.

Injection should be unhurried, with frequent aspirations for blood or CSF, and multiple test dosages are encouraged. Continuous conversation with the patient serves to assure the patient. It also alerts the physician to possible adverse reactions secondary to the drug misplacement. Monitoring for adverse reactions or delayed complications is required; see Table 1-8 for a list of possible reactions. A complete summary of the procedure, drug dosages, effects, and adverse reactions should be recorded. At the end of the procedure the patient should be debriefed about the experience and, if an untowarded reaction occurs, the patient should be informed.

SUGGESTED READINGS

Aldrete AJ, Johnson, DA: Allergy to local anesthetic, *JAMA* 207:356, 1969.

Arthur GR, Feldman HS, Covino BG: Acute IV toxicity of LEA-103, a new local anesthetic, compared to lidocaine and bupivacaine in the awake dog, *Anesthesiology* 65:724, 1986.

Bader AM, Datta S, Flanagan H: Comparison of bupivacaine and ropivacaine induced conduction blockade in the isolated rabbit vagus nerve, *Anesth Analg* 68:724, 1989.

Carpenter RL, Mackey DC: Local anesthetics. In Barash PG, Cullen BF, Stoelting RK, editors: *Clinical anesthesia*, Philadelphia, 1989, JB Lippincott.

Catchlove RFH: The influence of CO_2 and pH on local anesthetic action, *J Pharmacol Exp Ther* 181:291, 1972.

Clarkson CW, Hondeghem LM: Mechanism for bupivacaine depression of cardiac conduction: fast block of sodium channels during action potential with slow recovery from block during diastole, *Anesthesiology* 62:396, 1985.

Corke BC, Carlson CG, Dettbarn WD: The influence of 2-chloroprocaine on the subsequent analgesic potency of bupivacaine, *Anesthesiology* 60:25, 1984.

Covino BG: Pharmacology of local anesthetic agents, *Br J Anaesth* 5:701-706, 1986.

Covino BG: Clinical pharmacology of local anesthetic agents. In Cousins MJ, Bridenbaugh PO, editors: *Clinical anesthesia and management of pain*, Philadelphia, 1988, JB Lippincott.

Covino BG, Vassello HG: *Local anesthetics, mechanism of action and clinical use*, New York, 1976, Grune and Stratton.

Datta S, Lambert DH, Gregus J et al: Differential sensitivities of mammalian nerve fibers during pregnancy, *Anesth Analg* 62:1070, 1983.

DiFazio CA, Woods AM: Pharmacology of local anesthetics. In Raj PP, editor: *Practical management of pain*, ed 2, St. Louis, 1992, Mosby.

Englesson S: The influence of acid-base changes on central nervous system toxicity of local anesthetic agents, *acta Anaesthesiol Scand* 18:79, 1974.

Fagraeus L, Urban BJ, Bromage PR: Spread of epidural analgesia in early pregnancy, *Anesthesiology* 58:184, 1983.

Fisher MM, Pennington JC: Allergy to local anesthesia; *Br J Anaesth* 54:893-894, 1982.

Franz DN, Perry RS: Mechanisms of differential block among single myelinated and nonmyelinated axons by procaine, *J Physiol* (Lond) 236:193, 1974.

Hille BL: Local anesthetics: hydrophilic and hydrophobic pathways for the drug-receptor reaction, *J Gen Physiol* 68:497-575, 1977.

Kane RE: Neurologic deficits following epidural or spinal anesthesia, *Anesth Analg* 60:150, 1981.

Kim TC, Tasch MD: Effects of cimetidine and ranitidine on local anesthetic central nervous system toxicity in mice, *Anesth Analg* 65:840, 1986.

Kopacz DJ, Carpenter RL, Mackey DC: Effects of ropivacaine on uterine blood flow in pregnant sheep, *Anesthesiology* 71:69, 1989.

Littlewood DG, Buckley P, Covino BG et al: Comparative study of various local anesthetic solutions in extradural block in labour, *Br J Anaesth* 51:47, 1979.

Metha PM, Theriot E, Mehrotra D: A simple technique to make bupivacaine a rapid-acting epidural anesthetic, *Reg Anesth* 123:135, 1987.

Ravindran RS, Turner MS, Muller J: Neurologic effects of subarachnoid administration of 2-chloroprocaine-CE, bupivacaine, and low pH normal saline in dogs, *Anesth Analg* 61:279, 1982.

Raymond SA, Gissen AJ: Mechanisms of differential nerve block. In Strichartz GR, editor: *Local anesthetics*, Berlin, 1987, Springer-Verlag.

Rigler M, Drasner K, Krejcie T et al: Cauda equina syndrome after continuous spinal anesthesia, *Anesth Analg* 72:275-281, 1991.

Scott BD, McClure JH, Giasi RM et al: Effects of concentration of local anaesthetic drugs in extradural block, *Br J Anaesth* 52:1033, 1980.

Seeman P: The membrane expansion theory of anaesthesia. In Fink BR, editor: *Molecular mechanisms of anesthesia. progress in anesthesiology*, vol 1, New York, 1975, Raven Press.

Tucker GT, Mather LE: Clinical pharmacokinetics of local anaesthetic, *Clin Pharmacokin* 4:241, 1979.

Wagman IH, DeJong RH, Prince DA: Effects of lidocaine on the central nervous system, *Anesthesiology* 28:155, 1967.

Wang BC, Hillman DE, Spielholz NI et al: Chronic neurological deficits and nesacaine-CE: an effect of the anesthetic, 2-chloroprocaine, or the antioxidant, sodium bisulfite? *Anesth Analg* 63:445, 1984.

Winnie AP, LaVallee DA, DeSosa B et al: Clinical pharmacokinetics of local anaesthetics, *Canad Anaesth Soc J* 24: 252, 1977.

Regional Anesthetics

Part 2

CHAPTER 2

Guidelines for Local Anesthetic Techniques

P. Prithvi Raj

Introduction The performance of regional anesthesia techniques requires the same level of preparation and planning that would be needed to conduct general anesthesia. Essential monitoring that will enable the anesthetist to anticipate the effect of anesthetic agents on various organ systems must be available. It is necessary to be prepared for any emergency that may occur in the conduct of a block, and the preparation and performance of any regional anesthetic procedure must take place in an adequately prepared facility.

MONITORING

Preparation of the patient for regional anesthesia includes complete explanation of the procedure to be performed and informed consent before or while the patient is brought to the area where the block will occur. This room should be quiet, undisturbed, of adequate size, and have good lighting available. The characteristics and design of an ideal regional anesthesia block room have been described by Rosenblatt. Complete resuscitation facilities must be available and include equipment to provide positive-pressure oxygen and suction, intubation equipment with appropriate laryngoscope blades and handles already tested to be in working order, appropriate-sized endotracheal tubes and oral airways, and emergency drugs. Essential emergency drugs that should be available include succinylcholine, atropine, thiopental or diazepam, ephedrine, and lidocaine (Table 2-1). A functioning intravenous catheter is essential for all regional anesthesia procedures, except for small (2- to 3-ml) injections of local anesthetics into muscle trigger points

Table 2-1 Routine emergency drugs required during the performance of regional anesthesia procedures

DRUG	SUGGESTED DOSAGE (70-KG ADULT)	INDICATION
Atropine	0.2-0.4 mg IV increments	Bradycardia from vagal dominance
Diazepam	2.5-5 mg IV increments	Local anesthetic; seizure activity
Ephedrine	5-10 mg IV increments	Hypotension from sympathetic block
Lidocaine	50-100 mg IV bolus	Ventricular arrhythmias
Thiopental	50-100 mg IV increments	Local anesthetic; seizure activity
Succinylcholine	100 mg IV bolus	Muscle relaxation airway control

or single peripheral nerve blocks. Minimal monitoring should include continuous electrocardiographic (ECG) monitoring, heart rate, blood pressure, respiratory rate, oxygen saturation if sedative or narcotic analgesic medications will be given before or during the block, and level of consciousness.

NEEDLE BLOCK TRAY

A nerve block tray, whether it is commercially prepared or hospital prepared, should contain sufficient equipment to perform the regional anesthesia procedure intended (Box 2-1). Basic items on each nerve block tray should include items for sterile skin preparation and draping; containers for sterile antiseptic solution and local anesthetic; syringes for skin infiltration anesthesia and performance of the block; and an assortment of needles for skin infiltration and drawing up local anesthetic solutions, preparing the skin, and performing the block. Injection tubing should be available, and if continuous infusions are planned, appropriate catheters should also be available. If drugs are to be added to regional block trays, the hospital pharmacy should be consulted to ensure stability and potency of the drug, and ensure that sterility can be maintained during the sterilization process.

The choice between using reusable regional anesthesia trays or one of the commercially available trays is one of personal preference and the ultimate cost involved. Arguments can be made in favor of each.

Needles

Nerve injury can occur following injection of local anesthetic for regional anesthesia, and is thought to involve one of three mechanisms. The cutting edge of the needle may cause direct injury to the nerve; local anesthetic injection into the nerve sheath under high pressure can cause direct neural damage or ischemia of the nerve; and a toxic effect of the local anesthetic or its preservative may be responsible for neural toxicity.

During peripheral or plexus nerve block procedures, a needle having a short, blunt bevel has been shown to produce less nerve trauma than the conventional hypodermic needle, which has a long or cutting bevel (Fig. 2-1). The blunt-bevel needle also allows more precise perception of the different tissue planes encountered during the performance of regional anesthesia procedures. It is impor-

---

Box 2-1   Contents of multipurpose regional anesthesia block tray

Routine Items
Prep tray
Container for antiseptic solution (50 ml)
Antiseptic solution
Prep sponges (3)
4 × 4 gauze sponges
Ruler (15 cm)
Sterility indicator
Sterile drapes (4)
Intravenous extension tubing
Container for local anesthetic (2, 50 ml)
Local anesthetic solution for infiltration
 (1.5% lidocaine, 10 ml)
Epinephrine (1 mg/ml)
Syringes
 1 ml, to dispense epinephrine
 3 ml, for skin infiltration
 5 ml, glass to identify the epidural space
 10 ml, to inject local anesthetic
Needles
 25 × 2.5 cm (1 in) for skin infiltration of
 local anesthetic
 22 × 7.5 cm (3 in) for deeper skin infiltration
 22 × 11.8 cm (4.5 in) for deep skin infiltration
 18 × 3.8 cm (1.5 in) to pierce skin, and
 draw up solutions

Special contents added depending on the procedure
Specific block needles (see text)
 Spinal
 Spinal introducer needle
 Epidural
 Blunt-bevel needles, appropriate size
Catheter for continuous infusions; spinal, epidural,
 peripheral nerve
Local anesthetic for nerve block
Contrast agent and container
Neurolytic solution and container

---

tant to use the smallest diameter needle possible to avoid tissue trauma and undue discomfort; however, it is essential that the needle be large enough to inject local anesthetic and aspirate blood easily should an accidental intravascular injection occur. For this reason a 22-gauge needle is recommended for most nerve blocks. For procedures that require deep penetration, such as a celiac plexus or hypogastric plexus block, an 18- or 20-gauge needle is preferable to have better control in guiding the needle and for ease of aspiration.

A 25- or 27-gauge needle should be used for infiltration of the skin and subcutaneous tissue before proceeding with a larger needle for the nerve block. If a catheter is to be used for a continuous infusion technique, it is important to prepare the skin first by making

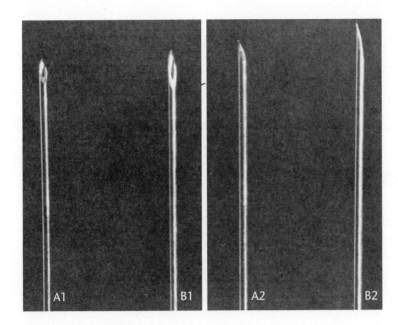

Fig. 2-1 *Needles used for peripheral block. **A1** and **A2**, Short, blunt, 45° needle bevel. **B1** and **B2**, Long, sharp, 14° needle bevel (conventional hypodermic needle).* (From Raj PP, editor: *Clinical practice of regional anesthesia,* New York, 1991, Churchill Livingstone.)

a nick with a larger (18-gauge) needle in order to avoid disrupting the catheter tip as it is inserted into the skin. If a styletted needle is used, ensure that the stylet fits flush with the bevel of the needle to avoid coring the tissue and possible obstruction of the needle tip during insertion. Translucent hubs are recommended, as they allow earlier observation of blood with aspiration in the event of an intravascular injection. Extension tubing can be beneficial when directly attached to the needle, as it allows the syringe to be changed when multiple injections are to be used, such as with confirmation of needle placement using contrast agents under fluoroscopy before injecting local anesthetic or neurolytic solutions, and avoids movement of the needle.

The incidence of spinal headache appears to be directly related to the size of needle used and the orientation of the needle in performing spinal anesthesia. It is thought that the spinal needle oriented parallel to the dura separates the fibers rather than cuts them, as a spinal needle oriented perpendicular to the dural fibers does, and produces a smaller defect in the dura mater (Fig. 2-2).

All spinal needles come with a removable stylet, which must be close-fitting to prevent coring of the skin and the resultant obstruction of the needle and contamination of spinal space with epidermal tissue and skin bacteria. Several spinal needle types and sizes are commercially available, although only two different needle tip points are available. The tip points can have either a beveled cut-

ting point or a noncutting, rounded, pencil point (Fig. 2-3). The commonly used spinal needles with a cutting point are the Quincke-Babcock spinal needle, which has a medium-length cutting bevel with a sharp point, and the Pitkin needle, which has a short bevel with cutting edges and a rounded heel. The cutting-point spinal needles appear to be associated with a high incidence of postspinal headache even when smaller-sized needles are used (25- and 26-gauge). Spinal needles with a noncutting, rounded, pencil tip seem to cause less trauma to the dura mater with splitting the dura fibers rather than cutting them, and appear to be associated with a lower incidence of postspinal headache when larger caliber (22- or 24-gauge) needles are used. The Greene, Whitacre, and Huber needles have a noncutting, rounded, pencil tip. The Greene spinal needle is available only in a reusable form and comes in two sizes, 22 and 26 gauge. The Whitacre spinal needle has a completely rounded noncutting bevel with a solid tip, and its opening is on the side, 2 mm proximal to the tip. It is available in 22- and 25-gauge disposable forms. The Huber spinal needle has a curved tip to allow introduction of a spinal catheter. Introducer needles are available to facilitate insertion of the smaller (25-, 26-, or 29-gauge) spinal needles, as these can be difficult to direct through the skin and subcutaneous tissues. Another advantage of using an introducer needle is that it avoids contact of the spinal needle with the skin and prevents coring of the skin and introduction of the epidermis or bacteria

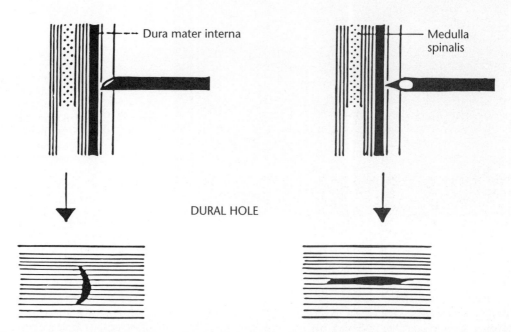

VERTICAL INSERTION

PARALLEL INSERTION

Dura mater interna

Medulla spinalis

DURAL HOLE

FIG. 2-2 *Types of needle insertion in lumbar puncture. In vertical insertion, the bevel of the spinal needle is inserted through the dura mater perpendicular, rather than parallel, to the longitudinal dural fibers. It is apparent that the number of fibers severed is greater using vertical insertion.* (From Raj PP, editor: *Clinical practice of regional anesthesia*, New York, 1991, Churchill Livingstone.)

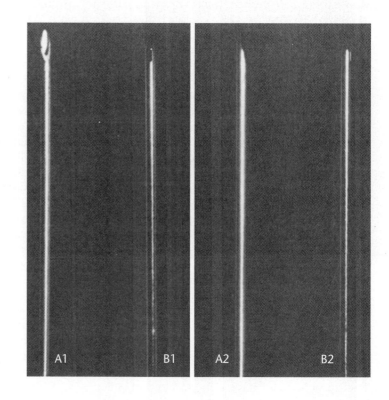

FIG. 2-3 *Spinal needles. A1 and A2, Beveled cutting point (Quincke-Babcock). B1 and B2, Noncutting, pencil-tip point (Whitacre).* (From Raj PP, editor: *Clinical practice of regional anesthesia*, New York, 1991, Churchill Livingstone.)

into the subarachnoid space. Introducer needles are usually 18 or 20 gauge, and a disposable 18-gauge needle can be used as an introducer if one is not available.

During epidural anesthesia, as in spinal anesthesia, it is essential that the needle have a close-fitted stylet in order to avoid coring the skin and obstructing the needle and to be able to recognize the loss of resistance necessary to identify entry into the epidural space. Epidural needles have rounded, noncutting tips that either have a bevel at the tip or are curved at the tip with the bevel facing sideways (Fig. 2-4). The Crawford epidural needle is an example of the latter; it is most often used for the paramedian approach, as it slides off of the lamina easily and a catheter can thread directly upward when a 45° to 60° angle is used to enter the epidural space. The Crawford needle is not recommended for the midline approach, as the obtuse angle of the tip does not penetrate the interspinous ligaments with ease. The Tuohy needle has a curved Huber point with the bevel facing sideways, and the tip can either be sharp or blunt at the end. The curved end helps to facilitate passage of the catheter, which can proceed in the direction of the needle curve.

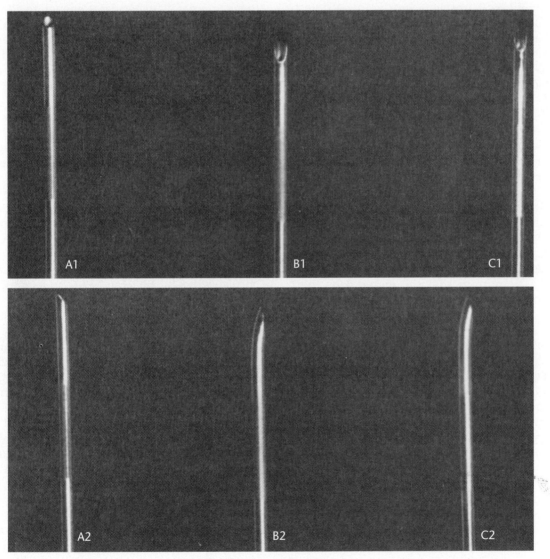

FIG. 2-4 *Epidural needles.* **A1** *and* **A2,** *A Crawford needle with a short bevel is best for a paramedian approach.* **B1** *and* **B2,** *A Tuohy needle with a curved Huber point and bevel facing sideways.* **C1** *and* **C2,** *A Hustead needle with reduced bevel angle. Note 1-cm shaft markings.* (From Raj PP, editor: *Clinical practice of regional anesthesia,* New York, 1991, Churchill Livingstone.)

A modification of the Tuohy needle is the Hustead needle, which has a reduced bevel angle to avoid shearing a catheter during passage and is the most commonly used disposable epidural needle. The Weiss needle, another modification of the Tuohy needle, has wings on the hub to facilitate handling of the hub. Calibrated depth markings are available on a large number of epidural needles to help estimate the depth of the epidural space and the length of epidural catheter threaded into the epidural space. The hub of an epidural needle should be translucent to allow rapid visualization of cerebrospinal fluid (CSF) or blood in the event of subarachnoid or intravascular placement of the needle, and should be lightweight with grooved sides to allow the user to easily sense differences in tissues and allow control during insertion. A bevel indicator should be present on the hub to indicate the orientation of the bevel and facilitate catheter placement.

Catheters

A wide variety of catheters is available for insertion through both spinal and epidural needles, as well as for placement on peripheral nerves and plexuses for continuous infusion techniques. The primary difference between them is the material they are made of and their physical properties. The ideal material for catheter construction should have the properties as described by Bromage. It is important that the material be inert, nonirritating, and supple enough to avoid cracking during placement. Its tensile strength should prevent breakage of the catheter when exposed to traction and during insertion, and also allow maneuverable rigidity. The length of the catheter should be adequate to allow it to reach up over the shoulder from the lumbar region and still have sufficient length to enter the epidural space. The external diameter should be small enough to allow it to easily pass through an epidural needle, and the internal diameter lumen must be large enough to allow injection of fluids and aspiration of blood and CSF. The wall of the catheter must be thick enough to avoid kinking and obstruction. The tip of the catheter should be smooth, dull, and flexible to prevent perforation of veins or dura. Radiopaque catheters can allow verification of correct placement with radiographic guidance, and graduated markings

facilitate control of the depth of catheter insertion into the epidural space.

Recently subarachnoid catheters have been introduced for continuous spinal infusions. Continuous spinal catheter infusion is not a new technique of regional anesthesia, as it was described by Tuohy in 1944. An epidural catheter can be used for continuous subarachnoid infusion; however, the incidence of spinal headache with an 18- to 20-gauge catheter would be too high in younger patients. The present technology has developed a subarachnoid catheter that is small enough to be used clinically without an unacceptably high incidence of spinal headache. These catheters are 27, 28, or 32 gauge, and have internal diameters large enough to allow for injection of medications. Although a stylet is necessary during insertion of these catheters, spinal catheters are available with a stylet built into the lumen of the catheter to increase tensile strength, allow radiopacity, and resist kinking.

Catheters are available for continuous peripheral nerve, plexus, and sympathetic ganglion infusions. They should have most of the properties of an ideal epidural catheter; however, they should be sufficiently rigid to maintain their initial placement and avoid migration away from the area to be blocked. The 18-gauge Longdwell thin-wall Teflon catheter (Becton Dickinson & Co.) has been used for prolonged infusions of sympathetic ganglia, peripheral nerves, and plexuses. It is available in 8.8-, 13.2-, and 17.6-cm lengths.

Syringes

The proper syringe aids the performance of regional anesthetic procedures by accurately delivering a given volume of local anesthetic with ease. It is important to select the right-sized syringe for the block to be performed; if it is too large it will be awkward to use, and if too small it will require frequent refilling, with possible movement of the needle during manipulation of the syringe-needle connection. If a large volume of local anesthetic or multiple injections of different solutions will be required, direct connection of the needle and syringe can be avoided by using a short length of intravenous tubing between the needle and syringe. If a large (10- to 20-ml) syringe is used, one with rings for the thumb and finger allows better control during injection of local anesthetics and control of the syringe with one hand. It is important that a syringe allow easy aspiration to avoid intravascular injection; this is best accomplished with a 3-, 5-, or 10-ml syringe.

Syringes used to identify the epidural space by the loss of the resistance technique require a tight-fitting barrel and a plunger that offers no resistance against the barrel. Glass syringes are most commonly used, and have no resistance between the barrel and plunger when wet. Glass syringes are available with a silicone lining that offers no resistance when dry, but if wet causes the plunger and barrel to stick together. One disadvantage of glass syringes is that the powder from sterile gloves can cause the plunger to stick in the barrel, which must be avoided. Plastic syringes with low friction can be used for the loss of resistance, but they have a different feel from glass and have not been as popular.

Tubing and Pumps

Continuous infusions of local anesthetics alone or local anesthetic-narcotic combinations are commonly used for providing anesthesia and for prolonged analgesia postoperatively, as well as for relief of chronic pain conditions. If these systems are used for postoperative pain management or chronic pain relief, it is essential that the patient be seen and examined daily to ensure adequate analgesia and to avoid any side effects.

Several commercial pumps are available that are capable of providing continuous infusions, including intravenous infusion pumps, patient-controlled analgesia pumps with basal rate capability, and syringe pumps. The pump must be capable of generating enough force to infuse the medication through the resistance of the narrow tubing without exceeding its limits and causing frequent high-pressure alarms. It should be easy to operate and have the capacity to set the rate delivered per hour, maximum volume to be delivered over a certain time period, and volume infused, as well as a locking capability to prevent tampering with the preset rate. Because these infusion volumes frequently are small, the pump must be capable of infusing small volumes (as little as 1 ml/hr with subarachnoid infusions). Alarm capabilities are important, and the unit should signal low infusion volumes, obstruction to flow, increased pressure, and tampering with the unit.

Fluoroscopy

Fluoroscopy is an invaluable adjunct in the performance of difficult regional anesthetic procedures in morbidly obese patients with poor anatomic landmarks or during celiac or hypogastric plexus blocks, and is essential to verify accurate needle placement and spread of opaque contrast material before injecting neurolytic agents.

CONTRAST AGENTS

The contrast agents that are commonly used have a fully substituted, triiodinated benzene ring structure, and may have an ionic or nonionic formulation (Table 2-2). The nonionic contrast agents are used to provide opacification of the central nervous system (CNS), as they have reduced CNS toxicity after subarachnoid injection. Metrizamide (Amipaque, Winthrop), the first of the clinically used nonionic formulations, has been used for years to provide state-of-the-art imaging during myelography; however, it comes in a powdered form that must be prepared before its use, and the frequency of seizures with its use is unacceptably high compared with newer agents available. When contrast agents are used near the central axis and the potential for subarachnoid injection exists, it is recommended that either iopamidol (Isovue, Squibb) or iohexol (Omnipaque, Winthrop) be used, as they have lower potential for CNS toxicity, are water soluble, and are provided in a liquid form that is easy to use. In other regions of the body, the ionic contrast agents diatrizoate (Renografin or Hypaque) or iothalamate (Conray) can be used without any significant clinical effects or adverse sequelae if the volume is limited to 10 to 15 ml.

Table 2-2 Radiologic contrast agents

AGENT	TYPE	USE
Diatrizoate (Renografin, Hypaque)	Ionic	Nerve plexus blocks
Iothalamate (Conray)	Ionic	Nerve plexus blocks
Metrizamide (Amipaque)	Nonionic	Central neural blockade
Iopamidol (Isovue)	Nonionic	Central neural blockade
Iohexol (Omnipaque)	Nonionic	Central neural blockade

Peripheral Nerve Stimulator

A nerve stimulator can locate a nerve by applying a small, adjustable amount of electric current to a searching needle to cause depolarization of the nerve when the needle is within close proximity. An understanding of a few concepts of basic electrophysiology is important for the proper use of a peripheral nerve stimulator in regional anesthesia. When a mixed nerve is stimulated, the motor component, A-α fibers, requires less current for stimulation and depolarization than the sensory element, A-δ and C fibers; this property allows a stimulating needle to elicit muscle contraction and avoid painful paresthesias. The distance between a nerve and the exploring needle is estimated by the current required to cause nerve stimulation, and maximal muscle contraction with minimal current is consistent with close proximity of the needle to the nerve. The choice of electrodes for stimulation of the needle is important. When the cathode (negative) terminal is connected to the needle, much less current is required to produce depolarization compared to when the anode (positive) terminal is used to stimulate the needle. This is due to preferential cathodal stimulation: when the stimulating needle is negative, it causes current to flow to the needle, and causes depolarization of the nerve; if the stimulating needle is positive (the anode terminal), the current will flow away from the needle tip and cause hyperpolarization of the nerve, which requires four times as much current (Figs. 2-5 to 2-8).

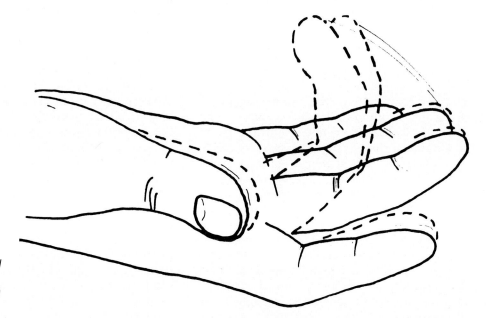

FIG. 2-5 *Flexion of medial 1½ digits is seen as the needle approaches the nerve trunk in brachial plexus block.* (From Raj PP, editor: *Illustrated manual of regional anesthesia,* Berlin, 1988, Springer-Verlag.)

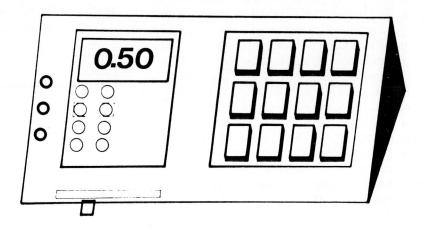

FIG. 2-6 *Current is reduced to 0.5 to 1 mA, and the needle is stabilized when maximal stimulation of the contracting muscles is achieved.* (From Raj PP, editor: *Illustrated manual of regional anesthesia,* Berlin, 1988, Springer-Verlag.)

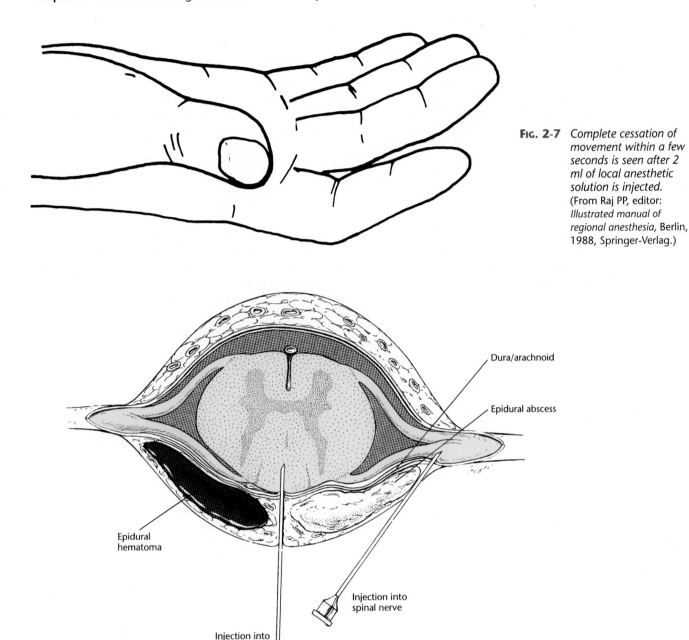

FIG. 2-7 *Complete cessation of movement within a few seconds is seen after 2 ml of local anesthetic solution is injected.* (From Raj PP, editor: *Illustrated manual of regional anesthesia,* Berlin, 1988, Springer-Verlag.)

Dura/arachnoid

Epidural abscess

Epidural hematoma

Injection into spinal nerve

Injection into spinal cord

FIG. 2-8 *Neurologic complications associated with spinal and epidural blockade.* (From Raj PP, editor: *Clinical practice of regional anesthesia,* New York, 1991, Churchill Livingstone.)

A nerve stimulator capable of monitoring neuromuscular blockade will be inadequate to aid needle placement adjacent to peripheral nerves unless it can deliver an adjustable and monitored stimulus of 1 to 2 seconds. A voltage of 1 to 2 V, or current of less than 0.5 mA, may be required to accurately locate a peripheral nerve. A peripheral nerve stimulator used for regional anesthesia should have several important characteristics to improve performance. It is important that a nerve stimulator have a constant current output, as resistance of the different tissues and needles can vary between 1 and 20Ω and variation of current will interfere with the accurate placement of the needle tip adjacent to the nerve. The current output should be clearly visible, preferably in a digital format to allow ease in determining the lowest current required for effective nerve stimulation. The output of the stimulator should have a large dial with easy adjustment, and it should have a linear output (the output equals the amount the dial is turned to deliver; for example, 50% current output with a 50% reading on the meter). The polarity of the leads should be clearly marked to ensure negative terminal attachment to the needle as previously described. The stimulation pulse width should be short (50 to 100 μsec is ideal) to distinguish needle proximity to peripheral nerves. High and low outputs allow greater adjustment; high current is used when distant from the nerve or to monitor neuromuscular block, and low current output when fine movement and adjustment is required, as when the needle tip is near the nerve. A battery indicator is necessary to avoid a faulty battery as a cause of an inadequate response to nerve stimulation. It is important that the connecting wires and clips be of high quality and have low resistance to prevent inaccurate current reading on the monitor. Additional information can be obtained in Pither and coworkers' review article, which has an in-depth discussion of experimental characteristics of nerve stimulators and a comparison of commercially available peripheral nerve stimulators and their properties.

Both insulated and uninsulated needles have been used with peripheral nerve stimulation for regional anesthesia nerve blocks. The electrical properties and characteristics of each needle type have been well defined. If the insulation of a sheathed needle extends to the tip, the current source will be localized to a point at the needle tip with a spherical zone of current density. An uninsulated needle differs in that it will have a maximal current density proximal to the needle tip extended up the needle shaft.

Many commercially produced insulated needles for regional anesthesia procedures are available. A catheter placed over a styletted needle with a metal hub can effectively function as an insulated needle and provide the capability to leave a catheter in place for prolonged infusions. If an uninsulated needle is chosen, preferably it should have a metal hub; however, a plastic hub can be used if it is of sufficient length to allow attachment of the alligator clip to the shaft of the needle. The most commonly used needles are a 25-gauge 3.75-cm (1.5-inch) needle, a 22-gauge 3.75-cm (1.5-inch) needle, a 22-gauge 8.75-cm (3.5-inch) spinal needle, and a 20- or 22-gauge 10-cm (4-inch), 15-cm (6-inch), or 20-cm (8-inch) standard block needle.

ADJUVANT TECHNIQUES TO IMPROVE THE SUCCESS OF REGIONAL ANESTHESIA
Mixtures

pH Adjustment. Various approaches have been used to facilitate and speed the onset of action of local anesthetic drugs. Most of these involve manipulating the pharmacologic factors involved in producing anesthesia of the nerves with local anesthetics. The commercially available local anesthetic solutions are all acidic (pH 3.0 to 6.5), and since the pK_a of the local anesthetics range from 7.6 to 8.9, the drugs in the commercial preparations will be predominantly in the cationic form according to the Henderson-Hasselbach equation, with only a small amount of drug present in the unionized lipid-soluble form. The cationic form, however, does not cross biologic membranes. Thus, to increase the amount in the lipid-soluble base form needed to cross the nerve membrane, one can either increase the pH of the solution or decrease the pK_a of the drug being injected. Still another means of increasing the amount of lipid-soluble drug outside the nerve membrane would be to increase the concentration of the drug in solution. At present, the most frequently used technique to improve onset of local anesthetic drugs is the adjustment of the pH of the local anesthetic solution. The increase in pH is accomplished by the addition of bicarbonate. While this is an old technique, a number of recent papers have reported improved onset times using multiple local anesthetics. DiFazio and coworkers demonstrated that a greater than 50% decrease in onset time for epidural anesthesia took place when the pH of the commercially available lidocaine with epinephrine was raised from a pH of 4.5 to a pH-adjusted level of 7.2 by the addition of bicarbonate. Similarly, Hilgier reported a marked improvement in onset time for brachial plexus anesthesia when bupivacaine with epinephrine (pH 3.9) was alkalinized to a pH of 6.4 before injection. Both of these relatively large changes in pH resulted in major increases in the amount of free base available in solution for nerve penetration and also resulted in a marked (~ 50%) improvement in the onset time for anesthesia. Smaller changes in pH and decreases in onset time using bupivacaine solutions without epinephrine for epidural analgesia in the parturient have been reported by McMorland and coworkers using 0.25% bupivacaine. Improved onset time with pH-adjusted mepivacaine has also been reported for brachial plexus anesthesia.

LOCAL ANESTHETIC CARBONATE

Another approach to shortening onset time for the production of surgical anesthesia has been the use of carbonated local anesthetic solutions. In these solutions, the local anesthetic salt is the carbonate (e.g., lidocaine carbonate rather than lidocaine hydrochloride), and CO_2 is added to the solution to maintain a high concentration of the carbonate anion. To date, carbonated local anesthetics still are not available in the United States. However, several past clinical studies by Bromage and coworkers found that onset time was shortened, the spread of anesthesia was more extensive, and a better quality of neural blockade took place when a carbonated rather than an uncarbonated lidocaine solution was used. On average, Bromage noted a 40% decrease in onset time using a carbonated lidocaine solution.

ALTERING LOCAL ANESTHETIC pK_a

Another way to modify latency is to warm the local anesthetic solution. Although the exact mechanism for this affect is not clear, it is very likely to be due to an increase in the pK_a of the local anesthetic that occurs with increases in temperature.

IMPROVING INTENSITY AND DURATION

Opiate Addition

Another major advancement aimed at improving the success of regional anesthesia has come about with the use of adjunct drugs with spinal and epidural anesthesia. These drugs act at a secondary site of action that is different from the site of action of the local anesthetic. The primary drugs used with local anesthetics at the spinal cord level have been opiates such as fentanyl or α_2 drugs such as clonidine. Clinical use of epidural and spinal opiates to ameliorate postoperative pain is widespread and has been extensively investigated. These drugs are felt to act by suppression of sensory input at Rexed lamina II and V of the dorsal horn in the substantia gelatinosa of the spinal cord. Combining fentanyl with local anesthetics with initially reported by Justins and coworkers as a means of producing more complete anesthesia with the epidural application of local anesthetics. The activity of opiates as local anesthetics has also been evaluated. Meperidine and methadone have been noted to have local anesthetic properties, whereas other opiates such as morphine and its derivatives do not have local anesthetic activity.

At present, the combination of opiate with local anesthetic for epidural use is widespread in obstetrics and for acute pain management postoperatively. Using this combination, it may be observed clinically that a marked increase in analgesic activity takes place by means of a synergistic effect in decreasing pain input by these two drugs at very low concentrations. Chestnut and coworkers, for instance, demonstrated that low concentrations of fentanyl (1 µg/ml) added to extremely dilute solutions of bupivacaine (0.0625%) produce effective analgesia without the production of motor blockade in laboring patients. The typical side effects of perispinal narcotics, such as itching and urinary retention, do occur, however, and can be managed by the administration of low doses of naloxone.

Monoamines

Other endogenous analgesic systems at the spinal cord level include those mediated by neurotransmitters such as monoamines (epinephrine). In this area, improved analgesia has been shown to occur by using an α_2-adrenergic agonist such as clonidine combined with minimal doses of local anesthetic or opiates applied to the spinal cord.

Epinephrine Addition

In general, the duration of local anesthetics is thought to be proportional to the time that the drug remains in contact with the nerve. The clinical observation is that drugs added to the local anesthetic solution that delay absorption of the local anesthetic increase both intensity of blockade and duration of anesthesia. The most commonly added drug is epinephrine in a concentration of 1:200,000 (5 µg/ml). Such a solution can decrease local tissue blood flow and retard drug absorption from the site of drug injection. In general, this will increase the duration and intensity of local anesthetic blockade of the nerve, very likely due to increased nerve penetration by the local anesthetic and thus increased local anesthetic concentration in the nerve. Addition of epinephrine at the same time will also result in a significant decrease in blood levels of the local anesthetics secondary to decreased drug absorption (Table 2-3). This effect of combining epinephrine with local anesthetics takes place with *all* local anesthetics when they are used for peripheral nerve blockade, such as for infiltration and nerve conduction blocks. When local anesthetics are used for epidural anesthesia, epinephrine will reduce absorption and prolong the block produced by the local anesthetic for all except the very lipid-soluble drugs, bupivacaine and etidocaine. As a result, when lidocaine and mepivacaine are used, a 75% to 90% increase in duration of brachial plexus blockade will occur when epinephrine is added. With bupivacaine and etidocaine, an increase in duration of brachial plexus blockade of approximately 50% occurs with the addition of epinephrine; however, an increase in the duration of epidural blocks of only 10% to 15% occurs when epinephrine is added to these drugs.

LOCAL ANESTHETIC TOXICITY

Toxicity following local anesthetic administration can be classified into two major categories: (1) allergic reactions, and (2) system toxicity, including CNS and cardiovascular toxicity.

Allergic Reactions

Allergic reactions to local anesthetics are extremely rare. Such reactions may be manifested by dermatitis, urticaria, anaphylaxis, pruritus, and bronchospasm. Close examination of the circumstances and events surrounding local anesthetic allergic reactions usually reveals the coadministration of epinephrine or a steroid such as Depo-Medrol. In patients who present with a history of allergy to local anesthetics, skin sensitivity testing can be rapidly accomplished. The procedure involves the administration of a series of local anesthetics and additives as skin wheals followed by assessment at 30 minutes. Size and extent of any localized reaction can be easily scored and

the patient's allergy to local anesthetics accurately assessed. Suggested grading criteria are as follows: − (no visible change at injection site); + (1-cm wheal with erythema); ++ (2-cm wheal with erythema); +++ (3-cm wheal with erythema). Usually a response of ≤ 1 cm (+) is due to localized histamine release rather than an antigen-antibody response. Negative skin tests should be treated with caution, since protein of the skin is different from other protein in the body, and the antigen may be a metabolite rather than the parent drug. In patients exhibiting a negative of +1 response, an intravenous challenge can be given using 50 mg of 1% lidocaine, 1% mepivacaine, 0.125% bupivacaine, or 0.1% tetracaine. A minimum of 30 minutes should be allowed between each injection. A negative response indicates that the local anesthetic in question can be safely administered in larger doses. Patients exhibiting any positive response to the intravenous challenge should be subjected to more extensive and precise immunologic testing, such as the Prausnitz-Küstner test. In this test, serum from the suspected sensitive patient is injected intradermally in either normal human subjects or monkeys.

Allergy to the amide local anesthetics is exceedingly rare. Almost all reported reactions have been found to be due to methylparaben. Thus use of preservative-free amide local anesthetic solutions would appear to be preferable in the effort to preclude allergic reactions.

Systemic Toxicity

The primary pharmacologic action of local anesthetic agents is the inhibition of the excitation conduction process in peripheral nerves. However, the ability of these agents to stabilize membranes is not limited to peripheral nerves. Any excitable membranes, such as those that exist in heart, brain, and at the neuromuscular junction, will be altered by local anesthetic agents if they achieve a sufficient tissue concentration. Regional anesthesia, properly performed, usually does not result in blood concentrations of local anesthetics sufficient to cause systemic effects. However, the accidental intravascular injection or the use of an excessive extravascular amount of local anesthetics can result in blood and tissue concentrations that will cause profound systemic effects. In general, the primary systemic effects of local anesthetic agents are manifest in the central nervous and cardiovascular systems.

Table 2-3   Comparable safe doses* and duration of epidural local anesthetics

Drug	Dose (mg/kg)	Average Duration (min)
2-chloroprocaine	20	60
Lidocaine with 1:200,000 Epinephrine	9	100
Mepivacaine with 1:200,000 Epinephrine	9	120
Bupivacaine	2	200
Etidocaine	4	200

*Safe dose estimated to produce plasma levels that on average are less than half of the plasma levels at which seizures could occur

Effects on the Central Nervous System

The central nervous system appears to be particularly susceptible to the systemic actions of local anesthetic agents. Since these agents are relatively lipid-soluble, low-molecular weight compounds, they readily cross the blood-brain barrier. Table 2-4 summarizes the available threshold blood concentrations required to produce CNS toxicity in humans. Initially, local anesthetic agents produce signs of CNS excitation. Objective signs of excitatory CNS effects include shivering, muscular twitching, and tremors initially involving muscles of the face and distal parts of the extremities. Ultimately, generalized convulsions of a tonic-clonic nature occur. If a sufficiently large dose of a local anesthetic agent is administered, the initial signs of CNS excitation are rapidly followed (and even masked) by a state of generalized CNS depression. Seizure activity ceases and respiratory depression followed by respiratory arrest ensue. The excitatory effect of local anesthetics in the brain involves the selective blockade of inhibitory pathways in the cerebral cortex. The specific site of action may involve either inhibitory cortical synapses or inhibitory cortical neurons. This effect is believed to be a membrane-stabilizing action of local anesthetics rather than an effect on inhibitory neurohumoral agents such as γ-aminobutyric acid. The initial blockade of inhibitory pathways by local anesthetic agents would permit facilitory neurons to function in an unopposed fashion, which would result in an increased CNS activity. Increased concentrations of local anesthetics would then tend to block both the inhibitory and facilitory pathways, resulting in a generalized state of CNS depression.

Bupivacaine is approximately eight times more potent than procaine when used for production of regional anesthesia; it is approximately seven times more toxic than procaine with regard to the dose required to produce convulsive activity in cats. Similar studies in dogs indicated that an intravenous dose of approximately 20 mg/kg lidocaine was required to produce convulsions compared with doses of 8 mg/kg etidocaine and 5 mg/kg bupivacaine. The relative CNS toxicity of bupivacaine, etidocaine, and lidocaine is approximately 4:2:1, which is similar to the relative potency of these agents observed in the clinical setting.

Table 2-4   Threshold for production of central nervous system toxicity by local anesthetics in humans and monkeys

Agent	Threshold Dose (in mg/kg) Producing CNS Symptoms in Humans	Approximate Serum Level (in g/ml) Producing Convulsive Activity in Monkeys
Procaine	19.2	—
Chloroprocaine	22.8	—
Lidocaine	6.4	18-26
Mepivacaine	9.8	22
Prilocaine	>6.0	20
Bupivacaine	1.6	4.5-5.5
Etidocaine	3.4	4.3
Tetracaine	2.5	—

Effects on the Cardiovascular System

Local anesthetic agents can produce profound effects on the cardiovascular system. The systemic administration of these agents can exert a direct action both on cardiac muscle and peripheral vascular smooth muscle. In general, the cardiovascular system appears to be more resistant than the CNS to the effect of local anesthetic agents. As noted above for CNS toxicity, cardiovascular toxicity appears to be related to the relative potency of the local anesthetic agent. Animal studies have indicated that the dose of local anesthetic agents needed to cause significant cardiovascular effects is approximately three times higher than the dose of these agents needed to have distinct effects on the CNS.

As the blood concentration of local anesthetic agents approaches the cardiotoxic level, a fall in blood pressure is usually the first sign of a systemic effect on the cardiovascular system. The initial drop in blood pressure appears to be related primarily to a fall in cardiac output, which is transient in nature and spontaneously reversible in most patients. However, if the amount of local anesthetic administered is excessive or if additional local anesthetic agent continues to reach the circulation, a profound and irreversible state of cardiovascular depression results. The profound hypotension and cardiovascular collapse seen before death is related not only to the negative inotropic action of the local anesthetics, but also to the extensive peripheral dilation known to occur with local anesthetics. At high concentrations, the depressant effect of these agents on the excitability of cardiac tissue also becomes evident as a decrease in sinus rate and onset of atrioventricular conduction block. Ultimately the combined peripheral vasodilation, decreased myocardial contractility, and depressant effects on rate and conductivity will lead to cardiac arrest and circulatory collapse.

More potent highly lipid-soluble and protein-bound local anesthetic agents such as bupivacaine may be relatively more cardiotoxic than the less potent, less lipid-soluble and protein-bound local anesthetics such as lidocaine. Several case reports have appeared in the literature in which bupivacaine and etidocaine were associated with rapid and profound cardiovascular depression.

Changes in acid-base status will alter the potential cardiovascular toxicity of local anesthetic agents. Hypercarbia and acidosis will decrease the threshold of local anesthetic agents for convulsive activity. Similarly, hypercarbia, acidosis, and hypoxia will tend to increase the cardiodepressant effect of local anesthetic agents.

Methemoglobinemia. The administration of large (>10 mg/kg) doses of prilocaine during regional anesthetic procedures may lead to the accumulation of a metabolite (O-toluidine), an oxidizing agent capable of converting hemoglobin (Hb^{2+}) to methemoglobin (Hb^{3+}). When sufficient methemoglobinemia (3 to 5 g/100 ml) is present, the patient may appear cyanotic and the blood may acquire a brownish discoloration. Such levels of methemoglobinemia are safe in healthy individuals, but any such slight impairment of oxygen transport in subjects with cardiac or pulmonary disease or in infants (whose erythrocytes are relatively deficient in methemoglobin reductase) may warrant immediate treatment. Reducing agents such as methylene blue (1 to 5 mg/kg) or, less satisfactorily, ascorbic acid (2 mg/kg), may be given intravenously to rapidly convert methemoglobin to hemoglobin.

Tissue Toxicity

Local anesthetic agents that are employed clinically rarely produce localized nerve damage. Neither local anesthetics themselves nor commonly included antibacterial preservatives such as methylparaben have been shown to produce any neurotoxic effect when administered at recommended doses with recommended clinical concentrations. Studies on isolated frog sciatic nerves revealed that the concentrations of procaine,

cocaine, tetracaine, and dibucaine required to produce irreversible conduction blockade are far in excess of the concentration of these agents used in the clinical setting.

Some concern has been expressed regarding the potential neurotoxicity of chloroprocaine. An inadvertent injection of relatively large volumes of 2% or 3% chloroprocaine into the subarachnoid space during the intended performance of epidural block has recently been reported to result in sensory and motor deficits persisting for several weeks (after the initial total spinal anesthesia had subsided). The reported sequelae were most probably due to the low pH (3.12 to 3.16) of these solutions of 2-chloroprocaine hydrochloride, rather than to any effect of the drug itself. The poor buffering capacity of cerebrospinal fluid may also have contributed to this complication, since this factor must have prolonged the exposure of the fibers within the subarachnoid space to this rather acidic medium. The possibility that this agent can cause localized neural damage is based on the report of prolonged sensorimotor deficits in four patients following the epidural or subarachnoid injection of large doses of this particular drug.

Subsequent studies in animals have proved somewhat contradictory regarding the potential neurotoxicity of chloroprocaine. Studies involving an isolated rabbit vagus nerve preparation have shown that chloroprocaine was associated with signs of neural irritation, whereas the use of lidocaine under similar conditions failed to cause local toxic effects. However, histologic examination of rabbit sciatic nerves exposed to chloroprocaine for a period of 6 hours did not reveal any signs of histologic damage. Investigations in dogs in which chloroprocaine and bupivacaine were administered intrathecally in doses sufficient to cause total spinal anesthesia demonstrated that chloroprocaine produced total paralysis in approximately 30% of the animals, whereas none of the bupivacaine-treated dogs showed evidence of permanent neurologic sequelae. Studies of a similar nature in sheep and monkeys have failed to show any difference in neurotoxicity between chloroprocaine and other local anesthetics or control solutions. More recently, it has been reported that paralysis has been observed in rabbits in which intrathecal chloroprocaine solutions were administered intrathecally. However, the paralysis was believed to be related to the sodium bisulfite, which was employed as an antioxidant in chloroprocaine solutions. The use of pure solutions of chloroprocaine without sodium bisulfite did not cause paralysis, whereas the sodium bisulfite alone was associated with paralysis.

COMPLICATIONS

Neurologic complications of central neural blockade due to hematoma or infection are extremely rare. Patients with bacteremia and intrinsic clotting disorders are theoretically at higher risk for these problems and should be identified in the preoperative period. The role of antiplatelet drugs and low dose heparin, and that of the presence of a localized infection at a site distant from the site of needle insertion in the etiology of epidural or intrathecal complications, are less well understood. Reported isolated cases of problems attributed to low doses of antiplatelet or anticoagulant drugs are balanced by reports of large numbers of epidural and spinal blocks in such patients without incident. Because of the rarity of these complications and the known spontaneous occurrences in nonsurgical populations, a large series would be required to answer this question. The clinician must weigh the risk against the known advantages, and may wish to obtain appropriate laboratory documentation before making the anesthetic choice.

Epidural and Subarachnoid Hematomas

Epidural and subarachnoid hematomas may also present as neurologic deficits in the postoperative period. Epidural needles and catheters often cause vascular trauma associated with minimal bleeding that usually resolves without sequelae. However, patients with abnormal clotting abilities may be at increased risk for development of epidural hematoma formation. Reports of spontaneous epidural hematomas in anticoagulated patients and in normal patients point out the risk of coincidental hematoma development as well. One large study reports the safe use of epidural catheters in patients undergoing anticoagulation for major vascular surgery. The catheters were inserted before beginning heparin treatment and removed postoperatively without incident. Allowing the epidural blockade to wear off before instituting continuous postoperative infusions permits evaluation of the patient's neurologic status. Postoperative complaints of back pain or an

increase in intensity of epidural blockade, particularly the development of new paresis, require immediate and aggressive evaluation to rule out hematoma formation.

Anterior Spinal Artery Thrombosis

Anterior spinal artery thrombosis or spasm causes a syndrome consisting primarily of paresis with a variable sensory deficit, usually occurring in the early postoperative period. The etiology is unknown, though direct trauma and hypoperfusion may be causative factors. Patient factors such as age and presence of peripheral vascular disease may also be important. While the addition of vasoconstrictors to intrathecal local anesthetics has been implicated, it is unlikely to be a primary etiologic factor in this problem. Though spinal cord perfusion studies do not show a deleterious effect with epinephrine, risk management would suggest that vasoconstrictors be avoided in high-risk patients unless indicated.

Persistent Paresthesias

Persisting paresthesias following peripheral nerve blocks can result in symptoms varying from mild dysesthesias lasting a few days to severe aching pain and permanent paresis. The mechanism is presumably direct nerve trauma from needle insertion or intraneural injection of local anesthetic. Selander and coworkers have shown axonal degeneration and damage to the blood nerve barrier with intrafascicular injections of local anesthetic and saline solutions. Conventional sharp-bevel needles have also been associated with increased nerve damage compared to blunt-bevel needles. Prevention of peripheral nerve injury includes gentle techniques when paresthesias are being sought; avoidance of intraneural injection; and appropriate choice of needle, agent, and patient. Persistent paresthesias often do not become evident until the second or third postoperative day. Other causes, such as positioning, ischemia due to prolonged tourniquet inflation or tight casting, and surgical trauma, as well as underlying coincident medical problems such as undiagnosed peripheral neuropathies, should be considered. A neurologic evaluation including electromyography (EMG) can be helpful in determining the level of neural injury. Fortunately, the outcome of these complications is usually good, with full recovery within a few days to weeks being the norm.

Postdural Puncture Headache

The most common postoperative complications of subarachnoid and epidural blocks are relatively minor and include postdural puncture headache, backache, and urinary retention. Postspinal headache is a minor but relatively common complication of subarachnoid blockade. Methods to prevent this problem by performing autologous blood or saline patches at the time of dural puncture have not been consistently successful. The most reliable preventive factors are the use of small needles and selection of older patients for this technique. Interestingly, intrathecal catheters placed through large gauge (18- or 20-gauge) needles do not have the high incidence of headache that would be anticipated with this size needle. The reasons for this discrepancy are not known, though a theoretical mechanism involving fibroblastic reaction at the catheter site has been suggested. Early detection and aggressive management of postdural puncture headache is recommended. Conservative treatment with hydration and bedrest should be followed by autologous blood patch using 10 to 15 ml of blood at 2 to 3 days if unsuccessful. Treatment should not be delayed inordinately; case reports of intracerebral hematoma following postdural puncture headache suggest that significant loss of cerebrospinal fluid (CSF) may result in serious morbidity in rare cases.

Faulty Equipment and Technique

Faulty equipment and technique can cause complications during the performance of a block. Attempted withdrawal of an epidural or intrathecal catheter through the needle can result in shearing of the catheter, leaving a portion of it in the epidural or intrathecal space. Occasionally the catheter will break off at the skin during removal. Most current catheters are made of inert materials and can theoretically be left in place. Surgical exploration need not be routinely undertaken, though the patient should be informed of the presence of the catheter remnant. Inserting the catheter beyond the recommended 2 to 3 cm may result in coiling and subsequent knotting in the epidural space and should be avoided. One report describes knotting of the catheter around the L2-3 nerve root, causing pain and difficulty in removing the catheter. Breakage of needles was more common in earlier days when the manufacturing process resulted in structural weakness at the juncture of the needle hub and shaft. Recommendations concerning surgical exploration in the event of a broken needle remain valid because of the propensity for needle points to migrate and cause potentially serious tissue damage.

MAJOR INFECTIOUS COMPLICATIONS

Complications of Spinal and Epidural Anesthesia

Cutaneous infection, epidural abscess, bacterial meningitis, and chronic adhesive arachnoiditis have followed after spinal and epidural anesthesia. Of these complications, cutaneous infections can be treated with topical treatment and rarely cause serious sequelae. The other three are serious and are considered here.

Epidural Abscess. Epidural infection usually arises endogenously from hematogenous spread secondary to infection elsewhere in the body. *Staphylococcus aureus* is the most common infection. The infection may cause thrombosis, spinal cord compression, and subsequent paraplegia. The abscess should be diagnosed early, promptly drained, and treated with antibiotic therapy (Table 2-5).

Meningitis. Meningitis developing after spinal anesthesia may be aseptic or septic. Thorsen states that the onset of symptoms in both forms of meningitis usually occurs 24 to 48 hours after the anesthetic is administered, but may be delayed as long as 10 days. Differentiation of septic from aseptic meningitis following spinal anesthesia may be very difficult. Classically, cerebrospinal fluid changes in aseptic meningitis following spinal anesthesia consist of mononuclear cells, normal glucose and protein concentration, and absence of organisms. Kamsler, however, reported a marked leukocyte response in cerebrospinal fluid in 31 of his 35 patients. In some instances, pleocytosis persisted for 1 week. Only four were symptomatic and none developed septic meningitis. Studies by Merritt and Fremont-Smith showed a consistent elevation of spinal fluid protein, normal or elevated glucose, and variable pleocytosis following spinal anesthesia. Aseptic meningitis following spinal anesthesia may be caused by the trauma of the procedure or by the introduction of sterile, irritating contaminants into the spinal fluid.

Septic meningitis is characterized by low spinal fluid glucose, predominantly polymorphonuclear leukocyte response, and organ-

Table 2-5   Differential diagnosis of epidural abscess, epidural hemorrhage, and anterior spinal artery syndrome

	EPIDURAL ABSCESS	EPIDURAL HEMORRHAGE	ANTERIOR SPINAL ARTERY SYNDROME
Age of patient	Any age	50% over 50 years	Any age
Previous history	Infection*	Efforts—anticoagulants	Arteriosclerosis
Onset	13 days	Sudden	Sudden
Generalized symptoms		None during epidural block; sharp, transient pain otherwise	None
Sensory involvement	None or paresthesias		
Motor involvement	Flaccid paralysis, later spastic	Flaccid paralysis	Flaccid paralysis
Segmental reflexes	Exacerbated—later obtunded	Abolished	Abolished
Queckenstedt's sign and myelogram	Signs of extradural compression	Signs of extradural compression	Normal
Cerebrospinal fluid	Increased cell count	Normal	Normal
Blood data	Rise in erythrocyte sedimentation rate	Prolonged coagulation time*	Normal

Infrequent findings.
From Usubiaga JE: Neurological complications of spinal and epidural analgesia. In Saidman LJ, Moya F, editor:
Complications of anesthesia, *Springfield, IL, 1970, Charles C. Thomas.*

isms on smear or culture or both. Organisms most commonly implicated in purulent iatrogenic meningitis are *S. aureus*, coliform species, and pseudomonads, although diplococcus, meningococcus, and even tubercle bacillus have been reported. Antibiotic therapy before diagnostic lumbar puncture may alter the usual spinal fluid picture of septic meningitis. Cellular and biochemical characteristics, as well as the growth behavior of the organisms, may be profoundly affected. Diagnosis of septic meningitis in a patient partially treated with antibiotics is, therefore, notoriously difficult.

Chronic Adhesive Arachnoiditis. Chronic adhesive arachnoiditis is a serious sequela to spinal anesthesia. A wide variety of agents have been found to be responsible for arachnoiditis, including Lysol, detergents, pyrogen-contaminated dextrose, and even pyrogen-free distilled water. Adhesive arachnoiditis may be found with numerous kinds of infection, including sepsis in gynecologic patients, as well as with spinal trauma and hemorrhage. Wadia and Dastar found 38 cases of arachnoiditis in 70 patients suffering from tuberculous infection. Adhesive arachnoiditis per se is not an absolute contraindication to spinal anesthesia. In patients with adhesive arachnoiditis and local or generalized infection, however, spinal anesthesia is not recommended.

SUGGESTED READINGS

Abouleish E, Vega S, Blendinger I et al: Long-term follow-up epidural blood patch, *Anesth Analg* 54:459-463, 1975.

Alpers BJ, Mancall EJ: *Clinical neurology*, ed. 6, Philadelphia, 1971, FA Davis.

Baron HC, LaRaja RD, Rossi G et al: Continuous epidural anesthesia in the heparinized vascular surgical patient: a retrospective review of 912 patients, *J Vasc Surg* 6:144-146, 1987.

Bashein G, Ready LB, Haschke RH: Electrolocation: insulated versus noninsulated needles, *Reg Anesth* 9:31-36, 1984.

Bert AA, Laasberg LH: Aseptic meningitis following spinal anesthesia: a complication of the past? *Anesthesiology* 62:674-677, 1985.

Bromage PR: *Epidural analgesia*, Philadelphia, 1978, WB Saunders.

Bromage PR: A comparison of the hydrochloride and carbon dioxide salts of lidocaine and prilocaine in epidural analgesia, *Acta Anesth Scand* Suppl XVI:55-69, 1965.

Bromage PR, Burfoot MF, Crowell DE et al: Quality of peridural blockade III: carbonated local anaesthetic solutions, *Br J Anaesth* 39:197-208, 1967.

Brown RE, Johnston L, Raj PP, Evans D: Continuous peripheral nerve of local anesthetic for management of pain due to reflex sympathetic dystrophy, *Reg Anesth* 15, 1S:88, 1990.

Chestnut DH, Owen CL, Bates JN et al: Continuous infusion epidural analgesia during labor: a randomized double-blind comparison of 0.0625% bupivacaine/ 0.0002% fentanyl versus 0.125% bupivacaine, *Anesth* 68:754-759, 1988.

Cousins MJ, Bromage PR: Epidural neural blockade. In Cousins MJ, Bridenbaugh PO, editors: Neural blockade in clinical anesthesia and pain management, Philadelphia, 1988, JB Lippincott.

Covino BG: Pharmacology of local anaesthetic agents, *Br J Anaesth* 58:701-716, 1986.

DiFazio CA, Carron H, Grosslight KR et al: Comparison of pH-adjusted lidocaine solutions for epidural anesthesia, *Anesth Analg* 65:760-764, 1986.

Eckstein KL, Rogacev Z, Vincente-Eckstein A et al: Prospective comparative study of postspinal headaches in young patients (less than 51 years), *Reg Anesth* 5:57, 1982.

Hancock DO: A study of 49 patients with acute spinal extradural abscess, *Paraplegia* 10:285-88, 1973.

Hilgier M: Alkalinization of bupivacaine for brachial plexus block, *Reg Anaesth* 10:59-61, 1985.

Hurley RJ, Lambert DH: Continuous spinal anesthesia with a microcatheter techniques: the experience in obstetrics and general surgery, *Reg Anaesth* 14:S3, 1989.

Justins DM, Francis D, Houlton PG et al: A controlled trial of extradural fentanyl in labour, *Br J Anaesth* 54:409-414, 1982.

Justins DM, Knott C, Luthman J et al: Epidural versus intramuscular fentanyl: analgesia and pharmacokinetics in labour, *Anaesth* 38:937-942, 1983.

Kamsler PM: Study of changes in the spinal fluid cell count during spinal anesthesia, *Anesth Analg* (Cleveland) 30:103-109, 1951.

Kieffer SA, Binet EF, Davis DO et al: Lumbar myelography with iohexol and metrizamide: a comparative multicenter prospective study, *Radiology* 151:665-670, 1984.

Kliemann FA: Paraplegia and intracranial hypertension following epidural anesthesia: report of four cases, *Arq Neuropsiquiatr* 33:217-29, 1975.

Kozody R, Palahniuk RJ, Wade JG et al: The effect of subarachnoid epinephrine and phenylephrine on spinal cord blood flow, *Can Anaesth Soc J* 31:503, 1984.

Lamb JT: Iohexol vs. iopamidol for myelography, *Invest Radiol* 20:537-543, 1985.

Mayumi T, Dohi S: Spinal subarachnoid hematoma after lumbar puncture in a patient receiving antiplatelet therapy, *Anesth Analg* 62:777-779, 1983.

McMorland GH, Douglas MJ, Jeffery WK et al: Effect of pH-adjustment of bupivacaine on onset and duration of epidural analgesia in parturients, *Can Anesth Soc J* 33:5, 537-541, 1986.

Merritt HH, Fremont-Smith F: *The cerebrospinal fluid*, Philadelphia, 1937, WB Saunders.

Moore DC: *Regional block, a handbook for use in the clinical practice of medicine and surgery*, Springfield, IL, 1965, Charles C. Thomas.

Moote CA, Varkey GP, Komar WE: The incidence of headache is similar after both continuous spinal anaesthesia and conventional spinal anaesthesia, *Reg Anaesth* 15, 1S:59, 1990.

Owens EL, Kasten GW, Hessel EA: Spinal subarachnoid hematoma after lumbar puncture and heparinization: a case report, review of the literature, and discussion of anesthetic implications, *Anesth Analg* 65:1201-1207, 1986.

Peterson DO, Borup JL, Chestnut JS: Continuous spinal anesthesia: case review and discussion, *Reg Anaesth* 8:109-113, 1983.

Pither CE, Ford DJ, Raj PP: Peripheral nerve stimulation with insulated and uninsulated needles: efficacy of characteristics, *Reg Anaesth* 9:9-12, 1984.

Pither CE, Raj PP, Ford DJ: The use of peripheral nerve simulators for regional anesthesia: a review of experimental characteristics, technique, and clinical applications, *Reg Anaesth* 10:49-58, 1985.

Rao TLK, El Etr AA: Anticoagulation following placement of epidural and subarachnoid catheters: an evaluation of neurologic sequelae, *Anesthesiology* 55:618-620, 1981.

Ready BL, Oden R, Chadwick HS et al: Development of an anesthesiology-based postoperative pain management service, *Anesthesiology* 68:100-106, 1988.

Rosenblatt RM, Shal R: The design and function of a regional anesthesia block room, *Reg Anaesth* 9:12-16, 1984.

Sarrell WG, LA Fia DJ: Acute lumbar epidural abscess: report of a case, *N Engl J Med* 250:318-20, 1954.

Selander D, Dhuner KG, Lundberg G: Peripheral nerve injury due to injection needles used for regional anesthesia, *Acta Anaesth Scand* 21:182-188, 1977.

Sidhu MS, Asrani RV, Bassell GM: An unusual complication of extradural catheterization in obstetric anaesthesia, *Br J Anaesth* 55:473-475, 1983.

Siegel RS, Alicandri FP, Jacoby AW: Letter: subgluteal infection following regional anesthesia, *JAMA* 229:268, 1974.

Smith DC, Crul JF: Oxygen desaturation following sedation for regional anesthesia; *Br J Anesth* 62:206-209, 1989.

Srecrama V, Ivan LP, Dennery JM et al: Neurosurgical complications of anticoagulant therapy, *Can Med Assoc J* 108:305, 1973.

Svancarek W, Chirino O, Schaefer Jr G et al: Retropsoas and subgluteal abscesses following paracervical and pudendal anesthesia, *JAMA* 237:892-4, 1977.

Thorsen G: Neurological complications after spinal anesthesia, *Acta Chir Scand* 95 (Suppl 121):138-45, 1947.

Tuohy EB: Continuous spinal anesthesia: its usefulness and technic involved, *Anesthesiology* 5:142, 1944.

Wadia NH, Dastur DK: Spinal meningitides with radiculomyelopathy. Part I. Clinical features, *J Neurol Sci* 8:239-60, 1969.

Wedel DJ, Mulroy MF: Hemiparesis following dural puncture, *Anesthesiology* 59:475-477, 1983.

Wenger DR, Gitchell RG: Severe infections following pudendal block anesthesia: need for orthopaedic awareness, *J Bone Surg* (Am)55:202-7, 1973.

Winchell SW, Wolfe R: The incidence of neuropathy following upper extremity nerve blocks, *Reg Anaesth* 10:12-15, 1985.

Anatomy for Neural Blockade of the Head and Neck

Part

3

Gasserian Ganglion

Steven D. Waldman

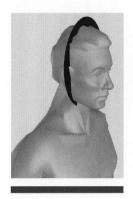

Introduction   The trigeminal nerve is the largest of the cranial nerves containing both sensory and motor fibers. Somatic afferent impulses carried by the trigeminal nerve transmit pain, light touch, and temperature sensation. Sensation from the skin of the face, the mucosal lining of the nose and mouth, the teeth, and the anterior two thirds of the tongue is transmitted to the central nervous system via the trigeminal nerve. The trigeminal nerve also carries both proprioceptive impulses and afferent impulses from stretch receptors from the teeth, oral mucosa, muscles of mastication, and temporomandibular joint to aid in mastication. In addition to the just-mentioned sensory innervation, visceral efferent fibers innervate a variety of muscles of facial expression, the tensor tympani, and some muscles of mastication.

ANATOMIC RELATIONSHIPS

The gasserian ganglion is formed from two roots that exit the ventral surface of the brainstem at the midpontine level. These roots pass in a forward and lateral direction in the posterior cranial fossa across the border of the petrous temperal bone. These roots enter a recess called *Meckel's cave*, which is formed by an invagination of the surrounding dura mater into the middle cranial fossa. The dural pouch that lies just behind the ganglion is called the *trigeminal cistern* and contains cerebrospinal fluid (CSF). The ganglion is canoe-shaped with the three peripheral branches—ophthalmic, maxillary, and mandibular—exiting the anterior convex aspect of the ganglion. The mandibular nerve exits Meckel's cave via the foramen ovale (Figs. 3-1 and 3-2).

INDICATIONS

Gasserian ganglion block is useful in the management of painful conditions of the face and head, including trigeminal neuralgia, pain of malignant origin, intractable cluster headache, and, rarely, other neuropathic pain syndromes, including postherpetic neuralgia.

REGIONAL ANESTHETIC TECHNIQUE

The patient is placed in the supine position with the cervical spine extended over a rolled towel. The skin approximately 2.5 cm lateral to the corner of the mouth is carefully prepped with povidone-iodine solution and sterile drapes are placed. The skin and subcutaneous tissues are then anesthetized with 1% lidocaine with epinephrine. A 13-cm, 22-gauge needle is then advanced through the anesthetized area, traveling in a plane perpendicular with the pupil of the eye (when the eye is midposition) in a cephalad trajectory toward the auditory meatus (Fig. 3-3). The needle is advanced until contact is made with the base of the skull at a depth of approximately 5 cm. The needle tip is then walked posteriorly an additional 1 to 1.5 cm into the foramen ovale (Fig. 3-4). Paresthesia of the mandibular nerve may be encountered upon entering the foramen ovale. The stylet is then

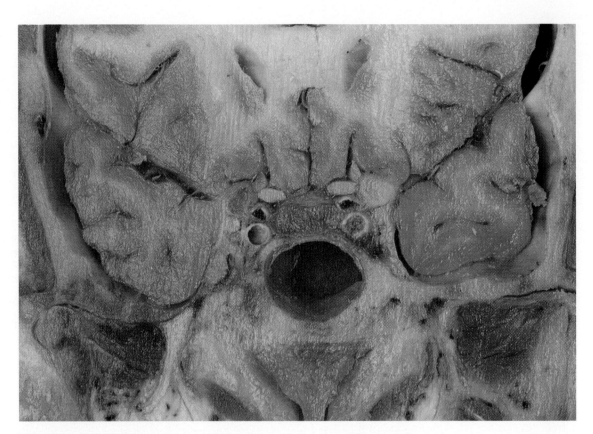

FIG. 3-1 *Coronal anatomic section through the head, revealing the gasserian ganglion.*

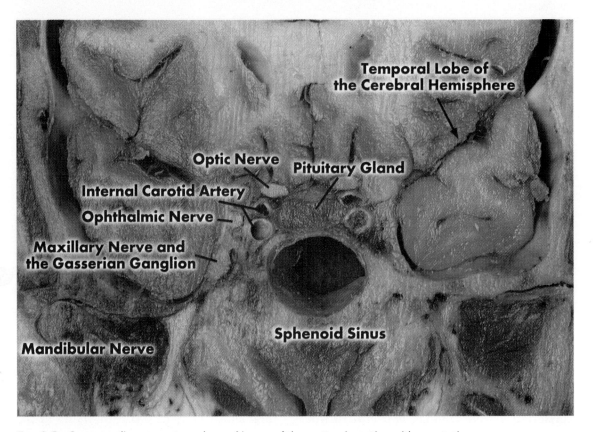

FIG. 3-2 *Corresponding computer-enhanced image of the anatomic section with annotation.*

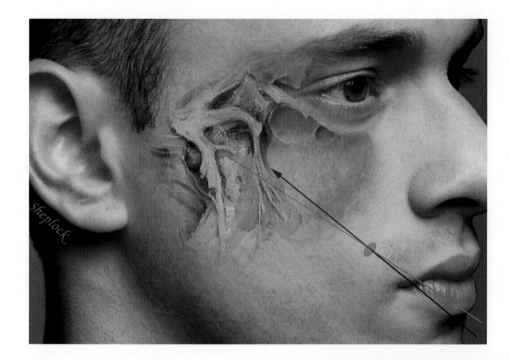

Fig. 3-3 *Dissection of the gasserian ganglion superimposed over the surface anatomy. The dissection is with much of the right side of the skull removed, leaving the medial sides of the right orbit and maxillary sinus. Behind the sinus are seen the three branches of the trigeminal nerve: ophthalmic (superior), maxilary (middle), and mandibular (inferior). The* blue arrow *indicates the initial direction for needle insertion. The* green arrow *indicates the final placement for the needle.*

removed. Careful aspiration for blood and CSF should be carried out. Failure to observe a free flow of CSF does not necessarily mean that the needle tip is not within the central nervous system. After the needle is in place, 0.25-ml increments of local anesthesia may be given to a total of 1 to 2 ml as a therapeutic or diagnostic and prognostic maneuver to assess the adequacy and anatomic distribution of anesthesia (Fig. 3-5).

Radiographic confirmation of the needle position should be carried out before injection of any neurolytic substance (Fig. 3-6). After needle position is confirmed, 0.1 ml aliquots of sterile glycerine or 6.5% phenol in glycerine may be injected for neurolysis.

SIDE EFFECTS AND COMPLICATIONS

Because of the higher vascular nature of the path of the needle, significant hematoma of the face and subscleral hematoma of the eye are not uncommon. The patient should be warned of the probability of this complication before institution of the block. As mentioned, because the ganglion lies within the CSF, even a very small amount of local anesthetic injected through the needle may lead to total spinal blockade. The neurolytic gasserian ganglion block should be carried out only by those familiar with the anatomy, as well as the technique of gasserian ganglion block, and then only under radiographic guidance.

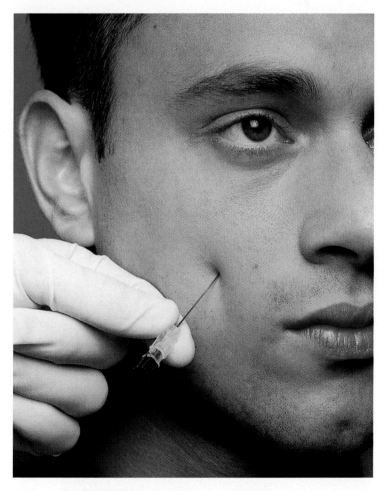

Fig. 3-4 *Blockade of the gasserian ganglion, with the needle in its final position.*

SUGGESTED READINGS

Bonica JJ: Gasserian ganglion block. In Bonica JJ: *The Management of pain* (1985-1990), Philadelphia, 1990, Lea & Febiger.

Feldstein G: Percutaneous retrogasserian glycerol rhizotomy. In Racz G, editor: *Techniques of neurolysis*, Boston, 1989, Kluwer Publishers.

Waldman SD: Evaluation and treatment of common headache and facial pain syndromes. In Raj PP, editor: *Practical management of pain*, St. Louis, 1992, Mosby.

Waldman SD: Management of acute pain, *Postgrad Med* 87:15-17, 1992.

Waldman SD: The role of neural blockade in the management of headaches and facial pain, *Headache Digest* 4:286-292, 1991.

Waldman SD: Trigeminal nerve block. In Weiner RS, editor: *Innovations in pain management*, Orlando, 1990, PMD Press.

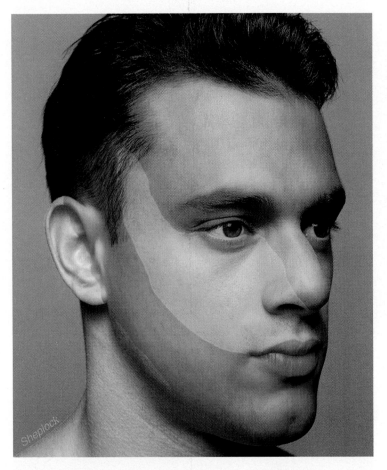

Fig. 3-5 *Sensory distribution of the branches of the trigeminal nerve. V₁ is green, V₂ is yellow, and V₃ is red.*

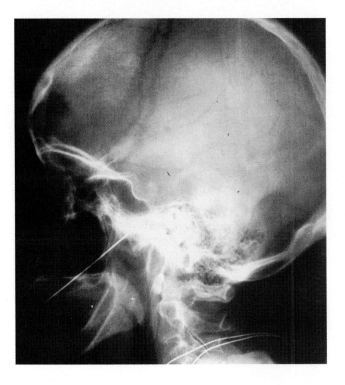

Fig. 3-6 *Lateral radiograph of the skull, revealing the needle tip with radioopaque contrast injected into Meckel's cave.*

CHAPTER 4

Distributions of the Trigeminal Nerve

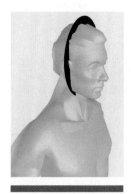

Marc B. Hahn

Introduction Blockade of the various divisions of the trigeminal nerve produces discrete anesthesia for superficial surgical procedures of the face and oral cavity. Blockade of these distributions may also prove helpful in the diagnosis and treatment of various pain syndromes.

ANATOMIC RELATIONSHIPS

The three divisions of the trigeminal nerve, the ophthalmic, maxillary, and mandibular, exit the gasserian ganglion from its anterior aspect (see Chapter 3) (Figs 4-1 and 4-2).

Ophthalmic Division (V₁)

The ophthalmic nerve (V_1) is the smallest and most superior of the three divisions. It runs lateral to the cavernous sinus and exits the cranium through the medial aspect of the superior orbital fissure. It supplies sensory afferents to the meninges, eyelids, lacrimal glands, conjunctiva, and eye (see Chapter 5). The major branch of the ophthalmic nerve is the frontal nerve, which divides into the supraorbital and supratrochlear nerves. The supraorbital nerve exits the orbit via the supraorbital foramen and divides into medial and lateral branches. These branches supply sensation to the upper eyelid, forehead, and scalp as far posterior as the vertex. The supratrochlear nerve passes over the trochlear of the superior oblique muscle and exits the orbit medial to the supraorbital nerve. The

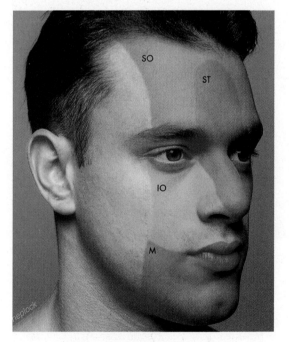

FIG. 4-1 *Sensory distribution of the terminal branches of the trigeminal nerve. Supratrochlear nerve distribution is in purple, supraorbital nerve distribution is in green, infraorbital nerve distribution is in yellow, and mental nerve distribution is in red.*

supratrochlear nerve supplies the inferomedial section of the forehead and the medial part of the upper eyelid.

Maxillary Division (V₂)

The maxillary nerve (V$_2$) also gives off a meningeal branch before leaving the cranium through the foramen rotundum and entering the sphenopalatine fossa. In the fossa, the maxillary nerve gives off branches—the zygomatic nerve, which supplies the superiolateral face (V$_2$), and the superior posterior alveolar nerve, which supplies the maxillary portion of the oral mucosa, maxilla, and upper dentition. The maxillary nerve then loops through the inferior orbital fissure, exiting through the infraorbital foramen as the infraorbital nerve (Figs 4-3 and 4-4). The infraorbital nerve supplies sensation to the skin from the lower eyelid to the upper lip. This includes the underlying mucosa and nasal alae.

Mandibular Division (V₃)

The mandibular nerve (V$_3$) is the largest division of the trigeminal nerve. In addition to its sensory function, the mandibular nerve also has a motor component. The mandibular nerve, after supplying a meningeal branch, exists the cranium via the foramen ovale just posterior to the lateral pterygoid muscles (Figs 4-3 and 4-4). The nerve then bifurcates into anterior and posterior branches. The anterior branch contains mainly motor fibers to the muscles of mastication. The only sensory component of the anterior branch, the buccal nerve, supplies the lateral face and the underlying mucosa. The posterior branch divides into the auriculotemporal, lingual, and inferior alveolar nerves, which supply respectively the temporal mandibular joint, the external ear, and the tympanic membrane; the anterior two thirds of the tongue, the floor of the mouth, and some of the lower dentition; and the lower dentition, mandible, and surrounding mucosa. The posterior branch also gives rise to some motor fibers off the inferior alveolar nerve. The inferior alveolar nerve terminates as the mental nerve, which exists the mental foramen and supplies the skin over the anterior aspect of the mandible.

INDICATIONS
Blockade of the Maxillary Division (V₂)

Blockade of the maxillary division of the trigeminal nerve produces anesthesia for superficial surgical procedures of the face in the V$_2$ distribution and to the upper teeth and gums. Blockade of the maxillary nerve may also prove helpful in the assessment, diagnosis, and treatment of various pain syndromes and for postoperative or post-trauma analgesia.

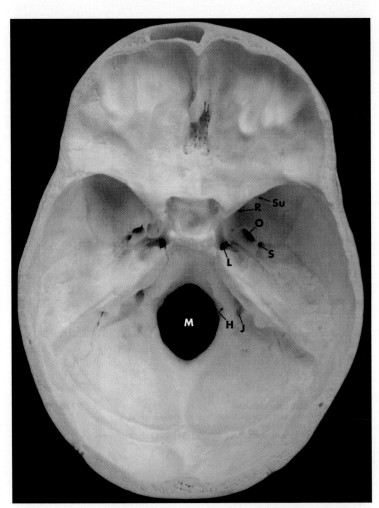

FIG. 4-2 *Intracranial view of the base of the skull, demonstrating the various foramen and the structures that exit through each. O, ovale, traversed by mandibular nerve, accessory meningeal artery; R, rotundum, traversed by maxillary nerve; SU, superior orbital fissure, traversed by the ophthalmic nerve; S, spinosum, traversed by recurrent branch of the mandibular nerve; L, lacerum, traversed by internal carotid artery; J, jugular, traversed by internal jugular vein and cranial nerves IX, X, and XI; H, hypoglossal, traversed by hypoglossal nerve; M, magnum, traversed by medulla oblongata, spinal accessory nerve, vertebral and spinal arteries.*

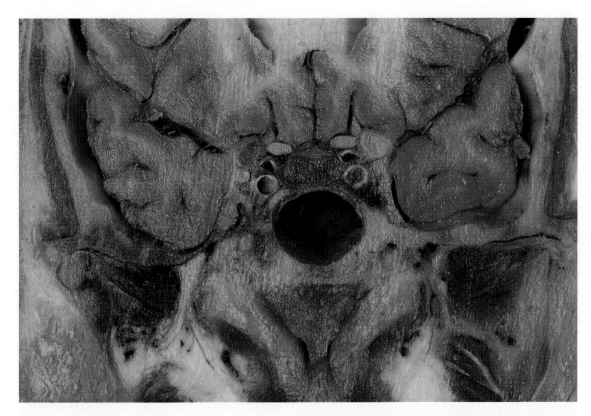

Fig. 4-3 *Coronal anatomic section through the head, revealing the maxillary and mandibular nerves.*

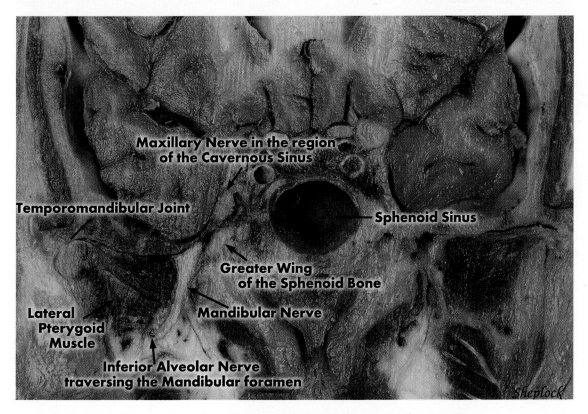

Fig. 4-4 *Corresponding computer-enhanced image of the anatomic section with annotation.*

Blockade of the Mandibular Division (V₃)

Blockade of the mandibular division of the trigeminal nerve produces anesthesia for superficial surgical procedures of the face in the V₃ distribution, the lower teeth, gums, and the anterior ⅔ of the tongue. Blockade of the mandibular nerve may also prove helpful in the assessment, diagnosis, and treatment of various pain syndromes and for postoperative or posttrauma analgesia.

Blockade of the Distal Branches

The supraorbital (supratrochlear), infraorbital, and mental nerves represent the most distal branches of the ophthalmic, maxillary, and mandibular divisions, respectively, of the trigeminal nerve. Blockade of these distal branches of the trigeminal nerve produces discrete anesthesia for superficial surgical procedures of the face and scalp. Blockade of these distributions may also prove helpful in the diagnosis and treatment of various pain syndromes.

REGIONAL ANESTHETIC TECHNIQUE
Blockade of the Maxillary Division (V₂)

The patient is placed in the supine position, with the head rotated contralateral to the side

of the block. Following local anesthesia to the overlying skin, a 22-gauge, 8-cm needle is inserted posterior to the coronoid process of the mandible, under the zygomatic arch (Fig. 4-5). The needle is advanced in a plane perpendicular to the skin until the lateral pterygoid plate is contacted, usually at a depth of approximately 4 to 5 cm. The needle is then withdrawn to the subcutaneous tissue and reinserted in an anterior-superior direction to a point 1 cm deeper than the depth at which the lateral pterygoid plate was encountered. The needle tip should ideally be both 1 cm anterior and superior to the point of bone contact (Fig. 4-6). The use of a sterile depth marker or calibrated needle is helpful for this technique. Once the needle has been positioned, 2 to 4 ml of local anesthetic may be injected.

Blockade of the Mandibular Division (V₃)

The patient is placed in the supine position with the head rotated contralateral to the side of the block. Following local anesthesia to the overlying skin, a 22-gauge, 8-cm needle is inserted at a point just inferior to the midpoint of the zygomatic arch, in the mandibular notch (Fig. 4-5). The needle is advanced in a plane perpendicular to the skin to a depth of less than 4 to 5 cm until a

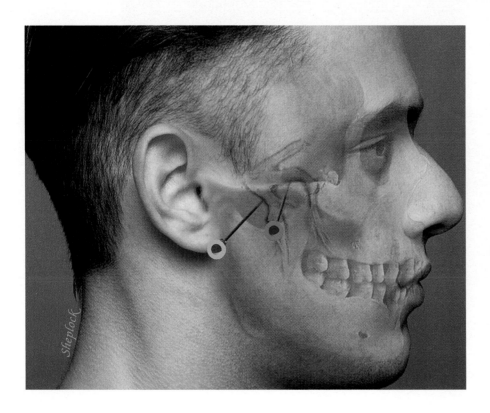

FIG. 4-5 *Dissection of the maxillary and mandibular nerves and bony landmarks superimposed over the surface anatomy. The* green needle *represents the direction of the needle for a maxillary nerve block. The* yellow needle *represents the direction of the needle for a mandibular nerve block.*

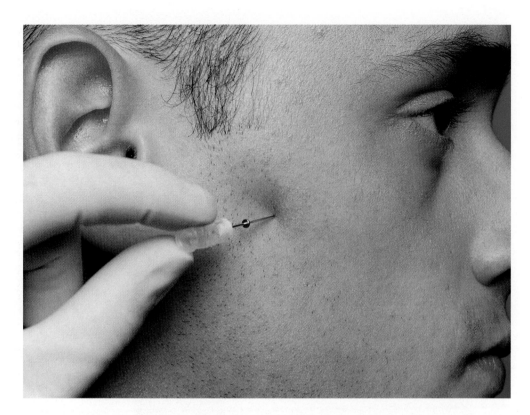

Fig. 4-6 *Blockade of the maxillary nerve, with the needle in its final position.*

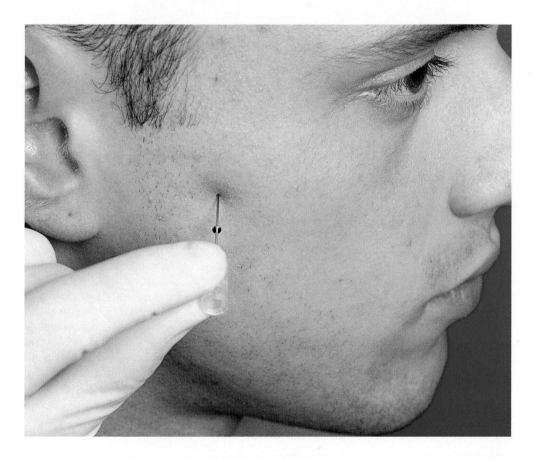

Fig. 4-7 *Blockade of the mandibular nerve, with the needle in its final position.*

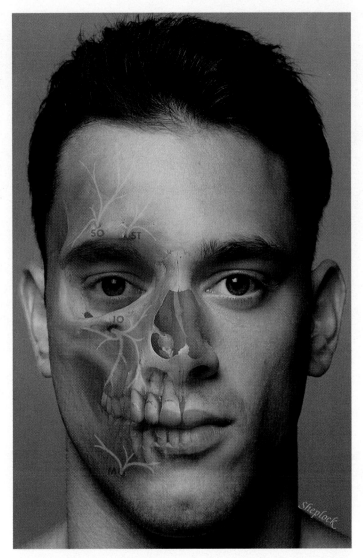

Fig. 4-8 *Computer-enhanced image of the supraorbital (supratrochlear), infraorbital, and mental nerves superimposed over the surface anatomy.*

paresthesia is produced or the pterygoid plate is contacted. If a paresthesia is not produced, the needle should be withdrawn to the subcutaneous tissue and redirected slightly posteriorly (Fig. 4-7). Once the needle has been positioned, 2 to 4 ml of local anesthetic may be injected.

The lingual and inferior alveolar nerves may be blocked intraorally at the point where the nerves enter the mandibular canal both 1 cm posterior and inferior to the lower third molar. Once the needle has been positioned at the ridge of the canal, 2 to 4 ml of local anesthetic may be injected.

Blockade of the Distal Branches

The supraorbital, infraorbital, and mental foramen are all in the same paramedian sagittal plane as the ipsilateral pupil (Fig. 4-8). With the patient in the supine position, the specific foramen is approached with a fine (25- to 30-gauge) needle until a paresthesia is produced. The foramen need not be entered for local anesthetic blockade. Once the needle is placed, 1 to 3 ml of local anesthetic is administered. Following local anesthetic blockade of the supraorbital nerve, the needle may be redirected medially for blockade of the supratrochlear nerve (Fig. 4-9).

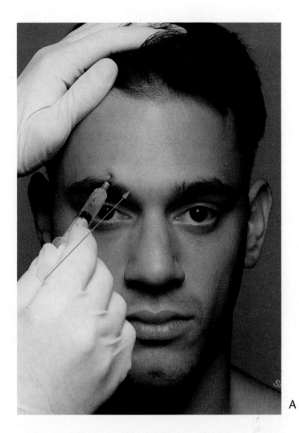

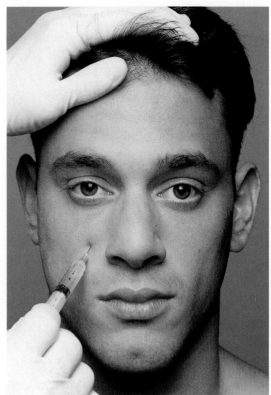

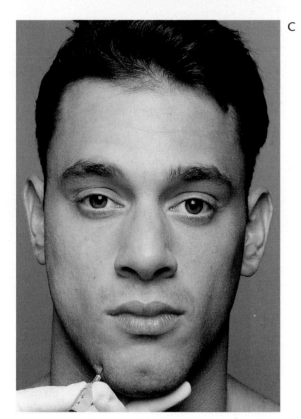

FIG. 4-9 *Blockade of the supraorbital (**A**), infraorbital (**B**), and mental (**C**) nerves. The green arrow in **A** represents the direction of the needle for supratrochlear nerve block.*

If a neurolytic technique is planned, the needle should enter the foramen and small doses of neurolytic agents (less than 1 ml) should be administered.

SIDE EFFECTS AND COMPLICATIONS

Blockade of the Maxillary Division (V₂)

Careful aspiration before injection will help prevent both inadvertent intravascular or subarachnoid administration.

Due to the increased vascularity of these tissues, ecchymosis or hematoma in the area of the block is quite common. It is also possible to enter the infraorbital fissure leading to orbital anesthesia, ophthalmoplegia, or visual changes.

Blockade of the Mandibular Division (V₃)

As with the block of the maxillary nerve, careful aspiration before injection will help prevent both inadvertent intravascular or subarachnoid administration.

Once again, due to the increased vascularity of these tissues, ecchymosis or hematoma in the area of the block is quite common.

Blockade of the Distal Branches

Due to the small volume of drug and the distal location of the nerves, complications are unlikely to be encountered with this technique. However, care should be taken to avoid intraneural injection, which may lead to nerve injury, when entering the various foramen.

SUGGESTED READINGS

Carron H: Control of pain in the head and neck. In Johns ME, Rice DH, editors: *Otolaryngologic clinics of North America*, vol 14:3, Philadelphia, 1981. WB Saunders.

Murphy TM: Somatic blockade of head and neck. In Cousins M, Bridenbaugh PO, editors: *Neural blockade*, ed. 2, Philadelphia, 1988, JB Lippincott.

Netter F, Mitchell GAG: Nerve plexuses and peripheral nerves. In Brass, A, editor: *The CIBA collection of medical illustrations*, New Jersey, 1983, CIBA.

Snell RS, editor: *Clinical anatomy for medical students*, Boston, 1973, Little, Brown.

CHAPTER 5

Ophthalmic Nerve (Retrobulbar Blockade)

Robert C. Hamilton

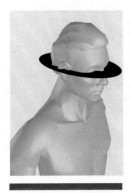

Introduction Regional anesthesia for ophthalmology, in addition to blockade of the three branches of the ophthalmic nerve, usually requires blockade of the three motor nerves to the extraocular muscles. In addition, the periorbital terminal rami of the facial (seventh) nerve that supply the orbicularis oculi muscle are often blocked.

ANATOMIC RELATIONSHIPS

The orbit rim, comprising the zygomatic, frontal, and maxillary bones, forms the rounded rectangular base of a pear-shaped pyramid that tapers posteriorly to form a tight apex (Figs. 5-1 and 5-2). The globe is in the shape of a sphere averaging about 23.5 mm in diameter (commonly 20 mm to 30 mm but rarely outside these limits) with an anterior bulge, the cornea, of smaller radius of curvature. The depth of the orbit from inferior orbit rim to the optic foramen ranges from 42 to 54 mm. The lateral orbit rim is set back 12 to 18 mm behind the cornea, allowing exposure of the globe to its equator (Fig. 5-3). Fig. 5-4 illustrates further orbit and globe relationships.

A network of orbital connective tissues permits the extraocular muscles to function and allows for movement of the optic nerve and ciliary vessels and nerves as the globe rotates. The fat of the posterior orbit has a macroarrangement into central and peripheral compartments, respectively inside and outside the cone of rectus muscles.

With the globe in primary gaze position, the intraorbital portion of the optic nerve lies totally on the medial side of the midsagittal plane (visual axis), running in the transverse plane towards the optic foramen (Fig. 5-5). The nerve enters the globe 3 mm to the nasal side of its posterior pole. In primary gaze the intraorbital portion of the optic nerve is closer to the medial than the lateral rectus muscle (Figs. 5-1 and 5-2) and assumes a sinuous course between the posterior pole of the globe and the optic foramen. The intraorbital part of the optic nerve, about 4 mm in diameter, averages slightly more than 3 cm in length and has a winding course across the 2.5-cm gap between the optic foramen and the hind surface of the globe; within the orbit, therefore, the nerve has about 7 mm of "excess play" that is accommodated by its sinuosity. The dural covering of the nerve fuses with the sclera anteriorly and with the periorbita posteriorly at the optic foramen. Cerebrospinal fluid flows freely within the dura surrounding the nerve and is in continuity with the cerebrospinal fluid surrounding the midbrain (Fig. 5-6).

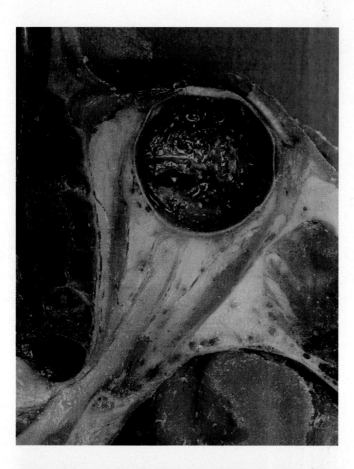

FIG. 5-1 *Transverse anatomic section through the skull, revealing the optic nerve, globe, branches of the ophthalmic nerve, and related structures.*

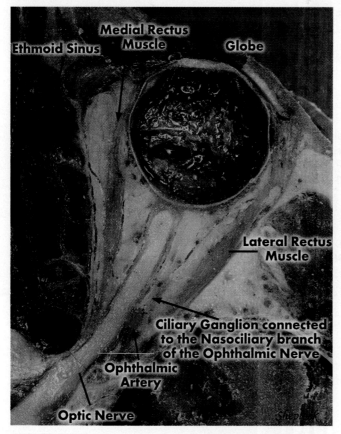

FIG. 5-2 *Corresponding computer-enhanced image of the anatomic section with annotation.*

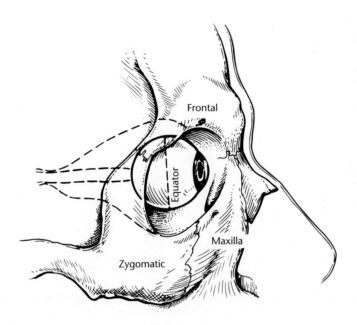

FIG. 5-3 *The lateral orbital rim is set back in line with the globe equator. The orbit, in sagittal section, is C-shaped rather than U-shaped, with a greater overhang superiorly. The globe is closer to the orbit roof than to its floor.* (From Grizzard WS: Ophthalmic anesthesia. In *Ophthalmology Annual 1989*, New York, 1989, Raven Press.)

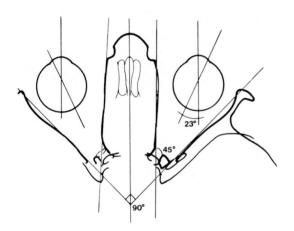

FIG. 5-4 *Line drawing of the globe and orbit. The globe occupies the front half of each orbit and projects anteriorly beyond it. The visual axis (eye in primary gaze) is sagittal; the anatomic axis of each orbit diverges from the visual axis by 23°. The medial wall of each orbit is in the sagittal plane of the skull and parallel to the contralateral medial orbit wall. The lateral wall of each orbit forms a 90° angle with the contralateral lateral orbit wall. The medial and lateral walls of each orbit make a 45° angle with each other. The optic foramen located at the apex is in the same sagittal plane as the medial orbit wall and therefore lies both posteriorly and medially in the orbit; thus the foramen is posterior and medial to the eyeball but not directly behind it.* (From Zide BM, Jelks GW: *Surgical anatomy of the orbit*, New York, 1989, Raven Press.)

The ophthalmic nerve, the smallest division of the trigeminal nerve, splits into three branches: lacrimal, frontal, and nasociliary (Figs. 5-7 and 5-8).

The three cranial nerves that supply motor function to the extraocular muscles are the oculomotor (III); the trochlear (IV); and the abducens (VI). The motor nerves to the four rectus muscles enter their respective bellies from the conal surface 1.0 to 1.5 cm from the apex of the orbit (Fig. 5-8). Local anesthetics in blocking concentration have to reach an exposed 5- to 10-mm segment of these motor nerves in the posterior intracone space for akinesia of their supplied muscles to occur. Injectate placed intraconally will achieve motor blocking concentration more easily and with smaller volume than when a pericone method is used.

The arterial blood supply of the orbit and its contents is predominantly from the ophthalmic artery, a branch of the internal carotid artery (Fig. 5-9). Regional anesthesia needles should not be introduced into the posterior 1.5 cm of the orbit, where the vessels are largest and a potential source of vision-threatening bleeding. Other vital structures (optic nerve and extraocular muscle origins) are tightly packed at the apex and also subject to serious damage. The supranasal orbital quadrant contains the end vessels of the ophthalmic artery system (Fig. 5-9), the medial end of the superior ophthalmic vein, and the trochlear mechanism of the superior oblique muscle (Fig. 5-9); it should be avoided as an injection site. Three relatively avascular adipose tissue compartments are in the anterior and midorbit; they are the preferred

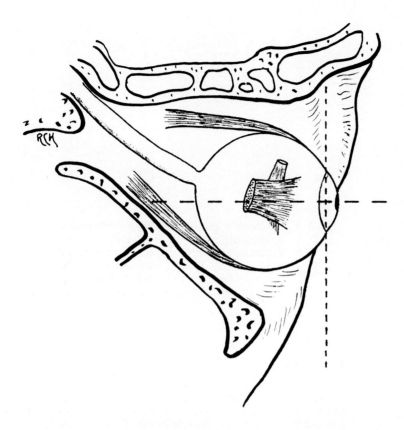

FIG. 5-5 *Globe in primary gaze. Fine dashed line indicates the plane of the iris (useful in gauging depth of needle advancement); coarse dashed line indicates the midsagittal plane of the eye and the visual axis through the center of the pupil. The optic nerve lies on the medial side of the midsagittal plane of the eye. (From Gimbel Education Services.)*

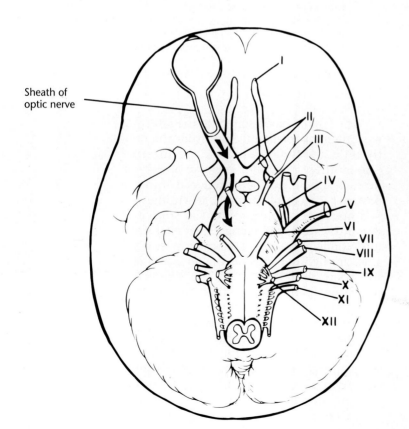

Sheath of optic nerve

FIG. 5-6 *Illustration of the base of the brain and the pathway for spread of local anesthetics inadvertently injected into the subarachnoid space surrounding the optic nerve. Note that this pathway includes the cranial nerves, pons, and midbrain. (From Javitt JC, Addiego R, Friedberg HL, et al: Brain stem anesthesia after retrobulbar block, Ophthalmology 94:721, 1987)*

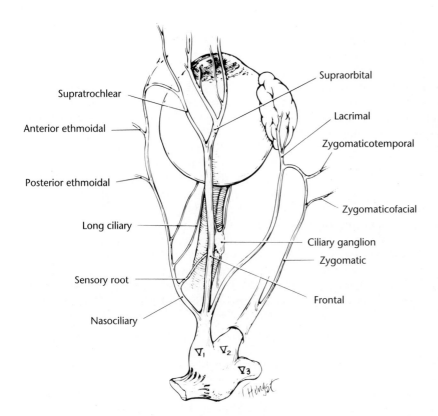

Supratrochlear

Anterior ethmoidal

Posterior ethmoidal

Long ciliary

Sensory root

Nasociliary

Supraorbital

Lacrimal

Zygomaticotemporal

Zygomaticofacial

Ciliary ganglion

Zygomatic

Frontal

V_1 V_2 V_3

FIG. 5-7 *Trigeminal nerve viewed from above. V₁, ophthalmic nerve; V₂, maxillary nerve; V₃, mandibular nerve. (From Doxanas MT, Anderson RL: Clinical orbital anatomy, Baltimore, 1984, Williams and Wilkins.)*

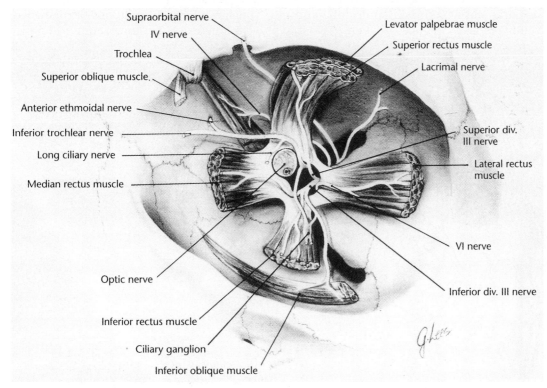

Supraorbital nerve

IV nerve

Trochlea

Superior oblique muscle

Anterior ethmoidal nerve

Inferior trochlear nerve

Long ciliary nerve

Median rectus muscle

Optic nerve

Inferior rectus muscle

Ciliary ganglion

Inferior oblique muscle

Levator palpebrae muscle

Superior rectus muscle

Lacrimal nerve

Superior div. III nerve

Lateral rectus muscle

VI nerve

Inferior div. III nerve

FIG. 5-8 *Detail of the motor innervation of the extraocular muscles. The four rectus muscles are innervated from their conal surfaces. Note the long course of the nerve to the inferior oblique (branch of inferior division III nerve). The trochlear nerve (IV) remains outside the muscle cone and enters the superior oblique at its superolateral edge. The three branches of the ophthalmic nerve are also shown: the lacrimal and frontal nerves remain outside the muscle cone; the nasociliary nerve (not labeled) is inside the cone. (From Miller NR: Walsh and Hoyt's clinical neuro-ophthalmology, vol. 1, ed. 4, Baltimore, 1982, Williams and Wilkins.)*

sites of local anesthetic injection and are located in the following positions: inferotemporal, superotemporal (Figs. 5-9 and 5-10) and medial (Fig. 5-11).

The principal vein of the orbit, the superior ophthalmic, runs backwards and laterally in a hammock-like connective tissue septum suspended under the superior rectus muscle, between it and the optic nerve (Fig. 5-12).

INDICATIONS

Surgery of the anterior and posterior segments, strabismus surgery, and oculoplastic surgery may all be performed under regional block anesthesia. In the United States, 1.3 million cataract extraction and intraocular lens implantation procedures are currently carried out each year under regional anesthesia. Blocks with lytic agents may be used in the management of chronic eye pain.

REGIONAL ANESTHETIC TECHNIQUE

The regional anesthesia requirements for intraocular surgery include globe and conjunctival anesthesia, extraocular muscle, and orbicularis muscle akinesia, and globe and orbital hypotony.

Atkinson's *cone injection technique*, described in 1934, of placing an inferotemporal needle within the cone of muscles with the globe elevated and adducted, became standard teaching to ophthalmology and anesthesiology residents and was, and continues to be, handed down verbally and in texts. However, its "up and in" globe positioning has been discredited. During inferotemporal needle insertion with the globe directed in this way, the optic nerve is brought closer to the needle tip and the macular area is more exposed to damage. It is much safer, during inferotemporal needle placement, to have patients direct their eyes in primary gaze.

In pericone (peribulbar or periocular) blocks, local anesthetic agents or mixtures are deposited within the orbit but not within the geometric confines of the cone of rectus muscles. Introduced as a safer method than intraconal blocking, serious complications nevertheless have been reported. Knowledge of orbital anatomy is every bit as important as with the intracone method, and there are disadvantages to using periconal blocking, such as a higher required supplementation rate and greater injectate volume if akinesia is to be achieved. Many variations of the pericone technique exist, a common one being place-

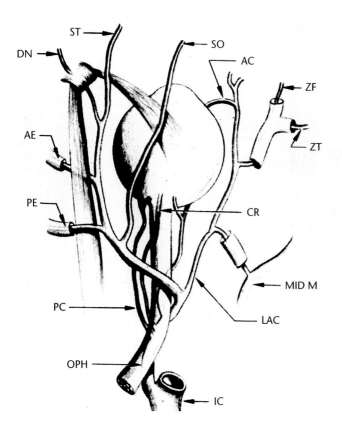

FIG. 5-9 *The ophthalmic artery system. Key:* IC, *internal carotid;* OPH, *ophthalmic;* PC, *posterior ciliary;* CR, *central retinal;* PE, *posterior ethmoidal;* AE, *anterior ethmoidal;* DN, *dorsal nasal;* ST, *supratrochlear;* SO, *supraorbital;* LAC, *lacrimal;* AC, *anterior ciliary;* ZF, *zygomaticofacial;* ZT, *zygomaticotemporal;* MID M, *middle meningeal.* (From Schorr N, Seiff SR: Central retinal artery occlusion associated with periocular corticosteroid injection for juvenile hemangioma, *Ophthalmic Surg* 17:231, 1986.)

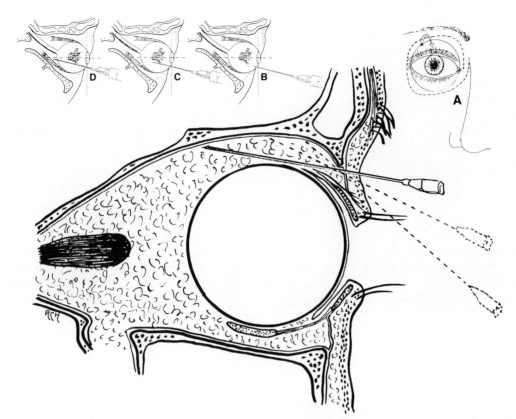

Fɪɢ. 5-10   *Superotemporal pericone block. The needle tip is inserted through the skin of the lid 3 mm lateral to the sagittal plane of the lateral limbus at the level of the superior orbit rim and aimed up markedly toward the roof of the orbit (**A**), with a medial component of about 5° in a plane lateral to the superior rectus/levator complex (**B**, **C**, **D**). The needle tip "walks" along the periorbita of the orbit roof (full-size illustration) in curvilinear fashion (**A**) until the needle tip is at a depth of 25 to 30 mm, at which point the injection is made with the usual precautions. (From Gimbel Educational Services.)*

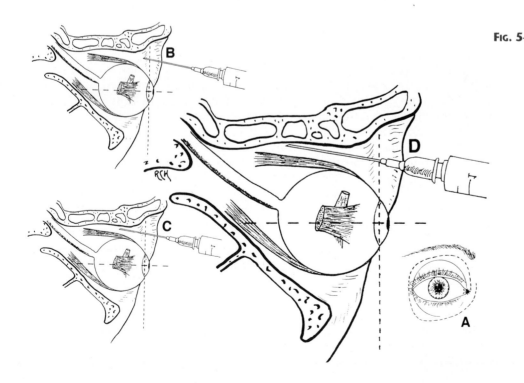

Fɪɢ. 5-11   *Medial pericone block. A 27-gauge, 25-mm sharp disposable needle enters transconjunctivally on the medial side of the caruncle at the extreme medial side of the palpebral fissure (**A**, **B**). With bevel facing the orbit wall, it passes backward in the transverse plane, directed at a 5° angle away from the sagittal plane and towards the medial orbit wall (**C**, **D**). For mainly lid akinesia effect, partial insertion suffices (**C**); for additional extraocular muscle akinesia, depth may be increased to a maximum of 25 mm as measured by observing the needle/hub junction reach the plane of the iris (**D**). (From Gimbel Educational Services.)*

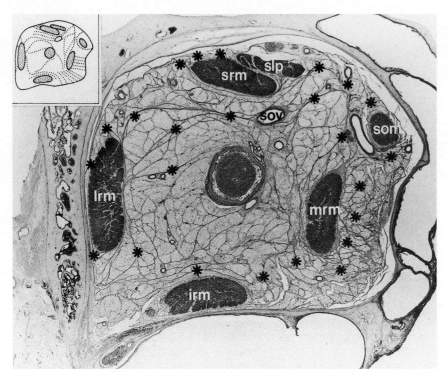

FIG. 5-12 *Cross-section of the orbit 2.6 mm posterior to the hind surface of the globe, showing the connective tissue hammock carrying the superior ophthalmic vein (sov) diagonally across the superior orbit from anteronasal to posterotemporal. Key:* slp, *levator palpebrae superioris muscle;* srm, *superior rectus muscle;* som, *superior oblique muscle;* lrm, *lateral rectus muscle;* irm, *inferior rectus muscle;* mrm, *medial rectus muscle;* *, *connective tissue septa.* (From Grizzard WS: Ophthalmic anesthesia. In *Ophthalmology Annual 1989*, New York, 1989, Raven Press.)

ment in two locations, one inferotemporal and the other in the superior orbit (supratemporal is preferable to supranasal; see Fig. 5-10). For those who wish to practice pericone blocking, the author suggests a two-needle technique as described in the legends of Fig. 5-13 and 5-11 respectively. Up to 5 ml injectate volume of 2% lidocaine (or equivalent) may be required at each site for anesthesia with muscle akinesia.

Performing *intracone* (retrobulbar) blocks implies needle tip and injectate placement within the geometric confines of the cone of rectus muscles. A straight needle, mounted on a syringe containing the chosen anesthesia mixture, is introduced either transconjunctivally or transcutaneously into the inferotemporal quadrant of the orbit, commencing at the junction of the inferior and lateral orbit rims (Fig. 5-14); details of the block are found in the legend of Fig. 5-15. Anesthesia and akinesia are more dependable than with pericone placement; 3 to 4 ml of lidocaine 2% (or equivalent) suffices. Complementary medial compartment blocking for lid akinesia may be added if necessary, using 2 to 4 ml injectate (Fig. 5-11).

Seventh nerve blockade for akinesia of the orbicularis muscle (to obtund blinking and squeezing of the eyelids) is less commonly practiced than in earlier eras. Methods used

included blocking the main trunk of the nerve after its emergency from the stylomastoid foramen or at one of several more peripheral sites. If solely intraorbital injections are given and the enzyme hyaluronidase is included in the injectate, however, significant spread occurs through the orbital septum to effectively obtund orbicularis muscle tone. The medial pericone block as depicted in Fig. 5-11 is particularly effective for blocking the eyelids in this way.

Absolute alcohol, following preliminary block with local anesthetic (to abolish the intense pain of alcohol injection), may be placed in small volume within the rectus muscle cone in the management of sightless or nearly sightless painful eyes, the goal being interruption of conduction in the sensory nerves and total sparing of the oculomotor nerves. Hyaluronidase should be omitted from lytic injectate mixtures in blocks for chronic eye pain.

SIDE EFFECTS AND COMPLICATIONS
Needle advancement within the confines of the orbit is essentially a blind procedure and has the potential for serious complications. In the literature a considerable lobby exists for the use of dull needles to reduce the inci-

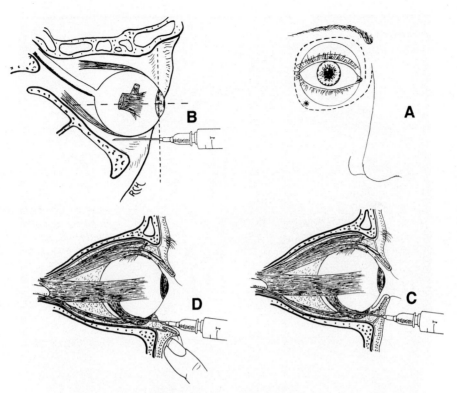

FIG. 5-13 *Inferotemporal pericone injection. A 27-gauge, 20- to 25-mm sharp disposable needle enters the orbit at the junction of the lateral and inferior rims (**A**) very close to the bone. The needle passes backwards in a sagittal plane (**B**) and parallel to the orbit floor (**C, D**), passing the globe equator to a depth controlled by observing the needle/hub junction reach the plane of the iris (**B**). The technique is equally applicable to the transcutaneous (**C**) or transconjunctival (**D**) route.* (From Gimbel Educational Services.)

FIG. 5-14 *Landmarks for an inferotemporal intracone injection. The outline of the globe equator is superimposed on a template of the orbital rim. A 27-gauge, 31-mm sharp disposable needle enters either transconjunctivally or transcutaneously at the junction of the lateral and inferior orbital rims (*) and is directed backwards in the sagittal plan with a 10° upward angle from the transverse plane until the globe equator is passed. At this point the needle is redirected upward and medially to approach but not pass the visual axis of the eye in primary gaze.* (From Gimbel Educational Services.)

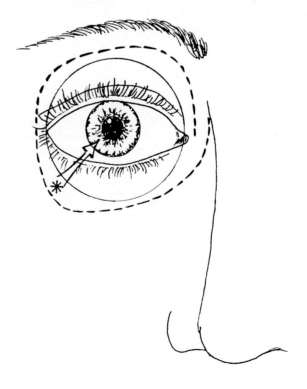

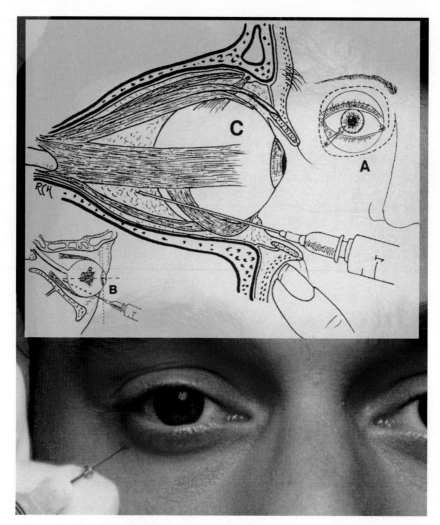

FIG. 5-15 *Recommended technique of retrobulbar block; may be transconjunctival as in line drawings, or transcutaneous as in the color photograph. Bony landmarks are identical for both techniques.* Line drawings: **A**, *viewed from in front;* **B**, *viewed from above;* **C**, *viewed from lateral side. A 31-mm needle enters the orbit at the junction of its inferior and lateral rims (**A***) and passes posteriorly, initially in the sagittal plane and parallel to the orbit floor, until its tip has passed the globe equator. Only then is the direction changed to upward and medially (arrow) as the tip is slowly moved towards a projected point behind the center of the pupil (**A** and **B**). During this passage inward, upward, and medially, the needle enters the intracone space by penetrating the intermuscular septum just inferior to the lower border of the lateral rectus muscle (**C**). When the needle/hub junction has reached the plane of the iris (**C**), the needle tip will be located in the anterior intracone space. Following negative test aspiration, injection of local anesthesia mixture as described in the test will result in effective blockade. Note the digital lower lid retraction that is required before a transconjunctival needle placement (**C**). The* color photograph *illustrates the final needle position for the transcutaneous technique when ready for injection.* (Line drawing from Gimbel Educational Services.)

dence of bleeding and the chance of scleral penetration. The superiority of blunt- over sharp-tipped needles has not been demonstrated in a controlled trial. Penetration of the eye from use of larger dull needles caused more serious damage than when fine disposable ones were implicated. Fine sharp needles cause less pain to the patient and allow the anesthesiologist much finer tactile discrimination. Maximum depth of needle penetration from the orbit rim should be 31 mm, a needle advancing from an inferotemporal entry should not be allowed to cross the midsagittal plane of the eye (Fig. 5-5).

The complications of regional anesthesia for ophthalmology fall into four main types: central spread, globe penetration, orbital hemorrhage, and myotoxicity.

With central spread, local anesthetics gain entrance through the optic nerve sheath to the dural cuff of the nerve and travel in the cerebrospinal fluid to produce a range of neurologic signs and symptoms that depend on the locus of spread and volume of injectate entering the sheath (Fig. 5-6). In a full-blown case the patient may be apneic, markedly hypotensive, and bradycardic. During initial needle tip placement, if increased resistance is felt, injection should be withheld and the needle tip relocated. It is mandatory that cardiopulmonary resuscitative equipment and appropriate drugs be immediately available in all locations where eyeblocks are administered.

Scleral penetration has been reported with both intracone and pericone injection techniques and has a higher incidence in patients with elongated myopic eyes. In these patients and patients with recessed eyes, pericone needle placement may be safer than intracone. Intravitreal bleeding commonly follows scleral penetration and may ultimately result in retinal detachment with loss of vision. The appropriate management of scleral penetration is complex and often drawn out over some weeks, involving difficult judgment calls on the part of the ophthalmologist. Erroneous injection of depot steroid medications or antibiotics into the vitreous is usually retinotoxic. In delivering steroids and antibiotics in an extraocular location, it is important to avoid intravascular placement of the needle tip. Reports exist

of retinal and ciliary arterial embolism of these medications, some with irreversible vision deterioration.

Serious impairment of the vascular supply to the globe may result from hemorrhage within the orbit. To reduce the incidence of bleeding it is essential to avoid needle insertion in the more vascular areas of the orbit, notably the apex itself which contains the largest vessels. Optic atrophy may be a late result of serious orbital bleeding. Direct trauma to the optic nerve may also arise from inappropriate needle placement.

Prolonged extraocular muscle malfunction may follow regional anesthesia of the orbit. Injection of local anesthetics directly into the extraocular muscle bellies should be avoided. Myotoxicity is more likely to result with agents used in higher concentration. The etiology of postoperative ptosis is multifactorial. Most postcataract ptosis occurs in patients in whom the levator aponeurosis was already unhealthy. Direct injection of local anesthetics into the levator muscle of the upper eyelid may account for certain cases.

SUGGESTED READINGS
Duker JS, Belmont JB, Benson WE et al: Inadvertent globe perforation during retrobulbar and peribulbar anesthesia, *Ophthalmology* 98:519-26, 1991.

Grizzard WS: Ophthalmic anesthesia. In Reinecke RD, editor: *Ophthalmology annual*, New York, 1989, Raven Press.

Grizzard WS, Kirk NM, Pavan PR et al: Perforating ocular injuries caused by anesthesia personnel, *Ophthalmology* 98:1011-6, 1991.

Hamilton RC: Brain-stem anesthesia as a complication of regional anesthesia for ophthalmic surgery, *Can J Ophthalmol* 27:323-5, 1992.

Katsev DA, Drews RC, Rose BT: An anatomic study of retrobulbar needle path length, *Ophthalmology* 96:1221-4, 1989.

Liu C, Youl B, Moseley I: Magnetic resonance imaging of the optic nerve in extremes of gaze: implications for the positioning of the globe for retrobulbar anaesthesia, *Br J Ophthalmol* 76:728-33, 1992.

Martin SR, Baker SS, Muenzler WS: Retrobulbar anesthesia and orbicularis akinesia, *Ophthalmic Surg* 17:232-3, 1986.

Rinkoff JS, Doft BH, Lobes LA: Management of ocular penetration from injection of local anesthesia preceding cataract surgery, *Arch Ophthalmol* 109:1421-5, 1991.

Shorr N, Seiff SR: Central retinal artery occlusion associated with periocular corticosteroid injection for juvenile hemangioma, *Ophthalmic Surg* 17:229-31, 1986.

Yagiela JA, Benoit PW, Buoncristiani RD et al: Comparison of myotoxic effects of lidocaine with epinephrine in rats and humans, *Anesth Anal* 60:471-80, 1981.

CHAPTER 6

Greater and Lesser Occipital Nerves

■

Marc B. Hahn

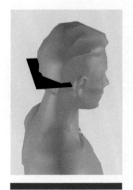

Introduction Blockade of the greater and lesser occipital nerves produces unilateral or bilateral anesthesia for minor surgical procedures of the scalp, and relief of headaches associated with muscular tension or spasm. The greater and lesser occipital nerves may be blocked separately or jointly, based upon the planned intervention. These blocks may be performed bilaterally.

ANATOMIC RELATIONSHIPS

The greater and lesser occipital nerves are derived from branches of the cervical nerves (Figs. 6-1 and 6-2).

The lesser occipital nerve, a branch of the cervical plexus (C2, C3), bends around the spinal accessory (XI) nerve. It then passes superiorly along the posterior border of the sternocleidomastoid muscle, dividing into cutaneous branches that supply the supralateral aspect of the neck, the upper pole of the ear, and the occipital region of the scalp.

The greater occipital nerve, a branch of the posterior ramus of the second cervical nerve, ascends over the posterior scalp from the insertion of the trapezius muscle onto the skull and supplies the scalp as far forward as the vertex (Fig. 6-3).

INDICATIONS

Surgical indications include soft tissue exploration and biopsy, repair of lacerations, or other minor procedures. Pain management indications include the diagnosis and treatment of headaches associated with muscular tension or spasm.

REGIONAL ANESTHETIC TECHNIQUE

The patient is seated, with the head and neck placed in a neutral or slightly flexed position for both the greater and lesser occipital nerve blocks.

Lesser Occipital Blockade

A fine 1.5- to 3.75-cm needle is introduced medial to the insertion of the sternocleido-

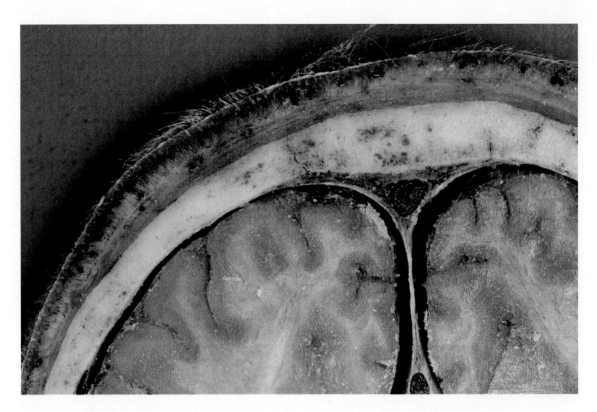

FIG. 6-1 *Transverse anatomic section through the base of the skull, revealing the greater and lesser occipital nerves.*

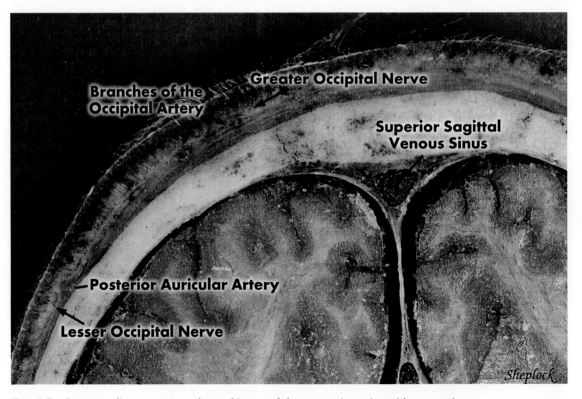

FIG. 6-2 *Corresponding computer-enhanced image of the anatomic section with annotation.*

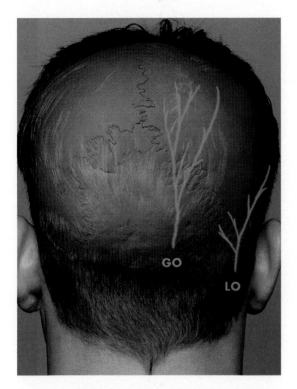

FIG. 6-3 *Distributions of the greater (GO) and lesser (LO) occipital nerves superimposed over the surface anatomy.*

mastoid muscle at the mastoid process. The needle is advanced in a medial and cephalad direction until the base of the skull is contacted and then withdrawn 1 to 2 mm. Following aspiration, 2 to 4 ml of local anesthetic is injected (Fig. 6-4).

Greater Occipital Blockade

A fine 1.5- to 3.75-cm needle is introduced lateral to the insertion of the trapezius muscle at the base of the skull. The needle is advanced in a cephalad direction until the base of the skull is contacted, and then withdrawn 1 to 2 mm. Following aspiration, 2 to 4 ml of local anesthetic is injected (Fig. 6-4).

Successful occipital blockade leads to prompt anesthesia in the distribution of the nerves (Fig. 6-5).

SIDE EFFECTS AND COMPLICATIONS

Intravascular injection may occur either in one of the many scalp veins or in the occipital artery. Due to the small volume of local anesthetic used, it is doubtful that this would be of any consequence.

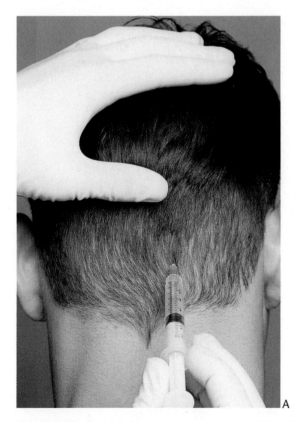
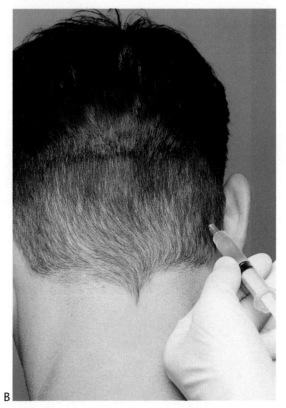

A   B

FIG. 6-4 *Blockade of the greater occipital nerve (A) and the lesser occipital nerve (B).*

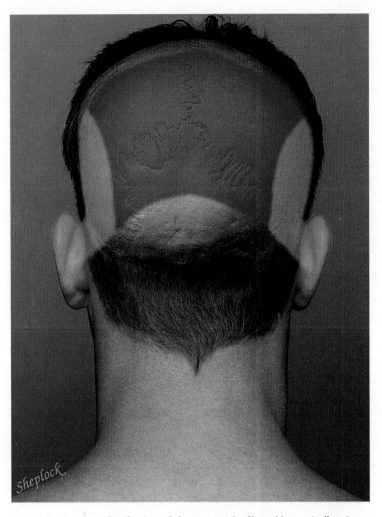

FIG. 6-5 *Sensory distribution of the greater (red) and lesser (yellow) occipital nerves.*

A subarachnoid injection may occur, leading rapidly to a total spinal blockade if the needle penetrates the dura through the foramen magnum or a cranial defect during the administration of local anesthesia. Injury to the brainstem may also occur. However, these complications are unlikely to occur with needles less than 3.75 cm in length.

SUGGESTED READINGS

Carron H: Control of pain in the head and neck. In Johns ME, Rice DH, editors: *Otolaryngologic clinics of North America,* vol 14:3, Philadelphia, 1981. WB Saunders.

Netter F, Mitchell GAG: Nerve plexuses and peripheral nerves. In Brass A, editor: *The CIBA collection of medical illustrations,* New Jersey, 1983, CIBA.

Snell RS, editor: *Clinical anatomy for medical students,* Boston, 1973, Little, Brown.

CHAPTER 7

Deep and Superficial Cervical (Plexus) Nerves

Marc B. Hahn

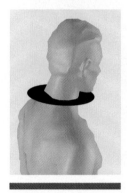

Introduction Blockade of the cervical plexus produces anesthesia for unilateral surgical procedures of the neck. Superficial and deep branches exist, and blockade of each may be selected based on the planned surgical procedure.

ANATOMIC RELATIONSHIPS

The cervical plexus is situated deep to the sternocleidomastoid muscle (Figs. 7-1 and 7-2). As the second, third, and fourth cervical nerves exit each respective intervertebral foramen, they pass posteriorly to the vertebral artery. The anterior branches pass in the sulci of the transverse process and then join to form the cervical plexus (Fig. 7-3).

The superficial branches (lesser occipital, great auricular, transverse cervical, and supraclavicular nerves) penetrate the cervical fascia posterior to the sternocleidomastoid muscle to supply cutaneous sensory innervation. The lesser occipital nerve (C2, C3) passes superiorly from the posterior border of the sternocleidomastoid muscle, dividing into cutaneous branches that supply the supralateral aspect of the neck, the upper pole of the ear, and the occipital region of the scalp. The great auricular nerve (C2, C3) passes antero-superiorly from the posterior border of the

sternocleidomastoid muscle before dividing into anterior and posterior branches. The anterior branch supplies cutaneous innervation to the posteroinferior face, whereas the posterior branch supplies cutaneous innervation over the mastoid process and the lower pole of the ear. The transverse cervical nerve (C2, C3) passes anteriorly from beneath the external jugular vein and supplies cutaneous innervation over the anterolateral aspect of the neck from the mandible to the sternum. The supraclavicular nerve (C3, C4) also exits posterior to the sternocleidomastoid muscle; it then passes inferolaterally and supplies cutaneous innervation over the lower neck to the acromioclavicular junction, as well as to the anterior chest to the level of the second rib.

The deep branches, although predominately motor nerves, also convey sensory and proprioceptive input from the deep structures of the neck (i.e., muscular, osseous, and articular structures).

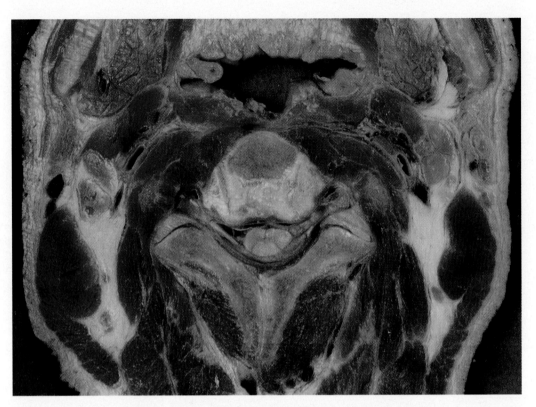

Fig. 7-1 *Transverse anatomic section through the cervical spine, revealing the relationship of the cervical nerve roots, spinal cord, vertebrae, muscles, and vascular structures.*

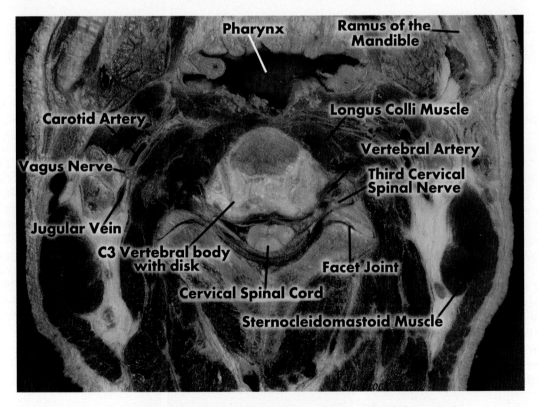

Fig. 7-2 *Corresponding computer-enhanced image of the anatomic section with annotation.*

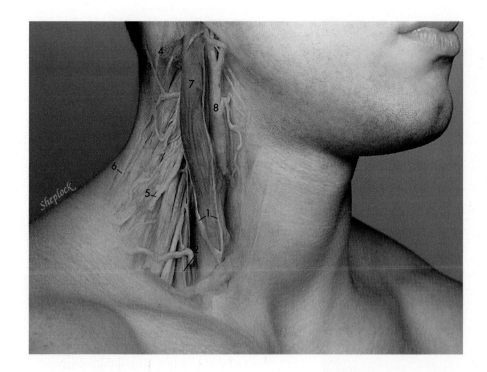

FIG. 7-3 *Dissection of the deep cervical plexus with the sternocleidomastoid muscle removed, superimposed over the surface anatomy. Key: 1, Superior and inferior rami of ansa cervicalis; 2, roots of phrenic nerve; 3, lesser occipital nerve; 4, great auricular nerve; 5, supraclavicular nerve origin; 6, spinal accessory nerve (CN XI); 7, internal jugular vein; 8, common carotid artery.*

INDICATIONS

Surgical indications include soft tissue exploration and biopsy, ipsilateral thyroid or parathyroid procedure, and carotid endarterectomy. Pain management indications include the diagnosis of any nociceptive process in the area of innervation.

REGIONAL ANESTHETIC TECHNIQUE

The superficial cervical blockade is performed first to reduce the discomfort the patient may experience with the deep cervical blockade.

Superficial Cervical Blockade

The head is extended and the neck is flexed, thus placing the patient in the "sniffing position" (Fig. 7-4). The head is then rotated contralateral to the side of the block. The posterior border of the sternocleidomastoid muscle and the external jugular vein are identified. An 8.75-cm fine needle (spinal needle) is inserted under the external jugular vein at the point where it intersects the posterior border of the sternocleidomastoid muscle. Ten to twenty ml of local anesthetic is injected behind the entire length of the posterior border of the muscle.

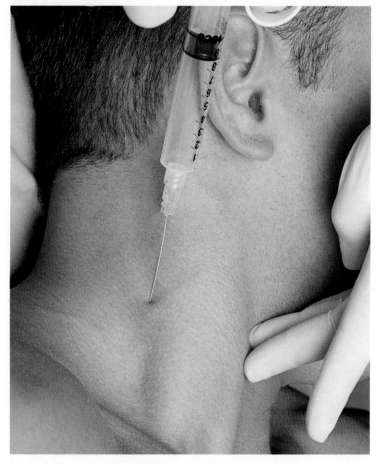

FIG. 7-4 *Blockade of the superficial cervical plexus.*

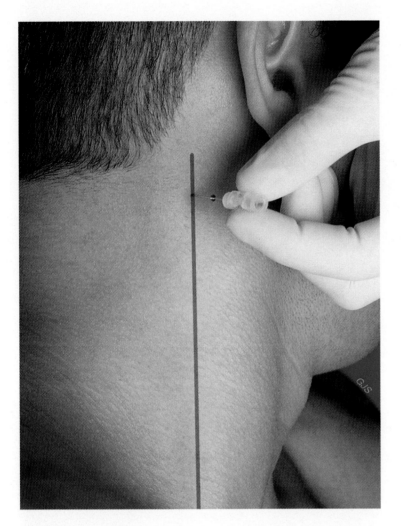

Deep Cervical Blockade

With the patient in the same position, a line is drawn from the mastoid process to the sternoclavicular junction (Fig. 7-5). The mastoid process is at the level of the transverse process of the first cervical vertebrae. The transverse processes of C2, C3, and C4 each lie under this line, approximately 1.5, 3.0, and 4.5 cm inferior to the mastoid process respectively. A 22-gauge blockade needle is inserted over the C2, C3, and C4 transverse processes perpendicular to all skin planes. The needle is inserted until either the transverse process is contacted, a paresthesia is produced, or the prevertebral fascia is penetrated (palpable click). If the needle is placed properly, it should remain perpendicular once support is removed. Following negative aspiration, 2 to 4 ml of local anesthetic is injected at each of the three sites.

Following the successful blockade of the cervical plexus, unilateral surgical procedures of the neck may be performed (Fig. 7-6).

FIG. 7-5 *Blockade of the deep cervical plexus.*

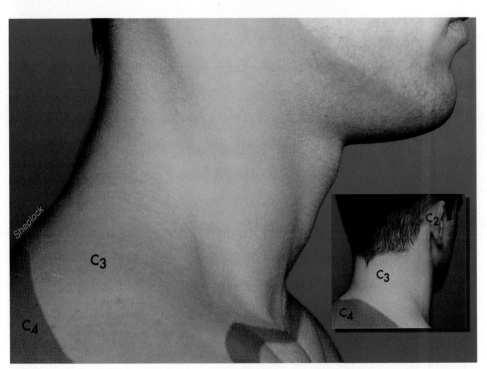

FIG. 7-6 *Sensory distribution of the deep and superficial cervical plexus. Dermatone key:* Red, *C2;* yellow, *C3;* purple, *C4.*

SIDE EFFECTS AND COMPLICATIONS

The most common complication of the deep cervical technique is blockade of both the cervical sympathetic chain and the recurrent laryngeal nerve. In rare instances this may lead to respiratory distress. Blockade of the ipsilateral phrenic nerve may lead to paralysis of the hemidiaphragm. Therefore bilateral deep cervical plexus blockade should be avoided. Intravascular injection may occur at either the external jugular vein or the vertebral artery. The latter leads more rapidly to signs of toxicity with as little as 0.25 ml of local anesthetic. A subarachnoid injection may occur if the needle penetrates a dural sleeve, leading rapidly to a total spinal blockade.

SUGGESTED READINGS

Bergeron P, Benichou H, Rudondy P et al: Stroke prevention during carotid surgery in high risk patients, *J Cardiovasc Surg* 32(6):713-9, 1991.

Carron H, Korbon G, and Rowlingson J, editors: Cervical plexus block. In *Regional anesthesia: techniques and clinical applications*, New York, 1984, Grune and Stratton.

Davies MJ, Murrell GC, Cronin KD et al: Carotid endarterectomy under cervical plexus block: a prospective clinical audit, *Anaesth Intensive Care* 18(2):219-23, 1990.

Fried KS, Elias SM, Raggi R: Carotid endarterectomy under local anesthesia, *N Engl J Med* 87(10):795-7, 1990.

Netter F, Mitchell GAG: Nerve plexuses and peripheral nerves. In Brass, A, editor: *The CIBA collection of medical illustrations*, New Jersey, 1983, CIBA.

CHAPTER 8

Glossopharyngeal Nerve

Marshall D. Bedder

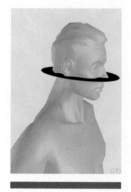

Introduction Blockade of the glossopharyngeal nerve has been described for both glossopharyngeal neuralgia and pain secondary to cancer of the throat. A successful diagnostic nerve block with local anesthetic is a prerequisite before proceeding with a neurolytic technique. A thorough understanding of the underlying anatomic relationships is critical for safe performance of any glossopharyngeal nerve block technique.

ANATOMIC RELATIONSHIPS

The glossopharyngeal nerve (IXth cranial nerve) originates from the rostral part of the medulla oblongata and leaves the skull through the jugular foramen anterior to the vagus and accessory nerves (Figs. 8-1 and 8-2). After leaving the jugular foramen, the nerve passes between the internal jugular vein and the internal carotid artery and then descends anterior to the internal carotid artery and deep to the styloid process (Fig. 8-3). It then arches toward the tongue, where it divides into a number of terminal branches.

The glossopharyngeal nerve contains both motor and sensory fibers. Sensory innervation is supplied to the middle ear and parts of the tongue and pharynx, with motor fibers innervating muscles of the pharynx. The branches include the tympanic branch; the carotid branch to the carotid sinus and carotid body; the muscular branch innervating the stylopharyngeus; the pharyngeal branches supplying sensory fibers to the mucous membranes of the soft palate, tonsils, and pharynx; and the lingual branch, which supplies sensory and taste fibers to the posterior third of the tongue, including the

circumvallate papillae. The glossopharyngeal nerve also communicates with the sympathetic trunk, vagus, and facial nerves.

INDICATIONS

Glossopharyngeal nerve block techniques have been well described as a useful diagnostic and prognostic procedure in patients with pain from cancer of the throat or glossopharyngeal neuralgias (GPN). Idiopathic GPN is an uncommon disease with tic-like lancinating pain in the neck, throat, or ear. It has been suggested that GPN is often secondary to tumors of the oropharynx and, less frequently, idiopathic. Long-term pain relief has been described with neurolytic alcohol blocks.

REGIONAL ANESTHETIC TECHNIQUE

A successful glossopharyngeal nerve block with local anesthetic, producing the desired pain relief with minimal or tolerable side effects, is necessary before proceeding to any neurolytic technique.

The patient is placed in the supine position with venous access and appropriate monitoring. The head is rotated contralater-

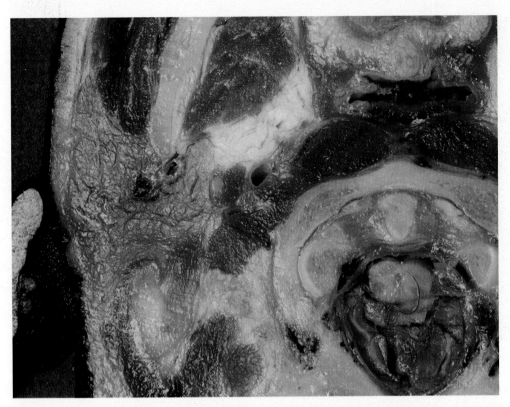

FIG. 8-1 *Transverse anatomic section through the head, revealing the glossopharyngeal nerve.*

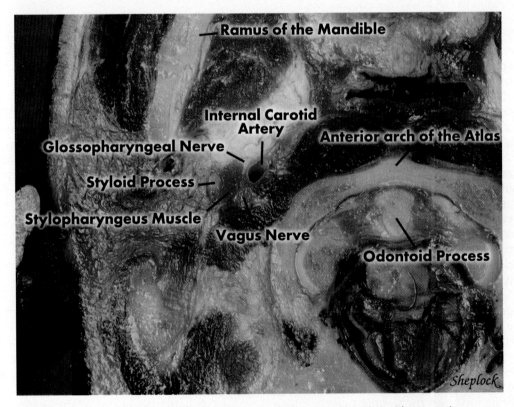

FIG. 8-2 *Corresponding computer-enhanced image of the anatomic section with annotation.*

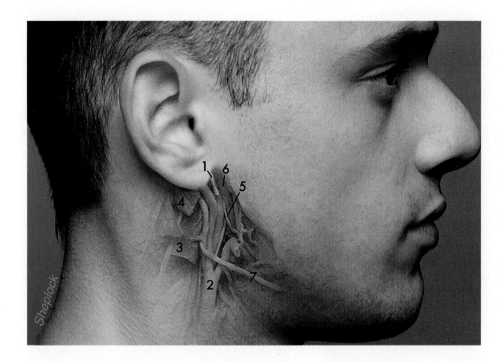

FIG. 8-3 *Dissection of the glossopharyngeal nerve and adjacent structures with the mandible, sternocleidomastoid muscle, posterior belly of digastric, stylohyoid, and infrahyoid muscles removed, superimposed over the surface anatomy. Key: 1, styloid; 2, external carotid artery; 3, internal jugular vein; 4, posterior belly of digastric muscle; 5, glossopharyngeal nerve; 6, stylopharyngeus muscle; 7, hypoglossal nerve.*

al to the side being blocked. The needle insertion site area is prepped with alcohol or povidone-iodine solution. A skin wheal of local anesthetic is formed approximately midway between the posterior border of the mandible and the tip of the mastoid process (Fig. 8-4). A 22-gauge blunt block needle is inserted through the skin and subcutaneous tissues and advanced until the bony styloid process is contacted. The needle is then withdrawn and redirected anterior to the styloid process.

The needle is advanced 0.5 to 1 cm past the depth of the styloid process. A volume of 2 to 4 ml of local anesthetic is then injected (Fig. 8-5). The problem with the standard anatomic approaches to blocking the glossopharyngeal nerve involves using the styloid process as an initial landmark. The styloid process, the calcified rostral end of the stylohyoid ligament, is variably calcified from person to person, and the length varies considerably, making it an uncertain endpoint.

A modification of the classic anatomic approach may improve accuracy and safety of the glossopharyngeal nerve block by using ultrasound guidance. This approach takes advantage of the anatomic proximity of the glossopharyngeal nerve as it runs anterior to the carotid artery. Color doppler ultrasound examination is used to visualize the carotid artery and the internal jugular vein. An echogenic ultrasound needle (Ultravue, BDtm) is inserted after ultrasound visualization of the

internal carotid artery. During ultrasound examination the needle tip is positioned on the anterior surface of the carotid artery (Fig. 8-6). This approach may minimize risk of puncturing either the internal carotid or the internal jugular vein. Blockade of the glossopharyngeal nerve at this level may also minimize vagal nerve blockade.

SIDE EFFECTS AND COMPLICATIONS

The most common side effect of glossopharyngeal nerve block is bleeding from penetration of either the internal jugular vein or the internal carotid artery. One must take extreme care before injecting local anesthetic solutions by confirming a negative aspiration for blood. Intravascular injection would cause convulsions and possible cardiovascular collapse.

The vagus and the glossopharyngeal nerve are in close proximity as they exit from the jugular foramen. Techniques of blocking the glossopharyngeal nerve at this level produce unilateral block of both nerves. Blockade of the vagus nerve has been shown to produce tachycardia, hypertension, and possible reduction in the hypoxic ventilatory drive.

Blockade of the glossopharyngeal nerve results in paralysis of the pharyngeal muscles; therefore a bilateral block is contraindicated. One may produce blockade of the accessory, facial, and hypoglossal nerve if large volumes of drug are used or if needle placement is not precise.

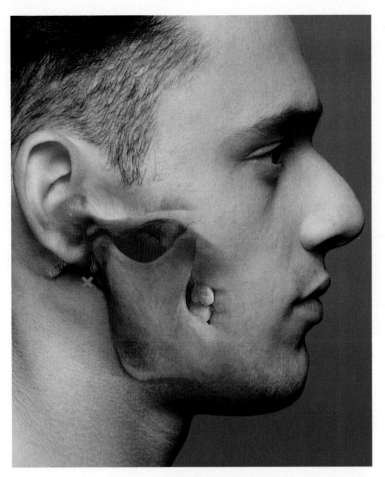

FIG. 8-4 *Computer-enhanced image of the needle insertion point (red X) for blockade of the glossopharyngeal nerve and lateral skull, superimposed over the surface anatomy.*

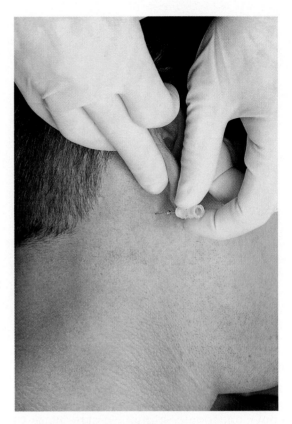

FIG. 8-5 *Blockade of the glossopharyngeal nerve, with the needle in its final position.*

SUGGESTED READINGS

Bedder MD: Glossopharyngeal nerve block using ultrasound guidance: a case report of a new technique, *Regional Anesthesia* 14(6):304-307, 1989.

Bonica JJ: Local anesthesia and regional blocks: In Wall PD, Melzack R, editors: *Textbook of pain*, London, 1984, Churchill Livingstone.

Eisely JH, Jain SK: Circulatory and respiratory changes during unilateral and bilateral cranial nerve IX and X block in two asthmatics, *Clin Sci* 40:117-125, 1971.

Fraioloi B, Esposito V, Ferrante L et al: Microsurgical treatment of glossopharyngeal neuralgia: case reports, *Neurosurgery* 25(4):630-32, 1989.

Katusic S, Williams DB, Beard CM et al: Epidemiology and clinical features of idiopathic trigeminal neuralgia and glossopharyngeal neuralgia: similarities and differences, Rochester, Minnesota, 1945-1984, *Neuroepidemiology* 10(5-6):276-81. 1991.

Murphy TM: Somatic blockade of head and neck. In Cousins MJ, Bridenbough PO, editors: *Neural blockade in clinical anesthesia and management of pain*, Philadelphia, 1988, JB Lippincott.

Netter FH: Cranial nerves. In Netter FH, editor: *The CIBA collection of medical illustration*, New Jersey, 1983, CIBA.

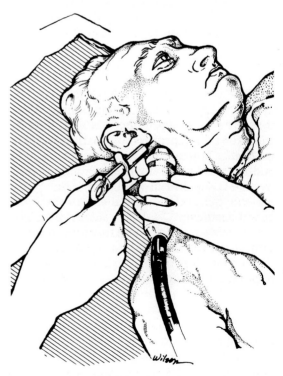

FIG. 8-6 *Blockade of the glossopharyngeal nerve using ultrasound guidance.*

CHAPTER 9

Sphenopalatine Ganglion

■

Steven D. Waldman

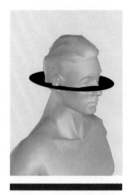

■

Introduction The sphenopalatine (pterygopalatine) ganglion is a 5-mm triangular structure comprising the largest group of neurons in the head, outside the brain. The ganglion receives afferent sensory input via fibers from the maxillary division of the trigeminal nerve. Motor input to the ganglion is carried via the greater superficial petrosal nerve, which is a branch of the facial nerve. Afferent sympathetic input is received from the carotid plexus. Efferent fibers from the sphenopalatine ganglion are divided into the orbital branch, which innervates the orbital periostium and lacrimal gland, and the nasal branch, which subdivides into the posterior superior nasal nerve, supplying the posterior septum, and the nasal palatine nerve, supplying the upper gingiva, hard and soft palate, and a portion of the tonsils. Efferent fibers from the sphenopalatine ganglion also interface with the carotid plexus, the trigeminal nerve, facial nerve, and the superior cervical ganglion.

ANATOMIC RELATIONSHIPS

The sphenopalatine ganglion (pterygopalatine, nasal, or Meckel's ganglion) is located in the pterygopalatine fossa, posterior to the middle turbinate. The ganglion is triangular and is covered by a 1 to 5 mm layer of connective tissue and mucous membrane (Figs. 9-1 and 9-2). Neural blockade of the sphenopalatine ganglion can be accomplished either via the transnasal approach, using application of topical local anesthetic, or via injection of local anesthetic through the greater palatine foramen (Fig. 9-3).

INDICATIONS

Blockade of the sphenopalatine ganglion with local anesthetic is useful in the management of acute migraine, acute cluster headache, and a variety of facial neuralgias. It may also be useful in status migrainous and chronic cluster headache. Neural blockade of the sphenopalatine ganglion may be used to provide regional anesthesia for nasal and dental surgery performed in the distribution of the sensory fibers of the ganglion.

REGIONAL ANESTHETIC TECHNIQUE
Transnasal Approach

Transnasal sphenopalatine ganglion block is accomplished by the application of local anesthetic to the mucous membrane overlying the ganglion. The patient is placed in the supine position. The cervical spine is then extended and the anterior naries is inspected for polyps, tumor, or foreign body. A small amount of 2% viscous lidocaine, 4% topical lidocaine, or 10% cocaine solution is then instilled into each nostril. The patient is asked to inhale briskly through the nose. This

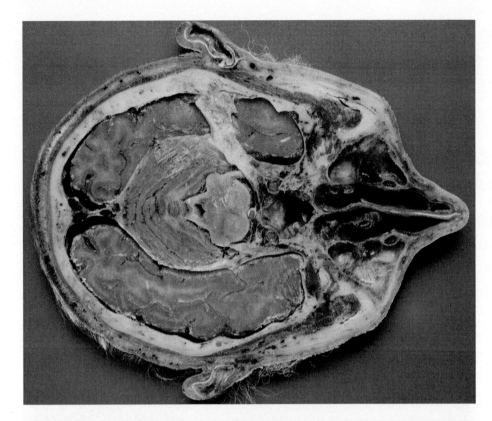

FIG. 9-1 *Transverse anatomic section through the head, revealing the sphenopalatine ganglion.*

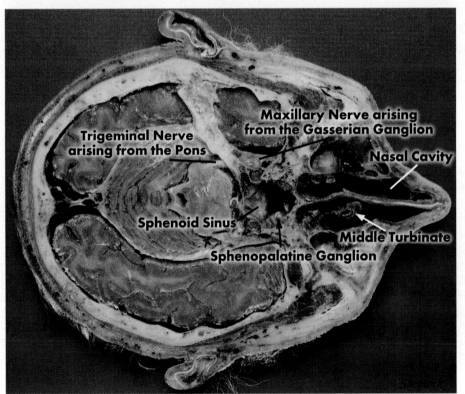

FIG. 9-2 *Corresponding computer-enhanced image of the anatomic section with annotation.*

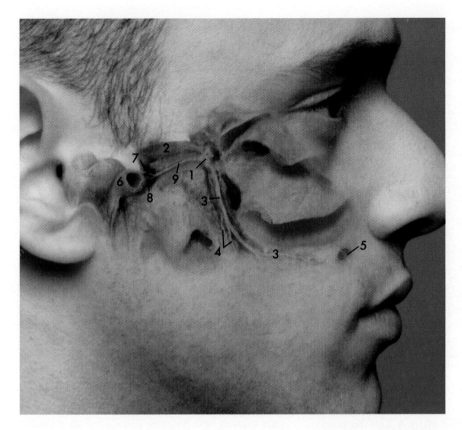

FIG. 9-3 *Dissection from behind the nasal cavity with the perpendicular plate of the palatine bone removed, which opens the greater palatine canal to reveal the sphenopalatine ganglion, the greater palatine nerve, and vessels superimposed over the surface anatomy. Key: 1, sphenopalatine ganglion; 2, maxillary nerve (V_2); 3, greater palatine nerve; 4, lesser palatine nerves; 5, lesser nasopalatine nerve; 6, internal carotid artery; 7, greater petrosal nerve; 8, deep petrosal nerve; 9, nerve of the pterygoid canal.*

draws the local anesthetic into the posterior nasal pharynx, serving the double function of lubricating the nasal mucosa and providing topical anesthesia, allowing easier passage of 10-cm cotton-tipped applicators. These applicators are saturated with the local anesthetic chosen and then advanced along the superior border of the middle turbinate until the tip comes in contact with the mucosa overlying the ganglion. One to two ml of local anesthetic is then placed along the cotton-tipped applicators in the nostril. The applicator acts as a tampon, allowing the local anesthetic to remain in contact with the mucosa overlying the ganglion and to then diffuse through the mucosa to the ganglion (Fig. 9-4). The applicators are removed after 20 minutes. The patient's pulse, blood pressure, and respirations are monitored for untoward effects secondary to sphenopalatine ganglion block.

Greater Palatine Foramen Approach

The patient is placed in the supine position with the cervical spine extended over a foam wedge. The greater palatine foramen is identified at the posterior portion of the hard

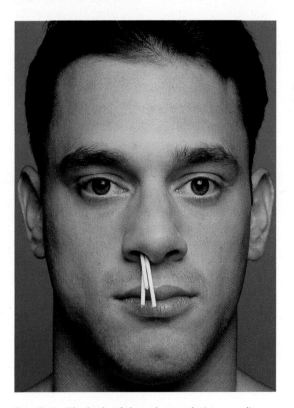

FIG. 9-4 *Blockade of the sphenopalatine ganglion via the transnasal approach.*

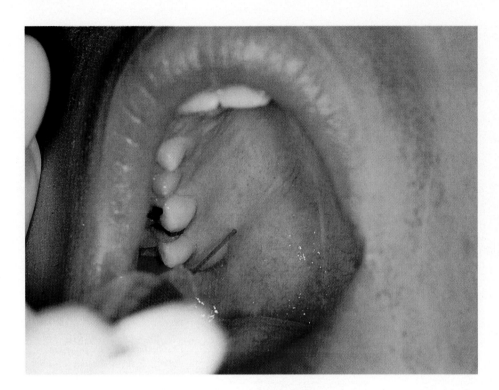

FIG. 9-5 *Blockade of the spheno-palatine ganglion via the intraoral approach through the greater palatine foramen.*

palate, just medial to the gumline of the third molar. A dental needle with a 120° angle is advanced approximately 2.5 cm through the foramen in a superior and slightly posterior trajectory. Since the maxillary nerve is just superior to the ganglion, a paresthesia may be elicited. After careful, gentle aspiration, 2 ml of local anesthetic is injected in incremental doses while observing the patient for signs of inadvertent intravascular injection (Fig. 9-5).

SIDE EFFECTS AND COMPLICATIONS

The major complication with these techniques is epistaxis. Because of the highly vascular nature of this anatomic region, local anesthetic toxicity may occur if attention is not paid to the total dose of local anesthetic used to carry out the sphenopalatine ganglion block. Occasionally patients will experience significant orthostatic hypotension fol-

lowing sphenopalatine ganglion block. For this reason the patient should be monitored carefully following the block, and moved to a sitting position and allowed to ambulate only with assistance.

SUGGESTED READINGS

Diamond S, Dalessio D: Cluster headache. In Diamond S, editor: *The practicing physician's approach to headache,* Baltimore, 1982, Williams and Wilkins.

Kitrelle JP, Grouse DS, Seybold M: Cluster headache: local anesthetic abortive agents, *Arch Neurol* 42:496-498, 1985.

Waldman SD: Evaluation and treatment of common headache and facial pain syndromes. In Raj PP, editor: *Practical management of pain,* St. Louis, 1992, Mosby.

Waldman SD: Management of acute pain, *Postgraduate Medicine* 87:15-17, 1992.

Waldman SD: Sphenopalatine nerve block. In Weiner RS, editor: *Innovations in pain management,* Orlando, 1990, PMD Press.

Waldman SD: The role of neural blockade in the management of headaches and facial pain, *Headache Digest* 4:286-292, 1991.

CHAPTER 10

Laryngeal (Superior and Recurrent) Nerves

Jeffrey S. Morrow

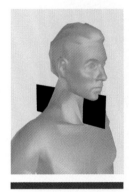

Introduction Sensory blockade of the airway mucosa plays a unique role in the armamentarium of the anesthetist. Although it produces no cutaneous anesthesia and, by itself, is not suitable for any surgical procedures, it should be mastered by any anesthetist practicing general anesthesia, where it will occasionally be useful in the examination and control of the airway. With suitable sedation and gentle sensory blockade of the airway, awake intubation can be performed, or the patient can be maintained in a very light plane of anesthesia with a controlled airway.

Mucosal anesthesia could theoretically be produced entirely by aerosolized topical local anesthetic. It can be difficult, however, to deliver an aerosol to the larynx, especially below ("behind") the true and false vocal cords.

Stimulation to the oropharynx and base of the tongue would not be attenuated without blockade of branches of the glossopharyngeal nerve.

ANATOMIC RELATIONSHIPS

Innervation of the mucosa of the airway from the epiglottis distally is a function of the vagus nerve by way of two branches: the superior laryngeal nerve and the recurrent laryngeal nerve. The superior laryngeal nerve descends in the neck posterior to the carotid artery. At a point just inferior to the lateral aspect of the hyoid bone, it divides into an internal and an external branch. The internal branch pierces the thyrohyoid membrane between the hyoid bone and the thyroid cartilage at a point lateral to the lesser cornu and medial to the greater cornu of the hyoid bone. After piercing the thyrohyoid membrane, this nerve divides into an ascending twig that supplies both sides of the epiglottis and the vestibule of the larynx, while a descending twig supplies mucosal sensation to the level of the vocal cords. The internal branch of the superior laryngeal nerve descends lateral to the larynx and innervates the cricothyroid muscles.

The recurrent laryngeal nerve, after looping beneath the innominate artery on the right and the aortic arch on the left, ascends lateral to the groove between the trachea and the esophagus to enter the caudal aspect of the larynx. It provides mucosal sensation below the cords and innervates all the intrinsic muscles of the larynx except for the cricothyroid muscle (Figs. 10-1, 10-2, and 10-3).

INDICATIONS

Anesthetization of the airway mucosa is useful in awake intubation, laryngoscopy, bronchoscopy, esophagoscopy, and transesophageal echocardiography (Fig. 10-4). The use of laryngeal nerve blocks reduces the blood level of local anesthetic produced, relative to an all-topical approach, and can easily be performed with the patient supine. It is also sometimes useful in pain control for the head and neck cancer patient.

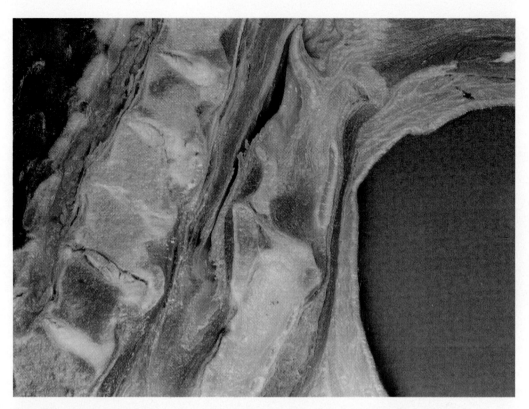

FIG. 10-1 *Sagittal anatomic section through the neck, revealing the laryngeal structures.*

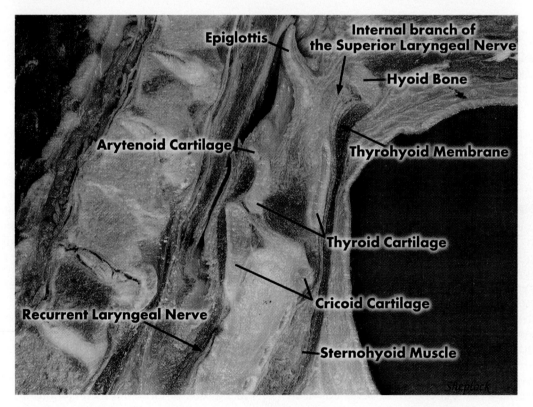

FIG. 10-2 *Corresponding computer-enhanced image of the anatomic section with annotation.*

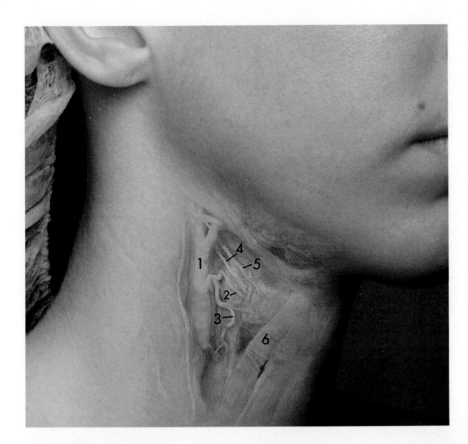

FIG. 10-3 *Dissection with parts of the mandible and sternocleido- mastoid muscle removed, superimposed over the surface anatomy. Key: 1, external carotid artery; 2, superior laryngeal artery; 3, superior thyroid artery; 4, internal branch of the superior laryn- geal nerve; 5, thyroidhyoid nerve; 6, superior belly of omohyoid muscle.*

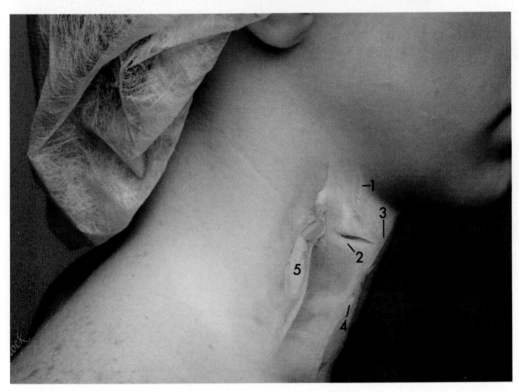

FIG. 10-4 *Sensory distribution of the superior and recurrent laryngeal nerves. Sagittal section of left side shown from right. Blue area represents innervation of superior laryngeal nerve; green area represents innervation of recurrent laryngeal nerve. Key: 1, epiglottis; 2, vocal cord; 3, lamina of thyroid cartilage; 4, arch of the cricoid cartilage; 5, lamina of cricoid cartilage.*

REGIONAL ANESTHETIC TECHNIQUE
Superior Laryngeal Nerve Block

With the patient supine, the anesthetist displaces the hyoid bone toward the opposite side with one hand, making the other greater cornu prominent and easily palpated. A three-ring syringe and a short 25-gauge needle are used to make contact with the lateral extent of the hyoid bone, and the needle is "walked" off of the inferior margin of the bone and advanced 1 to 2 mm until it pierces the thyrohyoid ligament (this may be more easily perceived with a 22-gauge needle). Aspiration should confirm that the airway has not been entered, and 2 to 3 ml of local anesthetic is injected. The hyoid bone can then be displaced to the opposite side and the other nerve blocked (Fig. 10-5).

Transtracheal Injection

Tracheal mucosa below the cords is most commonly anesthetized by injection of local anesthetic through the cricothyroid membrane. A midline approach is used. When air can be aspirated, and at the end of exhalation, 3 ml of local anesthetic is rapidly injected through a 22-gauge needle and the needle is quickly removed (Fig. 10-6).

Recurrent Laryngeal Nerve Block

The recurrent laryngeal nerve can be blocked at the level of the first tracheal ring if indicated for cancer pain. A 1.5 in, 22-gauge needle is passed, via an anterolateral approach, to the posterolateral margin of the tracheal ring, and 3 to 5 ml of local anesthetic is injected. Blockade of both nerves would produce bilateral vocal cord paralysis with airway obstruction and should not be performed (Fig. 10-7).

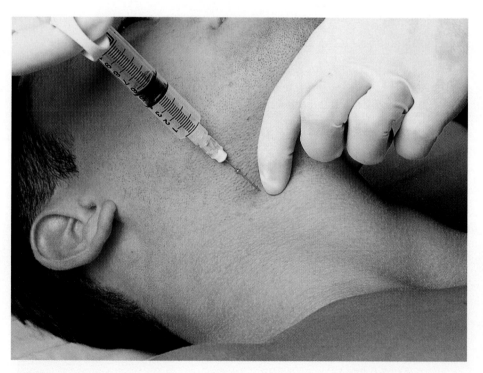

FIG. 10-5 *Blockade of the superior laryngeal nerve at the cornu of the hyoid bone.*

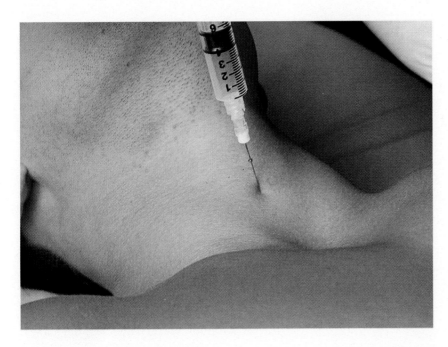

FIG. 10-6 *Sensory blockade of the tracheal mucosa (innervated by the recurrent laryngeal nerve) by topical application of local anesthetic through transtracheal injection.*

SIDE EFFECTS AND COMPLICATIONS

Superior laryngeal nerve block is essentially free of complications. When it is combined with transtracheal injection of local anesthetic, the airway can be so effectively anesthetized that one should be concerned about the possibility of aspiration without the protection of an early cough. The transtracheal injection itself will trigger a forceful cough and would present a problem for the patient where that would be undesirable (elevated intracranial pressure, for example). Vascular structures are also encountered if this injection is not performed in the midline.

SUGGESTED READINGS

Barton S, Williams JD: Glossopharyngeal nerve block, *Arch Otolaryngol* 93:186-188, 1971.

Curran J, Hamilton C, Taylor T et al: Topical analgesia before tracheal intubation, *Anesthesia* 30(6):765-768, 1975.

DeMeester TR, Skinne DB, Evan RH et al: Local nerve block anesthesia for peroral endoscopy, *Ann Thorac Surg* 24(3):278-283, 1977.

Fink RB: *The human larynx*, New York, 1975, Raven Press.

Gaskill JR, Gillies DR: Local anesthesia for peroral endoscopy: using superior laryngeal nerve block with topical application, *Arch Otolaryngol* 84(6):654-657, 1966.

Gotta AW, Sullivan CA: Anesthesia of the upper airway using topical anesthetic and superior laryngeal nerve block, *Br J Anaesth* 53(10):1055-1058, 1981.

Risk C, Fine R, D'Ambra MN et al: A new application for superior laryngeal nerve block: transesophageal echocardiography, *Anesthesiology* 72(4):746-747, 1990.

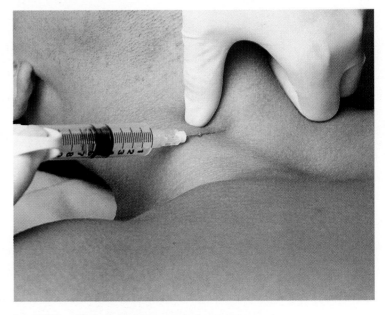

FIG. 10-7 *Blockade of the recurrent laryngeal nerve at the posterolateral margin of the first tracheal ring.*

Anatomy for Neural Blockade of the Upper Extremities

Part 4

A Brachial Plexus

CHAPTER 11

Anatomy of the Brachial Plexus

■

Michael F. Mulroy
Gale E. Thompson

■

Introduction The nerves to the upper extremity are easily anesthetized because of the close proximity of the nerve roots to each other and their relationship to easily identifiable bony and vascular landmarks. They can be approached at several levels, and multiple techniques have been described. The general anatomy will be reviewed first, then each specific block described separately.

ANATOMIC RELATIONSHIPS

The nerve roots of the C5 through T1 segments of the spinal column emerge from their intervertebral foramina and pass caudally through a sulcus in the transverse process of their respective vertebral bodies. This trough forms an anterior and a posterior tubercle, which nestle the nerves and provide a convenient bony landmark. The scalene muscles also provide a convenient envelope for these nerve roots, with the middle scalene attaching to the posterior tubercles and the anterior scalene attaching to the anterior tubercles of the transverse processes. The posterior fascia of the anterior scalene will lie anterior to the nerve roots as they emerge from the transverse processes, with the anterior fascia of the middle scalene lying posterior (Fig. 11-1). These muscles extend laterally to the first rib where they insert, and superiorly to the upper cervical levels of their proximal insertion on the third to the sixth cervical vertebrae. The fascial compartment thus created can function in some regards as an "envelope" that encourages spread of local anesthetic solution to nerves in the compartment.

As the nerves course laterally from their vertebral bodies, the upper (C5, C6) and lower (C8, T1) pairs merge and form the upper and lower trunks of the brachial plexus, with the middle C7 root forming the middle trunk. These trunks follow the scalene muscles laterally toward the rib, where they cross over the first rib and are joined at that point by the subclavian artery, which arises from the chest to cross the rib just anterior to the nerves. They rearrange themselves to surround the artery as it becomes the axillary artery distal to the rib. The trunks form two divisions which then recombine to form three cords; the lateral, medial, and posterior. The posterior cord forms the radial nerve, while the medial cord continues on as the ulnar nerve. The lateral cord continues on as the musculocutaneous nerve after it has sent a branch to join a branch from the medial cord to form the median nerve. These four main terminal branches provide sensation to the forearm and hand (Fig. 11-2). Smaller branches of the medial cord provide sensory

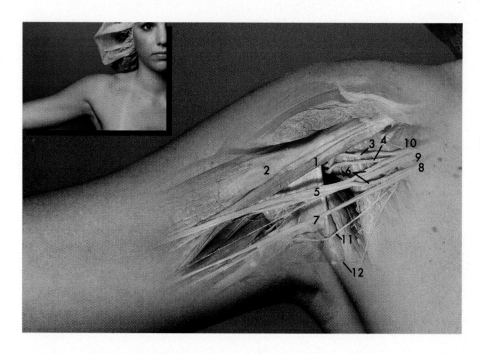

FIG. 11-1 *Dissection of the brachial plexus with all the blood vessels removed, superimposed over the surface anatomy. Key: 1, coracobrachialis; 2, biceps; 3, musculocutaneous nerve; 4, axillary nerve; 5, median nerve; 6, lateral and medial head of the median nerve; 7, ulnar nerve; 8, medial cord; 9, posterior cord; 10, lateral cord; 11, medial cutaneous nerve of the arm; 12, intercostabrachial nerve.*

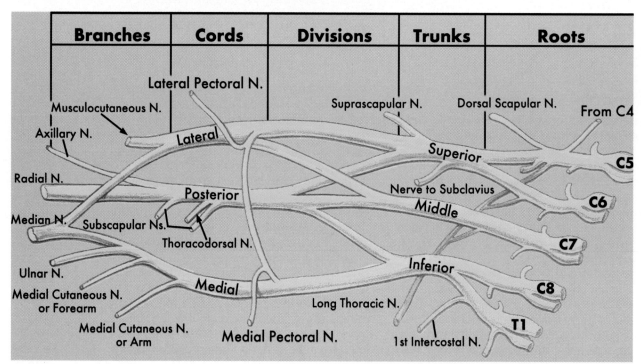

FIG. 11-2 *Brachial plexus anatomy, and the nerve roots that form the various peripheral nerves of the upper extremity.*

innervation to the medial aspect of the arm by means of the median antebrachial cutaneous nerve and the median brachial cutaneous nerve. These two smaller nerves leave the neurovascular bundle high in the axilla, as does the musculocutaneous nerve itself. This latter nerve travels through the body of the coracobrachialis muscle and provides motor fibers to it and to the biceps and sensory fibers to a variable area of distribution of the forearm. There are also sensory branches to the axilla itself that are not branches of the plexus, but arise from intercostal brachial branches (T2, T3) (Fig. 11-3 and 11-4).

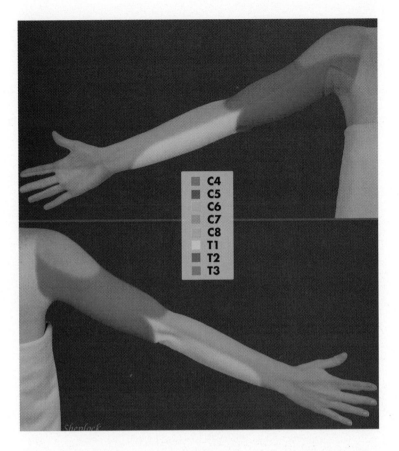

FIG. 11-3 *Sensory dermatome distribution of the anterior (top) and posterior (bottom) surfaces of the upper extremity.*

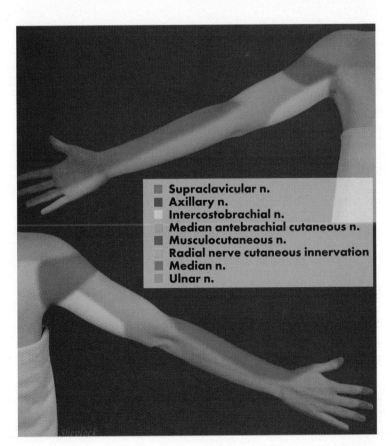

FIG. 11-4 *Peripheral nerve innervation of the anterior (top) and posterior (bottom) surfaces of the upper extremity.*

CHAPTER 12

Interscalene Approach

Michael F. Mulroy
Gale E. Thompson

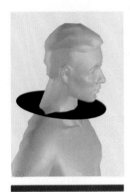

Introduction The interscalene approach to the brachial plexus is one of the simplest. A single injection here provides anesthesia of all the upper branches of the plexus. It can also conveniently produce anesthesia of the lower cervical plexus.

ANATOMIC RELATIONSHIPS

The first landmark for this block is the fleshy body of the anterior scalene muscle. The palpable groove between it and the middle scalene muscle can be used to identify the region of the nerve roots, and the fascial "envelope" at this level tends to encourage spread of the anesthetic solution to other roots. The prominent anterior tubercle of the sixth cervical process (one of the attachments of the anterior scalene) is another useful landmark. It is easily identified because of its prominence and reliable location lateral to the cricoid cartilage (Figs. 12-1 and 12-2).

Within the neck itself, several other anatomic structures of interest lie in close proximity to the nerve roots. The vertebral artery is anterior to the transverse process of C7, but then passes posteriorly into its own special channel, ascending through the transverse processes of each cervical vertebra into the base of the skull. It thus lies in very close proximity to the nerve roots, and can be entered if the needle is introduced directly perpendicular to the axial column. The sympathetic nervous system chain also lies on the anterior body of the cervical vertebrae, with the prominent stellate ganglion lying in a diffuse pattern along the bodies of C6 and C7. The phrenic nerve branches off the lower cervical plexus fibers and moves around the lateral border of the anterior scalene to descend along the anterior belly of this muscle in a caudad direction (Fig. 12-3).

INDICATIONS

The interscalene approach is particularly suited for anesthesia for shoulder procedures. It not only provides anesthesia of the upper portions of the brachial plexus, but the anesthetic solution also tends to spread to the lower cervical plexus, especially the C4 root that provides sensory anesthesia to the shoulder. Interscalene block is also effective for upper arm surgery, but frequently the inferior fibers of the plexus (the T1 root) are not anesthetized as well, and thus the ulnar side of the forearm may not obtain sensory anesthesia.

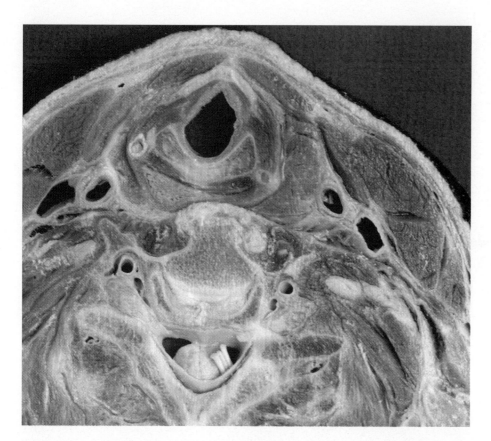

FIG. 12-1 *Transverse anatomic section through the neck at the level of the sixth cervical vertebra, revealing the relationship of the brachial plexus and related structures.*

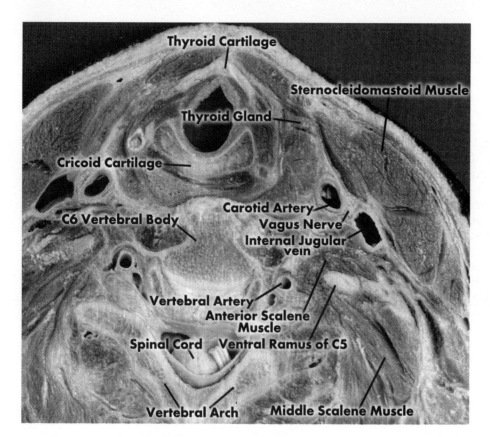

FIG. 12-2 *Corresponding computer-enhanced image of the anatomic section with annotation.*

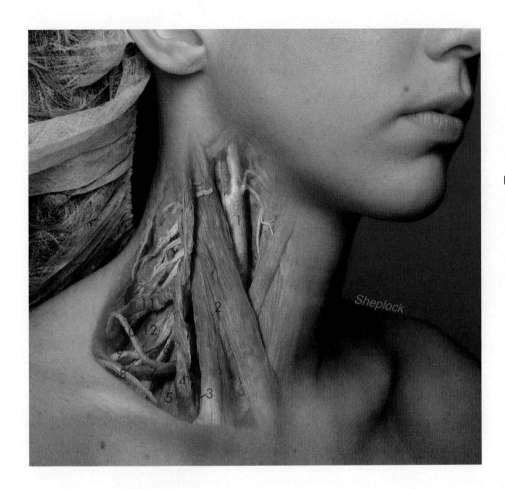

Fig. 12-3 *Dissection of the neck with the platysma and deep cervical fascia removed, revealing an unobstructed view of the brachial plexus superimposed over the surface anatomy. Key: 1, common carotid artery; 2, sternocleidomastoid muscle; 3, phrenic nerve; 4, external jugular vein; 5, anterior scaleneus muscle; 6, upper trunk of brachial plexus; 7, inferior belly of omohyoid muscle; 8, suprascapular artery; 9, suprascapular nerve; 10, superficial cervical artery; 11, superficial cervical vein; 12, middle scaleneus muscle.*

REGIONAL ANESTHETIC TECHNIQUE

The patient is placed in the supine position, with a small towel folded behind the head to provide some minor flexion of the neck and extension of the head. The head is turned slightly away from the operative side. The muscular landmarks are most easily identified by having the patient raise the head off the bed in a "sniffing" position. The most prominent muscle body anteriorly is the lateral border of the sternocleidomastoid; which should be noted, but the critical landmark is the palpable mass of the anterior scalene, which is usually less well defined and lies posterior to the sternocleidomastoid. If the palpating fingers are gently rolled posteriorly under the body of the sternocleidomastoid, the smaller anterior scalene can be felt, along with the 3- to 5-mm groove between it and the middle scalene muscle. This groove is the critical landmark and should be clearly marked on the skin. It is usually most effective to identi-

fy this groove at the level of the cricoid cartilage, which usually corresponds to the C6 transverse process (Fig. 12-4). The patient is then instructed to relax the muscles of the neck. A gentle probing in the interscalene groove at the C6 level will usually result in palpation of the transverse process itself. This is not particularly uncomfortable, particularly in the sedated patient. If the tubercle is felt, an X is marked on the skin overlying it (usually about 2.5 to 3.75 cm above the clavicle), since this is a critical landmark for performance of the block. Relaxation of the muscles is easier to obtain if the patient is instructed to hold the ipsilateral arm down at the side and pretend to reach for their own knee.

After these landmarks are identified and marked, the skin is prepped in an aseptic fashion and drapes applied. A skin wheal is inserted with a small-gauge needle at the point of the X, or where the interscalene groove lies at the level of the cricoid cartilage. A 3.75-cm, 22-gauge needle is then inserted through the

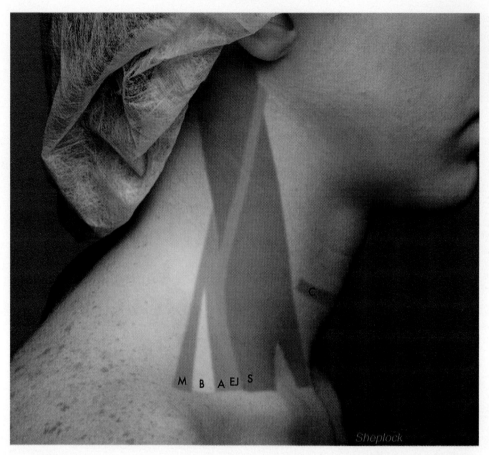

FIG. 12-4 *Landmarks needed to perform an interscalene blockade of the brachial plexus. Key: A, anterior scaleneus muscle; B, brachial plexus; M, middle scaleneus muscle; EJ, external jugular vein; C, cricoid cartilage.*

skin wheal perpendicular to the skin in all planes. (In many patients, a 1.5 cm-needle provides adequate length to reach the plexus.) This should produce an angle that is approximately 45° caudad and 45° posterior. The needle is advanced in the direction of the tubercle, which is constantly identified by the palpating index finger of the opposite hand (Fig. 12-5). If a paresthesia is obtained, 15 to 30 ml of local anesthetic solution is injected at this point. If a paresthesia is not obtained immediately, the needle is "walked" in and out with small steps in an anterior posterior direction (perpendicular to the plane at the nerves) until a paresthesia is elicited. The angle of the needle should remain about 45° caudad. A lower angle increases the likelihood of the needle entering the intervertebral foramina and potentially puncturing the dura itself (as a dural sleeve) or the vertebral artery, as mentioned above. Angling more steeply caudad than 45° increases the likelihood of contacting the dome of the lung and producing a pneumothorax.

Once paresthesia is elicited, a 0.5-ml test injection should be made to confirm that there is no cramping or discomfort indicating an intraneural injection. The risk of pinning the nerve root in the trough of the bone with the needle merits precautions to avoid intradural injection. Aspiration should also be performed frequently after every 3 to 5 ml of injection to avoid subarachnoid or intravascular injection.

SIDE EFFECTS AND COMPLICATIONS

Spread of local anesthetic to the cervical plexus is a frequent consequence of this technique. A 100% incidence of paralysis of the ipsilateral diaphragm occurs because of phrenic nerve involvement with this block. It is also not infrequent for the patient to develop a Horner's syndrome because of spillage onto the sympathetic chain. A significant complication is unintentional intravascular injection into the vertebral artery. Symptoms of CNS toxicity are almost immediate, and are produced with very small quantities of injectate. Pneumothorax is also possible, and is often hinted at by the presence of a cough and pleuritic chest pain during the search for paresthesias. Epidural spread of local anesthetic is also possible, as is subarachnoid injection. Spread of anesthesia into the epidural space can often produce some sensory changes in the opposite arm. Neuropathy may also result from direct intraneural injection or direct needle trauma.

SUGGESTED READINGS

Lanz E, Theiss D, Jankovic D: The extent of blockade following various techniques of brachial plexus block, *Anesth Analg* 62:55, 1983.

Peterson DO: Shoulder block anesthesia for shoulder reconstruction surgery, *Anesth Anal* 64:373, 1985.

Roch JJ, Sharrock NE, Neudachin L: Interscalene brachial plexus block for shoulder surgery: a proximal paresthesia is effective, *Anesth Analg* 75:386, 1992.

Rosenblatt RM, Cress JC: Modified Seldinger technique for continuous interscalene brachial plexus block, *Reg Anesth* 6:82, 1981.

Scammel SJ: Inadvertent epidural anesthesia as a complication of interscalene brachial plexus block, *Anesth Intensive Care* 7:56, 1979.

Winnie AP: Interscalene brachial plexus block, *Anesth Analg* 49:455, 1970.

Urmey WF, Talts KH, Sharrock NE: One hundred percent incidence of hemidiaphragmatic paresis associated with interscalene brachial plexus anesthesia as diagnosed by ultrasonography, *Anesth Analg* 72:498, 1991.

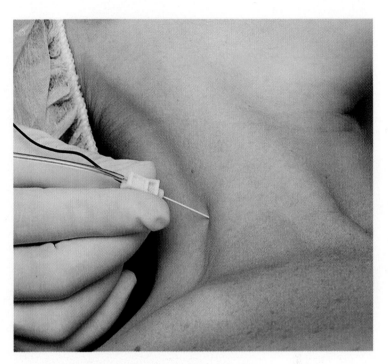

FIG. 12-5 *Blockade of the brachial plexus via the interscalene approach.*

CHAPTER 13

Supraclavicular Approach

Michael F. Mulroy
Gale E. Thompson

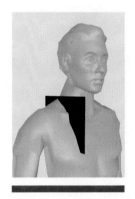

Introduction The supraclavicular approach is historically one of the earliest described approaches to anesthesia of the brachial plexus. It produces the most reliable blockade of all of the terminal branches of the plexus, although it is hampered by having significant potential for complications. Several authors have described variations of the original technique of Kuhlenkampf in an attempt to reduce this risk.

ANATOMIC RELATIONSHIPS

The critical landmark at this level is the first rib, which the trunks of the plexus cross as they enter the axilla to join the axillary artery (Figs. 13-1 and 13-2). The lateral portion of the rib lies approximately at the level of the midpoint of the clavicle in a frontal plane. The three trunks emerge from between the two scalene muscles and lie just posterior to the artery, in close proximity to each other. As the nerves cross the first rib, this bone runs in an anterior posterior direction and lies just above the dome of the lung. The pleura is directly under the medial border of this rib (Fig. 13-3).

Shortly after crossing the rib, the plexus gives off branches posteriorly as the suprascapular nerve, as well as anteriorly to form the long thoracic nerve to the chest wall. The subclavian and supraclavicular nerves also branch here, and supply the posterior shoulder. These nerves are sometimes encountered by a laterally placed needle before contact with the actual trunks, and may elicit paresthesias to the chest or scapular area.

INDICATIONS

The supraclavicular approach allows blockade of the plexus at the level where there are three trunks. Historically, this approach has been the one most reliable in producing anesthesia of *all* of the terminal branches of the brachial plexus. It avoids the sparing of the ulnar side that frequently accompanies interscalene block, and also provides good musculocutaneous sensory anesthesia, which is frequently missed with the axillary approach. Supraclavicular anesthesia is theoretically the technique of choice for any surgery of the upper arm, forearm or hand. On the other hand, it also has the highest associated incidence of pneumothorax.

REGIONAL ANESTHETIC TECHNIQUE

The patient is placed in the supine position with a small towel under the head and the head turned away from the side of surgery, just as for the interscalene approach. Again, the arm is held at the side, and the patient encouraged to envision that he or she is

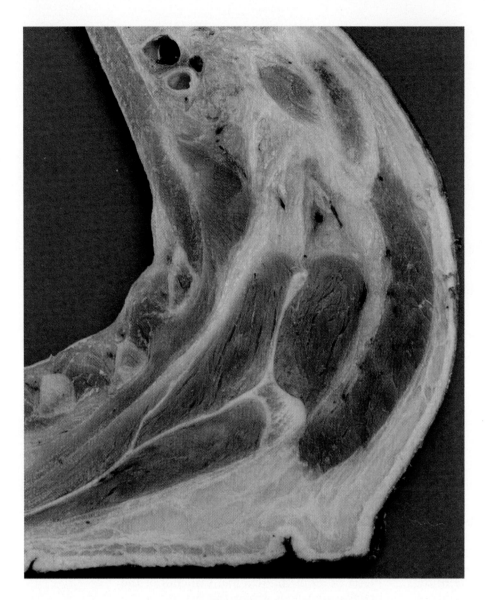

Fig. 13-1 *Sagittal anatomic section through the shoulder, revealing the relationship of the brachial plexus, the first rib, and related structures.*

reaching for the kneecap. The muscles of the neck can be identified as for the interscalene block, and the interscalene groove drawn. The medial and lateral borders of the clavicle are also identified and marked. The midpoint of the clavicle can then be measured and an X marked at this point. The first rib will generally lie just beneath this X, and the nerves can be expected to be identified at a point where the interscalene groove crosses the rib (Fig. 13-4). There are three approaches to the nerves at this level.

Classic Technique

The classic approach starts with a skin wheal 0.5 to 1 cm posterior to the midpoint of the clavicle. A 3.75-cm 22-gauge needle is introduced in a direction parallel to the spinal column so that the needle will be exactly perpendicular to the first rib when contact is made. The needle is inserted slowly, avoiding medial angulation (Fig. 13-5). If the first rib is not contacted by the time the needle is inserted 2.5 cm, the needle tip is redirected in small steps laterally to make sure that the rib has not been missed in that direction. If the rib is

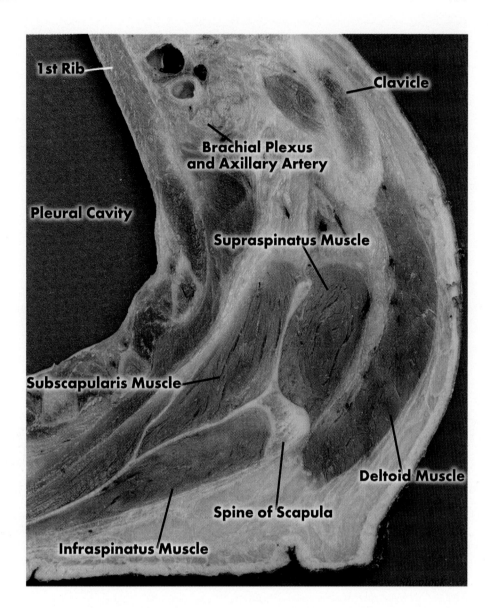

Fig. 13-2 *Corresponding computer-enhanced image of the anatomic section with annotation.*

not found laterally, it will be found with a small advancement of the needle medially. The medial direction of the needle obviously carries the risk of pneumothorax, and should be pursued in small, deliberate steps until the bone is contacted. Once contact is made with the first rib, the direction of search for the nerves is directly anterior and posteriorly, perpendicular to the path of the nerves at this point. The needle is walked along the rib until it drops off either anteriorly or posteriorly, at which time the direction of search is reversed. Small steps are required so as not to miss the

relatively narrow bundle at this level. It is also important to withdraw the needle almost completely to the skin in order to change direction. If the artery is contacted, it usually lies anterior to the neural bundle.

Once a paresthesia is elicited, the needle is withdrawn slightly and a test injection is made. If no cramping sensation or persistent paresthesia occur, then the total volume of anesthetic solution, usually 15 to 35 ml, is injected slowly around this point. Sensory anesthesia of the entire forearm should ensue within 5 minutes.

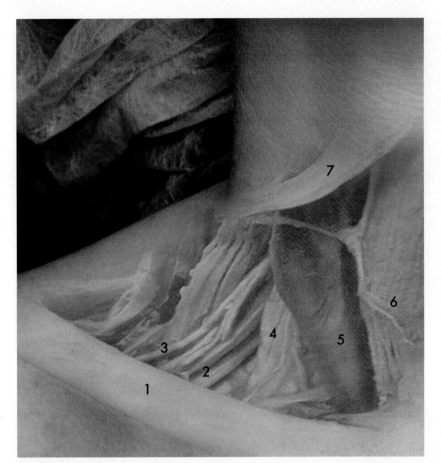

FIG. 13-3 *Dissection of the base of the neck, with the inferior belly of the omohyoid muscle displaced upwards to give an unobstructed view of the brachial plexus superimposed over the surface anatomy. Key: 1, clavicle; 2, trunks of the brachial plexus; 3, suprascapular nerve; 4, scalenus anterior muscle; 5, internal jugular vein; 6, sternohyoid muscle; 7, omohyoid muscle (displaced upwards).*

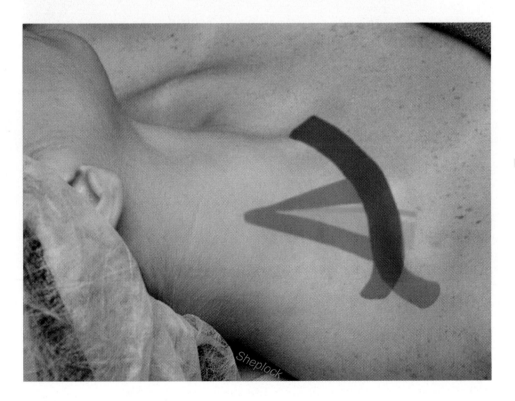

FIG. 13-4 *Landmarks needed to perform the blockade of the brachial plexus via the supraclavicular approach, highlighted and superimposed over the surface anatomy. Anterior and middle scalene muscles are in* brown, *brachial plexus is in* yellow, *subclavian artery is in* red, *first rib is in* green, *and clavicle is in* gray *(note overlap with first rib).*

Alternative Technique— "Subclavian Perivascular" Technique

Because of concern about the possibility of pneumothorax, alternative approaches have been advocated to avoid the need to advance the needle deep into the neck. Winnie has popularized the concept of the "perivascular sheath" as described previously, and advocates the introduction of the needle high in the interscalene space at the level of the first rib, but in a medial direction "dorsally tangential" to the axillary artery (Fig. 13-6). He describes a palpable click as the needle enters the sheath, and a paresthesia can be obtained just beyond this point, before contact with the first rib (or the lung). By not deliberately seeking contact with the rib, the potential for pneumothorax is theoretically reduced.

Injection is again a single-injection technique, with the cautions as mentioned.

Alternative Technique— "Plumb Bob" Technique

Another alternative approach addressing the same concerns is the "plumb bob" technique. Again, the needle is introduced at the midpoint of the clavicle but directed perpendicularly posterior, parallel to the rib rather than aimed towards it. With the patient supine, this direction would be moving directly towards the floor and would follow the line of insertion that a plumb bob would generate (Fig. 13-7). If the needle is inserted slowly at this point and then rotated in very small steps in a more caudad direction, it will encounter fibers of the brachial plexus before it encounters the dome of the lung.

SIDE EFFECTS AND COMPLICATIONS

The most common problem, as mentioned, is the risk of pneumothorax. This can be heralded by the development of pleuritic chest pain and cough during the insertion of the needle. If pneumothorax is suspected, a chest x-ray should be performed in the postoperative period. With a small-gauge needle, pneumothorax may be slow to develop and may not be readily seen unless erect films are taken in inspiration and expiration. A small pneumothorax may be tolerated by the patient without difficulty. If it is significant in size or is continuing to expand on follow-up chest x-ray, the pneumothorax should be treated by simple aspiration first, then with insertion of a chest tube in standard fashion if this is ineffective.

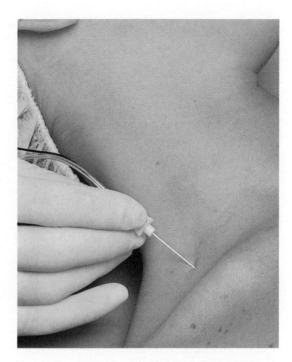

Fig. 13-5 *Blockade of the brachial plexus via the classic supraclavicular approach.*

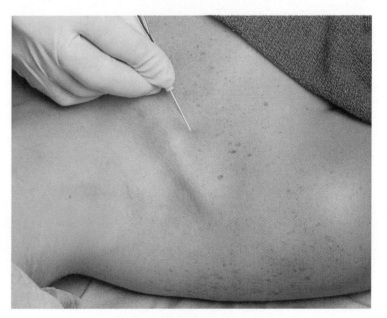

Fig. 13-6 *Blockade of the brachial plexus via the subclavian perivascular approach.*

Other complications are less frequent with this technique. There is less spread to the other nerve fibers such as the phrenic, but there is still the risk of unintentional intravascular injection because of the proximity of the artery and the veins anterior to the artery. Neuropathy is also possible if the nerve is pinned against the bone and an intraneural injection is made.

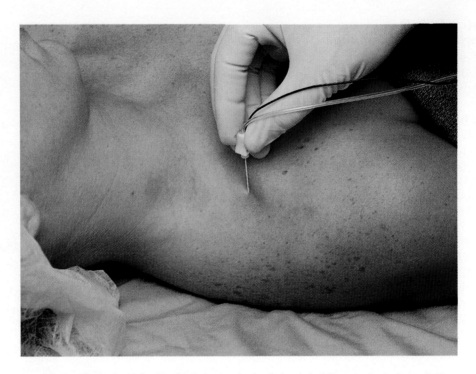

FIG. 13-7   *Blockade of the brachial plexus via the "plumb bob" supraclavicular technique.*

SUGGESTED READINGS

Brown DL, Cahill DR, Bridenbaugh DL: Supraclavicular nerve block: anatomic analysis of a method to prevent pneumothorax, *Anesth Anal* 76:530, 1993.

Kuhlenkampff D: Die anasthesierung des plexus brachialis, *Zentralbl Chir* 38:1337, 1911.

Lanz E, Theiss D, Jankovic D: The extent of blockade following various techniques of brachial plexus block, *Anesth Analg* 62:55, 1983.

Moore DC, Bridenbaugh LD: Pneumothorax: its incidence following brachial plexus block anesthesia, *Anesthesiology* 15:475, 1954.

Winnie AP, Collins VJ: The subclavian perivascular technique of brachial plexus anesthesia, *Anesthesiology* 25:353, 1964.

CHAPTER 14

Axillary Approach

Michael F. Mulroy
Gale E. Thompson

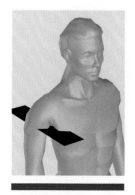

Introduction The axillary approach is the most commonly performed technique of brachial plexus anesthesia. Because anesthetic injection is made more distally, there is less risk of involvement of the central structures than with the interscalene approach and no chance of a pneumothorax as seen with the supraclavicular. Unfortunately, this technique often spares the musculocutaneous nerve, which escapes from the neurovascular bundle high in the axilla.

ANATOMIC RELATIONSHIPS

The axilla itself is formed by a muscular compartment. The fibers of the pectoralis major anteriorly and the latissimus dorsi posteriorly both insert on the upper part of the humerus, anteriorly and posteriorly to the neurovascular bundle, respectively. Although these muscles create a convenient compartment for the neurovascular bundle, they also limit the ability to palpate the structures or to introduce anesthetic high enough into the axilla to produce reliable anesthesia of the earlier branches.

At the level where the axillary artery can be most easily palpated (superficial to the humerus in the groove between the coracobrachialis and the triceps), three nerves surround it (Figs 14-1 and 14-2). The radial nerve usually lies posterior to the artery between it and the humerus. The median nerve usually lies on the superior side of the vessel, while the ulnar lies along the inferior or posterior border (Fig. 14-3). Anatomic dissection has shown that there continues to be a fascial "sheath" that surrounds the neurovascular bundle at this point. Although it is hoped that this fascial envelope will provide localization of the anesthetic solution and reliable single injection anesthesia, a significant incidence of incomplete anesthesia exists with axillary approach, ranging in the neighborhood of 15% in several series. It has been argued that septae subdivide the neurovascular bundle at this level and limit the circumferential spread of anesthetic solution. The septae have been demonstrated but arguments still prevail over their role in explaining unsatisfactory anesthesia with single-injection techniques.

INDICATIONS

Axillary anesthesia is ideal for any operation of the hand itself. It will provide reliable anesthesia of the three terminal branches that innervate the hand below the wrist. Some supplemental anesthesia is usually required if musculocutaneous blockade is mandatory.

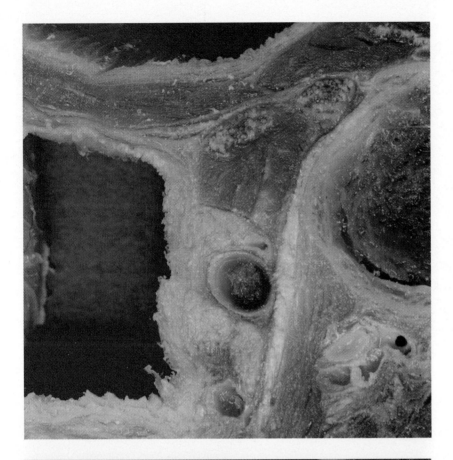

FIG. 14-1 *Transverse anatomic section through the upper arm revealing the relationship of the brachial plexus, axillary artery, humerus, and related structures.*

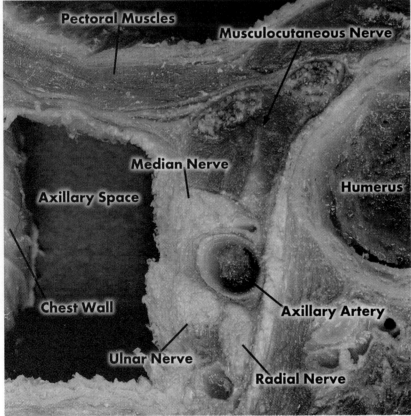

FIG. 14-2 *Corresponding computer-enhanced image of the anatomic section with annotation.*

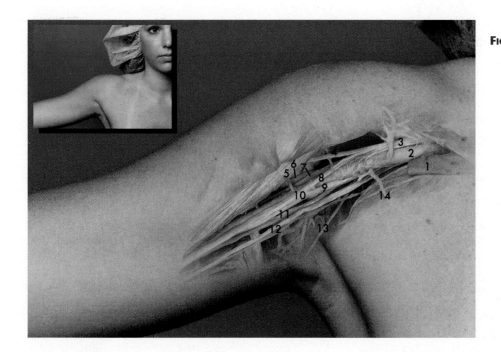

Fig. 14-3 *Dissection of the axilla with the pectoralis major and minor reflected and the axillary sheath and vein removed, revealing an unobstructed view of the brachial plexus superimposed over the surface anatomy. Key: 1, Axillary vein; **2**, axillary artery; 3, lateral cord; 4, musculocutaneous nerve; 5, coracobrachialis and short head of biceps muscles; 6, axillary nerve; 7, radial nerve; 8, lateral root of the median nerve; 9, medial root of the median nerve; 10, median nerve; 11, ulnar nerve; 12, medial cutaneous nerve of the forearm; 13, thoracodorsal nerve; 14, lateral thoracic artery.*

REGIONAL ANESTHETIC TECHNIQUE

The patient is placed in the supine position, with the head resting comfortably on a small pillow. The arm is extended 90° out from the body at the shoulder and flexed 90° at the elbow. The arm may be allowed to lie flat on the bed, but a slight anterior rotation (by placing a small towel under the wrist) can sometimes help identify the muscular structures in the axilla, as well as the neurovascular bundle. The patient is told to turn the head away from the side of the surgery, and the axilla is gently explored. If two fingers are placed in the groove between the coracobrachialis muscle and the triceps at the level of the pectoralis major insertion, the axillary artery can usually be felt fairly easily under the body of the coracobrachialis. The path of the artery should be marked on the skin as high up in the axilla as is feasible (Fig. 14-4).

After appropriate skin preparation and draping, a skin wheal is introduced directly over the artery as high up as is practical in the axilla. The position of the artery is then again identified with two fingers straddling the pulsation. A 1.25- to 2-cm small-gauge needle is then introduced. There are several modalities for identifying the neurovascular bundle. The traditional method is to seek to elicit paresthesias in the terminal nerves. If this technique is chosen, it is usually advisable to initiate the search in the nerve area

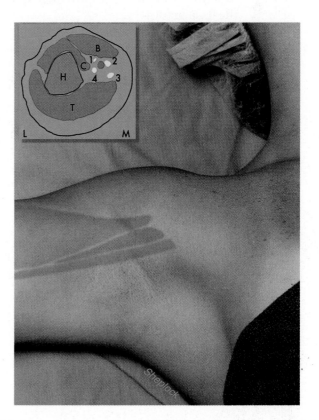

Fig. 14-4 *Landmarks needed to perform the blockade of the brachial plexus via the axillary approach, highlighted and superimposed over the surface anatomy. Illustration is cross-section at axilla. Axillary artery is in red, coracobrachialis muscle is in green; biceps muscle in in brown and triceps muscle is in yellow. Key: M, medial; L, lateral; B, biceps muscle; C, coracobrachialis muscle; T, triceps muscle; H, humerus; 1, musculocutaneous nerve; 2, median nerve; 3, ulnar nerve; 4, radial nerve.*

involved with the proposed surgery—in other words, on the superior side of the vessel if median nerve anesthesia is required.

An alternate approach is to directly seek entry into the axillary artery. Entry can be detected by aspiration of bright red blood through the needle. The needle can continue to be advanced during this aspiration until no further blood is obtained, and then the needle tip will lie within the neurovascular bundle posterior to the artery (Fig. 14-5). With both of these approaches, the entire volume of local anesthetic (15 to 35 ml) can be injected at this endpoint. During the injection, firm pressure can continue to be applied with the fingers that straddle the artery. This type of pressure will encourage the anesthetic solution to diffuse proximally along the sheath, and hopefully will include the musculocutaneous nerve at its site of origin. Alternatively, a tourniquet can be placed along the upper arm before the block is started to encourage proximal spread of the local anesthetic.

Both of these techniques imply an homogenous intact "sheath" and thus are described as single-injection techniques. Another variation is to simply feel the fascial "pop" as the needle is inserted and to inject the entire solution within this perceived sheath. As mentioned, evidence suggests that there are actually multiple sheaths in this area. Thus it has been recommended that an injection be made in at least two separate areas of the neurovascular bundle at this point in order to increase the probability for uniform spread of anesthetic solution. This can be done with either the paresthesia or the transarterial approach. With paresthesias, one half of the planned anesthetic solution is injected on the elicitation of the first paresthesia; a search for a second paresthesia on the opposite side of the artery is then immediately begun, and the remaining anesthetic solution injected on this second paresthesia. With the transarterial approach, half the anesthetic can be injected behind the artery, and the needle again withdrawn slowly through the artery until just anterior to it. The other half of the anesthetic solution can be injected here. Both these approaches provide for distribution of the anesthesia on at least two opposite sides of the artery.

A third approach is to use multiple small injections of local anesthetic by a fanning injection on both sides of the artery. This technique attempts to avoid direct contact with, or entrance into, the artery. The artery simply serves as the key guiding landmark for the beginning point of the fanning maneuver. If the palpating hand identifies, compresses, and fixes the artery in place, a 1.5-cm 25-gauge needle is usually of adequate length to reach the nerves if the fanning direction is perpendicular to the compressed artery. Occasionally a 3 to 4 cm 23-gauge needle must be used to infiltrate above the artery in the substance of the coracobrachialis muscle to anesthetize the musculocutaneous nerve. With this technique, 10 ml of local anesthetic is injected above and 10 ml below the artery in a fanning maneuver. Individual nerves may be supplemented with additional local anesthetic if needed (Fig. 14-6).

SIDE EFFECTS AND COMPLICATIONS

The most frequent side effect of axillary technique is incomplete anesthesia of the musculocutaneous nerve. If complete anesthesia was not obtained by the use of high volumes and distal compression, the musculocutaneous nerve can be blocked by injection of 5 ml of local anesthetic in a fanwise manner directly into the body of the coracobrachialis muscle.

The other common complication of axillary blockade is residual dysesthesias in the nerves. This complication occurs more frequently with the paresthesia technique, and may occur as often as 2% of the time. Obviously, direct intraneural injection should be avoided. A sharp angulation of the needle bevel has been implicated as a potential cause in the past, which has led to the widespread use of the blunter B-beveled needles for regional techniques.

The other major potential cause of complication with the axillary approach is intravascular injection. Administration of the anesthetic should be in small increments with frequent aspiration and testing to assess the patient's mental status.

SUGGESTED READINGS

Partridge BL, Katz J, Benirschke K: Functional anatomy of the brachial plexus sheath: implications for anesthesia, *Anesthesiology* 66:743, 1987.

Selander D: Axillary plexus block: paresthetic or perivascular (editorial), *Anesthesiology* 66:726, 1987.

Thompson GE, Rorie DK: Functional anatomy of the brachial plexus sheaths, *Anesthesiology* 59:117, 1983.

Vester-Andersen T, Christeansen C, Sorensen M et al: Perivascular axillary block: II. Influence of injected volume of local anesthetic on neural blockade, *Acta Anaesthesiol Scand* 27:95, 1983.

Winnie AP, Radonjic R, Akkineni AR et al: Factors influencing distribution of local anesthetic injected into the brachial plexus sheath, *Anesth Analg* 58:225, 1979.

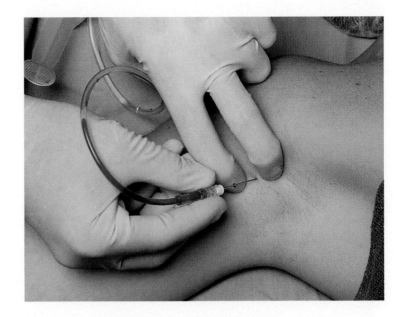

Fig. 14-5 *Blockade of the brachial plexus via the transarterial axillary approach.*

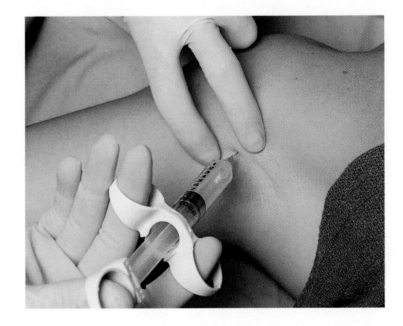

Fig. 14-6 *Blockade of the brachial plexus through multiple small injections via an axillary approach.*

CHAPTER 15

Blockade at the Elbow

Michael F. Mulroy
Gale E. Thompson

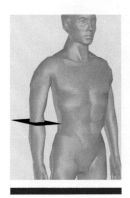

Introduction If a terminal nerve of the brachial plexus is not adequately blocked by one of the techniques described in earlier chapters, it can be blocked at the elbow or the wrist. At these two points there are adequate bony landmarks, and the nerves are somewhat superficial, so they can be approached relatively easily.

ANATOMIC RELATIONSHIPS

At the elbow, the ulnar nerve is the most superficial (Figs. 15-1 and 15-2). It lies in the groove between the medial condyle of the humerus and the olecranon process, and can be palpated itself. Palpation of this groove frequently produces paresthesias into the little finger. The median nerve lies on the opposite side of the joint, traveling across the joint just medial to the brachial artery at approximately the same depth. The radial nerve crosses the elbow joint on the opposite side of the skin crease, lying deep between the biceps tendon and the insertion of the brachial radialis. The least reliable anatomic localization is for the sensory branches of the lateral cutaneous nerve of the forearm. This nerve has already begun to ramify and lies superficially above the course of the radial nerve.

INDICATIONS

Blockade of the nerves individually at this point is less reliable than blockade of the plexus itself proximally. Blockade of the individual nerves, as mentioned, can supplement the partial brachial plexus anesthetic. Blockade at this point will produce anesthesia in the sensory distribution of the nerve distal to the elbow. For the radial, median, and ulnar nerves, the sensory distribution in the hand can just as easily be blocked at the

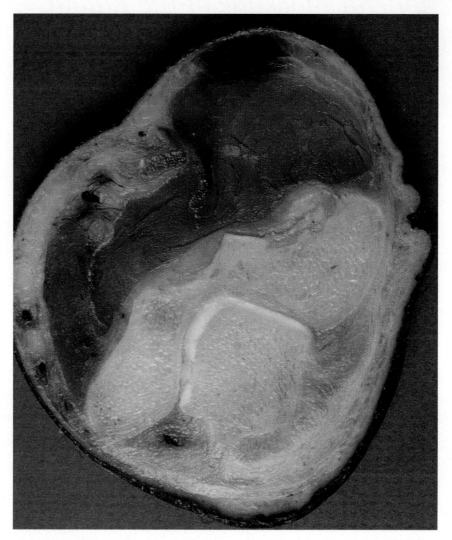

Fig. 15-1 *Transverse anatomic section through the arm at the elbow, revealing the relationship of the median, radial, and ulnar nerves, as well as related structures.*

wrist. It is only the terminal sensory branches of the musculocutaneous nerve that will provide better sensory anesthesia of the forearm itself between the elbow and the wrist, and this is the nerve that is most difficult to block at the elbow.

REGIONAL ANESTHETIC TECHNIQUE
Ulnar Nerve
The elbow should be flexed minimally, usually only to about 30º. Greater flexion will tend to restrict the nerve compartment and increase the potential for pressure on the nerve with injection in the groove. The nerve may also roll out of the groove with excessive flexion. The depression between the olecranon process and the condyle of the

humerus is easily identified. Three to five ml of local anesthetic can be injected subcutaneously with a small-gauge needle below the fascia into this groove parallel to the nerve. Direct intraneural injection or excessive pressure in this confined area should be avoided in order to reduce the chance of nerve damage (Fig. 15-3).

Median Nerve
On the opposite side of the elbow, the pulsation of the brachial artery can be identified along the medial side of the elbow joint. A 3.75-cm needle can be inserted above the artery on the ulnar side and directed towards the humerus (Fig. 15-4). This is most easily done about 2 cm above the antecubital

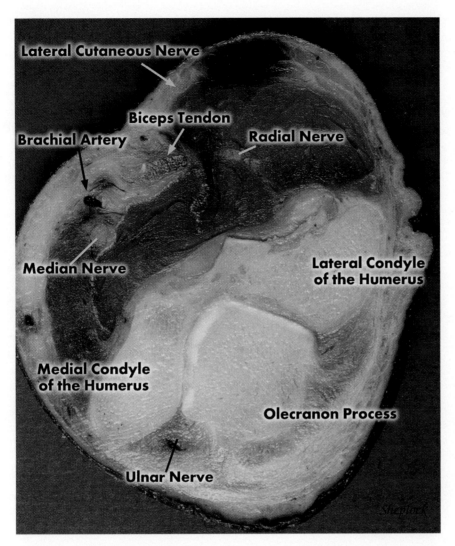

Fig. 15-2 *Corresponding computer-enhanced image of the anatomic section with annotation.*

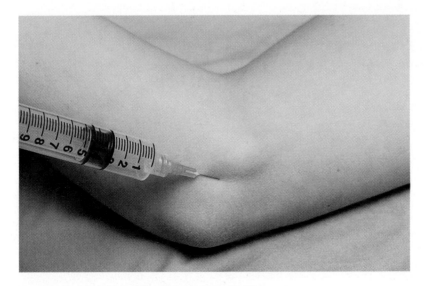

Fig. 15-3 *Blockade of the ulnar nerve at the elbow.*

crease. A "wall" of anesthesia can be created by injecting 5 to 7 ml of local anesthetic in this area about the depth of the brachial artery and somewhat deeper to it.

Radial Nerve

On the lateral side of the joint, the tendon of the biceps is identified at about the same level above the elbow crease. The needle is inserted lateral to the biceps tendon and advanced slightly cephalad and medial to contact the lateral condyle of the humerus. Again, 5 to 7 ml of solution is injected in a fan-like pattern as the needle is withdrawn.

Lateral Cutaneous Nerve of the Forearm

Subcutaneous injection over the course of the radial nerve will usually suffice to anesthetize these fibers. Local infiltration of the actual incision site is often just as effective.

SIDE EFFECTS AND COMPLICATIONS

The major concern in this area is direct injury to the nerve, especially the ulnar, by intraneural injection or by excessive pressure.

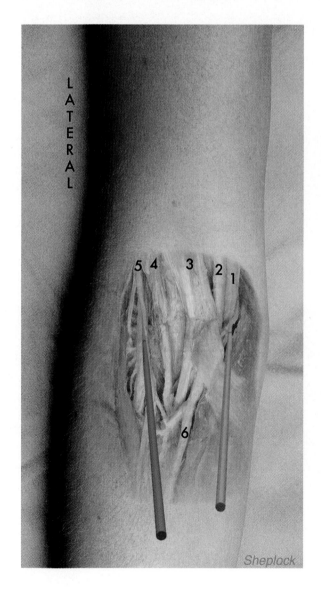

FIG. 15-4 *Blockade of the radial (green needle) and median (yellow needle) nerves at the elbow. The brachioradialis muscle is displaced laterally to show the radial nerve. Key: 1, median nerve; 2, brachial artery; 3, biceps muscle; 4, brachialis muscle; 5, radial nerve; 6, radial artery.*

CHAPTER 16

Wrist

Michael F. Mulroy
Gale E. Thompson

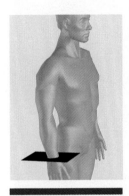

Introduction Blockade of the three terminal nerves to the hand at the level of the wrist provides anesthesia just as beneficial as blockade at the elbow, and it is somewhat simpler to perform. It is again useful in supplementing a partial brachial plexus block and can also be used for direct anesthesia to the hand.

ANATOMIC RELATIONSHIPS

At the wrist the three nerves lie predominantly on the palmar side (Figs. 16-1 and 16-2). They are easily found because of their superficial location near bony landmarks. The ulnar nerve lies at the ulnar side and is most easily approached at the level of the ulnar styloid, where it lies just lateral to the ulnar artery itself. The median nerve is in the middle of the wrist, deep between the tendons of the palmaris longus and the flexor carpi radialis, which are the two tendons must easily identified by asking the patient to flex the wrist. The radial nerve begins branching proximal to the wrist, but again can be in company with the radial artery. Several of its branches pass superficially and dorsally over the joint and through the anatomic snuff-box on the back of the hand.

INDICATIONS

As mentioned, these blocks are good for supplementing incomplete anesthesia of the forearm and can sometimes be used for independent anesthesia of the hand.

REGIONAL ANESTHETIC TECHNIQUE

Ulnar Nerve

A 25-gauge needle can be inserted on the ulnar side of the ulnar artery and advanced between it and the flexor carpi ulnaris to the level of the ulnar styloid. Three to five ml of solution are adequate to provide anesthesia in this area (Fig. 16-3).

Median Nerve

The tendons of the flexor palmaris longus and flexor carpi radialis are identified by gentle

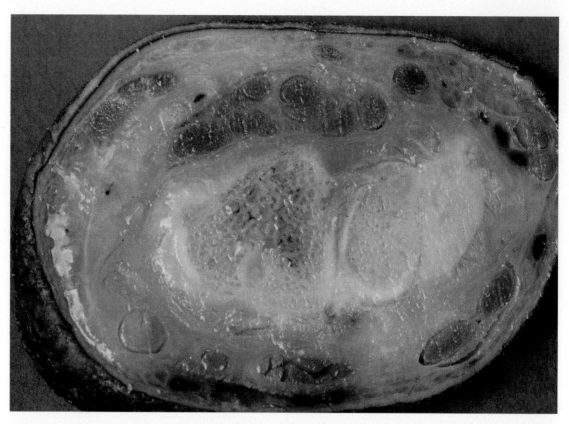

Fig. 16-1 *Transverse anatomic section through the arm at the wrist, revealing the relationship of the median, radial, and ulnar nerves, as well as related structures.*

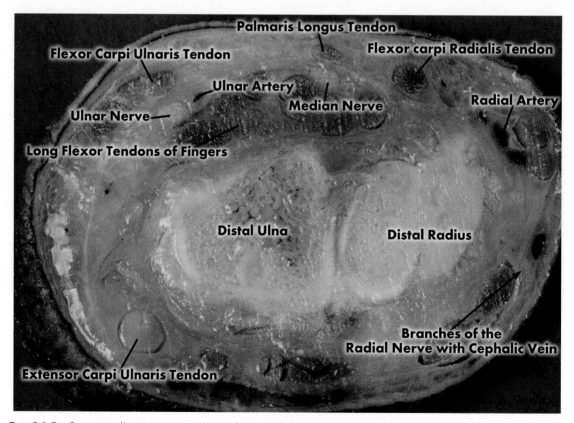

Fig. 16-2 *Corresponding computer-enhanced image of the anatomic section with annotation.*

flexion of the wrist. A needle inserted between them and through the deep fascia will lie in the vicinity of the nerve. Again, 3 to 5 ml of local anesthetic will provide anesthesia.

Radial Nerve

Three ml of local anesthetic should be injected along the lateral border of the radial artery just above the wrist. A superficial ring of sub-cutaneous injection must also be used to anesthetize the superficial branches that extend dorsally over the border of the wrist into the snuff-box area.

Side Effects and Complications

Again, neuropathy by direct intraneural injection is the major concern.

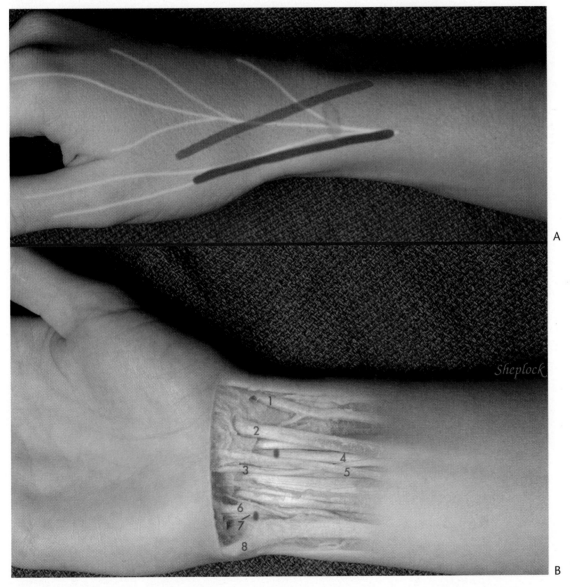

FIG. 16-3 *Blockade of the radial, median, and ulnar nerves at the wrist. A, Lateral wrist, showing blockade of the radial nerve. Distribution of the radial nerve is in* yellow. *The* green line *indicates tendons of the extensor pollicus longus. The* blue line *indicates tendons of the abductor pollicis longus and extensor pollicis brevis. The* light blue *area indicates the region of subcutaneous infiltration of local anesthetic for blockade of the radial nerve at the wrist. B, Anterior wrist with the skin and fascia removed to show blockade of the ulnar and median nerves. Red circles indicate the skin insertion sites for each block. Key: 1, radial artery; 2, flexor carpi radialis tendon; 3, palmar branch of median nerve; 4, median nerve; 5, palmaris longus tendon; 6, ulnar artery; 7, ulnar nerve; 8, flexor carpi ulnaris tendon.*

CHAPTER 17

Blockade of the Digital Nerves

Michael F. Mulroy
Gale E. Thompson

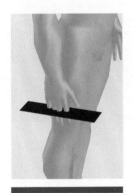

Introduction For surgery of the fingertip alone, digital nerve block is usually adequate.

ANATOMIC RELATIONSHIPS

There are two digital nerves along each digit (Figs. 12-1 and 12-2). They each have dorsal and ventral branches, but the main trunks lie alongside each phalanx at about the midpoint.

INDICATIONS

Anesthesia here is satisfactory for most procedures on the fingertips.

REGIONAL ANESTHETIC TECHNIQUE

The patient's hand is placed on a flat surface with the palm down and the fingers extended. The metacarpal heads can usually be palpated easily. The needle is introduced at the base of the web space on the finger to be blocked, usually at the level of the metacarpal head, which generally corresponds to the change in skin texture from the relatively rough character of skin dorsally to the smooth texture ventrally (Fig. 12-3). A 25-gauge needle is usually sufficient and does not require a skin wheal. The needle is directed somewhat downward towards the metacarpal head of the digit. One to two ml of local anesthetic is injected along the ventral head of the metacarpal, and a further 1 ml along the dorsal head to anesthetize both the branches. Obviously, both sides of the involved digit must be blocked. For the index and the little fingers, the lateral aspect of anesthesia is made by injections along the appropriate borders of the hand at the level of the metacarpal head. For the thumb, again, injections are made on either side of the metacarpal head at the same level. *No epinephrine is used in these solutions.*

SIDE EFFECTS AND COMPLICATIONS

The most significant problem with digital nerve blocks is the potential for producing ischemia of the fingertip if epinephrine is used in the local anesthetic solution, and thus it is avoided for this technique.

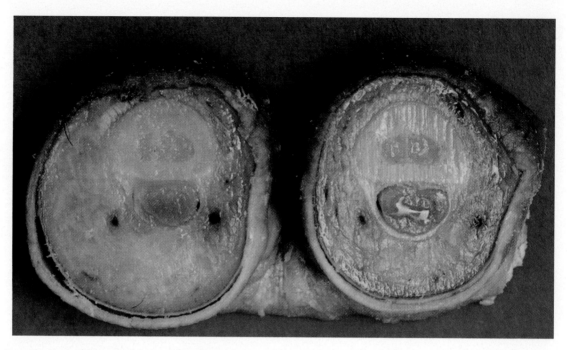

FIG. 17-1 *Transverse anatomic section through the hand at the base of the digits, revealing the relationship of the digital nerves and related structures.*

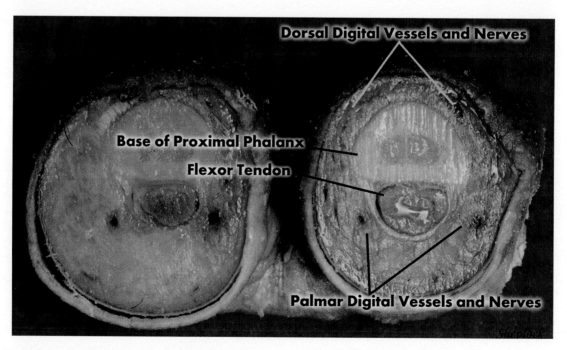

FIG. 17-2 *Corresponding computer-enhanced image of the anatomic section with annotation.*

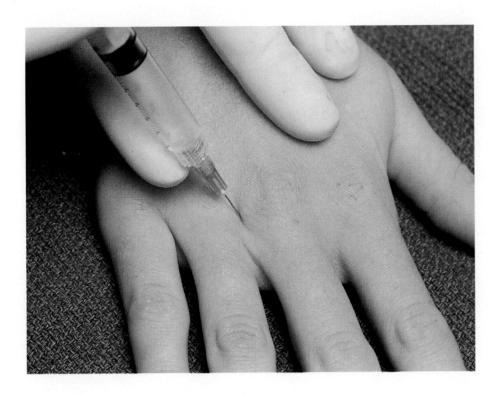

Fig. 17-3 *Blockade of the digital nerves at the metacarpal-phalangeal junction.*

Anatomy for Neural Blockade of the Lower Extremities

CHAPTER 18

Sciatic Nerve

Lynn M. Broadman

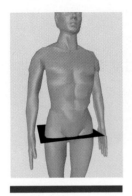

Introduction Blockade of the sciatic nerve may be used to provide anesthesia to the foot and the lower extremity distal to the knee. When used alone, the sciatic nerve block will provide anesthesia to all areas of the lower leg and foot except for the medial aspect of the calf and foot. The latter two areas are innervated by the saphenous nerve, a branch of the femoral nerve. When used in conjunction with the three-in-one paravascular block, one can obtain surgical anesthesia and postoperative analgesia for all lower extremity procedures.

ANATOMIC RELATIONSHIPS

The sciatic nerve arises from the sacral plexus. It is formed from the anterior divisions of L4, L5, and S1-3 nerves. These fused nerve roots then exit the pelvis through the greater sciatic foramen (notch) whereupon the sciatic nerve enters the leg by passing between the greater trochanter and ischial tuberosity (Figs. 18-1 and (18-2). The sciatic nerve provides sensory, motor, and some sympathetic innervation to the lower extremity (Figs. 18-3 and 18-4).

INDICATIONS

Surgical indications include soft tissue exploration and biopsy of the distal lower extremity and foot, with the exception of the medial aspect of the leg. More extensive surgical procedures of the lower extremity may be accomplished if blockade of the femoral, lateral femoral cutaneous, and obturator nerves are performed in conjunction with the sciatic block.

REGIONAL ANESTHETIC TECHNIQUE
Peripheral Approach

The sciatic nerve can be blocked using the classic Labat's technique; however, the peripheral approach is such easier to perform. The patient is placed in the lateral (Sim's) position with the leg to be blocked uppermost, flexed at the knee, and resting on the dependent lower extremity. One palpates the greater trochanter and ischial tuberosity and notes the notch between these two bony landmarks. The sciatic nerve lies in this notch, roughly midway between the two landmarks. A 8.5-cm, 22-gauge spinal needle is used to perform the block in adults, while a 3.5- to 5-cm, 22-gauge needle is employed in pediatric patients (Fig. 18-5).

A skin wheal is then raised over the needle entry point, using a 30-gauge needle and 1 to 2 ml of 0.5% lidocaine. The negative lead of the nerve stimulator is attached near the hub of the needle, and the tip is introduced into the notch of the anesthetized child or

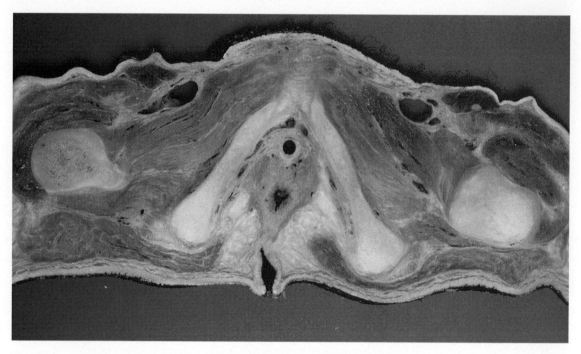

FIG. 18-1　*Transverse anatomic section through the pelvis, revealing the relationship of the sciatic nerve and related structures.*

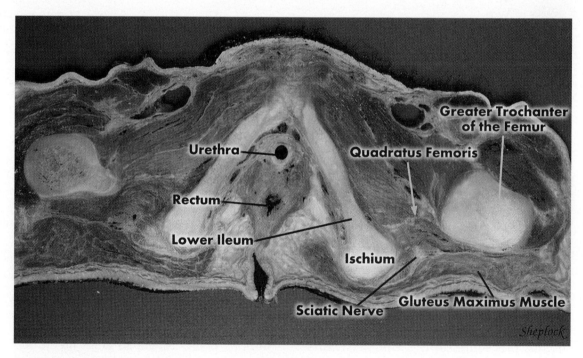

FIG. 18-2　*Corresponding computer-enhanced image of the anatomic section with annotation.*

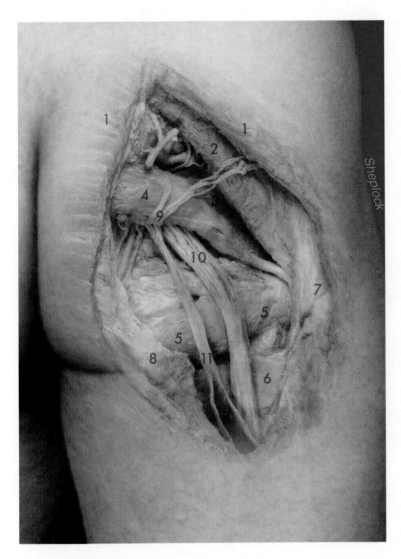

FIG. 18-3 *Dissection of the sciatic nerve with the central part of the gluteus maximus removed, superimposed over the surface anatomy. Key: 1, gluteus maximus muscle; 2, gluteus medius muscle; 3, gluteus minimus muscle; 4, piriformis muscle; 5, inferior gemellus muscle; 6, quadratus femoris muscle; 7, greater trochanter of the femur; 8, ischial tuberosity; 9, inferior gluteal nerve; 10, sciatic nerve; 11, posterior femoral cutaneous nerve.*

sedated adult. As the needle is advanced, stimulated dorsiflexion and plantar flexion should be noted in the foot of the extremity to be blocked. To confirm that the observed motor activity is due to the tip of the stimulating needle lying in close proximity to the sciatic nerve, 1 to 2 ml of local anesthetic solution should be injected. If all electrically stimulated motor activity is abolished, it may be assumed that the needle tip is in the correct fascial plane. The block is completed by injecting 0.15 ml/kg of local anesthetic solution. It is important to remember that before passing between the two prominent bony landmarks (the greater trochanter and the ischial tuberosity), a division of the sciatic nerve, the posterior cutaneous nerve of the thigh, has already branched off to provide

sensory innervation to the posterior aspect of the thigh and gluteal region. Theoretically the peripheral approach to neuroblockade of the sciatic nerve should not provide complete analgesia to tourniquet pain over the posterior aspect of the proximal thigh; however, this has not been my personal experience. It is hypothesized that this nerve also is blocked by the bolus injection of local anesthetic solution as the nerve passes between the ischial tuberosity and the sciatic nerve before it enters the posterior aspect of the leg.

Classic Approach
The patient is moved into the Sim's position as previously described for the peripheral approach. The classic approach of Labat uses

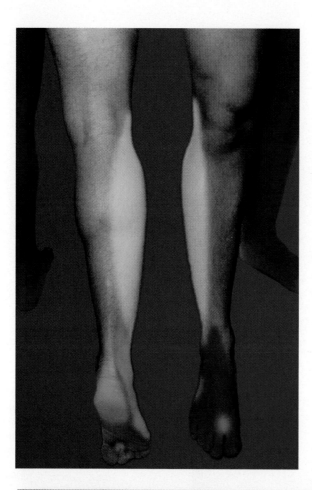

FIG. 18-4 *Sensory distribution of the sciatic nerve.* Yellow, *peroneal nerve;* blue, *calcaneal nerve;* orange, *sural nerve;* red, *deep peroneal nerve;* brown, *superficial peroneal nerve;* green, *medial plantar nerve.*

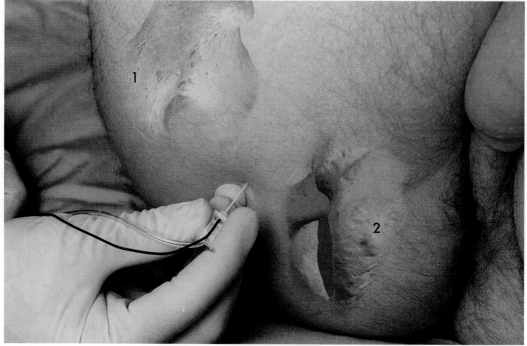

FIG. 18-5 *Blockade of the sciatic nerve via the peripheral approach. 1, Greater trochanter; 2, ischial tuberosity. Patients with lower extremity fractures should have their sciatic nerve block performed using the peripheral approach while they remain in the supine position. This will avoid painful fracture movement that would be caused by rotating them into the Sim's position.*

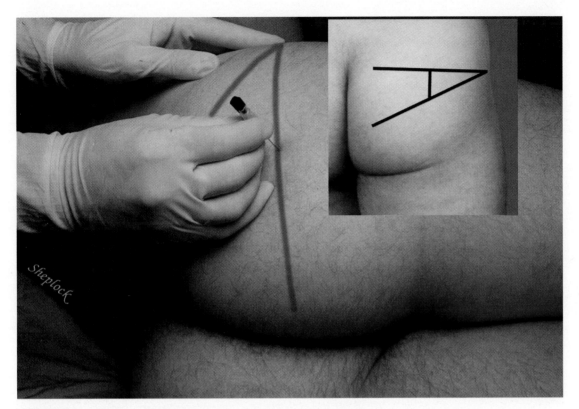

FIG. 18-6 *Blockade of the sciatic nerve via the classic (Labat) approach.*

the following bony landmarks to guide needle placement: a line is drawn from the greater trochanter to the posterior superior iliac spine. This line is bisected and a perpendicular line is drawn from the point of bisection over the surface of the gluteal muscle. A second line is drawn from the greater trochanter to the sacral hiatus. The point at which the latter line intersects the perpendicular line on the surface of the gluteal muscle marks the point of needle entry for the blockade of the sciatic nerve (Fig. 18-6). This spot is more proximal than the one used for the peripheral approach and is used to block the sciatic nerve as it exists the greater sciatic foramen. Once again, a nerve stimulator may be employed to localize the nerve, or the anesthetist may wish to elicit a paraesthesia.

SIDE EFFECTS AND COMPLICATIONS

In my experience the most common complication is block failure. However, the incidence of failure can be dramatically reduced with the use of a nerve stimulator. Other potential complications include hematoma formations in the gluteal region and dysesthesias following inadvertent interneuronal injections.

SUGGESTED READINGS

Boleau Grant JC: *Grant's atlas of anatomy*, Baltimore, 1972, Williams and Wilkins.

Broadman LM: Regional anesthesia for pediatric outpatients, *Anesthesiol Clin North Am* 5(1):53-72, 1987.

Katz J: *Atlas of regional anesthesia*, Norwalk, CT, 1993, Appleton and Lange.

Winnie AP: Regional anesthesia, *Surg Clin North Am* 55(4):861-892, 1975.

CHAPTER 19

Lumbar Plexus

John M. Stamatos
Patrick M. McQuillan
Marc B. Hahn

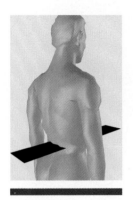

Introduction The lumbar plexus is responsible for sensation from the thigh to as far distal as the medial malleolus, as well as the anterior portions of the upper leg and lower abdomen. Blockade of the plexus usually is performed in conjunction with blockade of the sacral plexus for anesthesia of the lower extremity when central blockade is contraindicated. It is also used when anesthesia of a single lower extremity is needed, or when bilateral lower extremity sympathetic blockade is contraindicated.

ANATOMIC RELATIONSHIPS

The lumbar plexus is made up of the ventral roots of the first four lumbar nerves. In half of the population a small branch of the twelfth thoracic root is included. The plexus is located deep within the psoas muscle and anterior to the transverse process of each lumbar vertebrae (Figs. 19-1 and 19-2). The plexus divides into its component nerves immediately. They include the iliohypogastric, ilioinguinal, genitofemoral, lateral femoral cutaneous, obturator, accessory obturator, and femoral nerves (Fig. 19-3).

The iliohypogastric nerve is derived from T12 and L1. After exiting the psoas muscle laterally, it passes through the transverse abdominis muscle and provides sensory innervation to the suprapubic and anterior hip region. The ilioinguinal nerve, derived from L1, follows the inguinal canal and provides sensory innervation to the medial aspect of the thigh and the anterior scrotum or labia. In 35% of patients the ilioinguinal nerve is joined to the genitofemoral nerve. When this occurs, branches from the struc-ture follow the normal path of the ilioinguinal nerve. The genitofemoral nerve, derived from L1 and L2, divides into the genital and the femoral branches when it exits the psoas muscle. The genital branch innervates the skin and fascia of the scrotum or labia and the adjacent thigh. The femoral branches provide cutaneous innervation of the femoral triangle. The lateral femoral cutaneous nerve, derived from L2 and L3, passes under the lateral aspect of the inguinal ligament and provides innervation to the lateral aspect of the thigh. The obturator nerve comprises preaxial fibers from L2 through L4. It follows the obturator artery and vein through the obturator canal and medial aspect of the thigh. The accessory obturator nerve, L3-L4, is present in only 9% of patients and innervates the capsule of the hip joint. The femoral nerve comprises postaxial fibers from nerve roots L2 through L4. It is the largest division of the lumbar plexus and divides into multiple branches that innervate the anterior thigh and medial portions of the lower leg to the ankle (see Chapters 20, 21, 22, and 35).

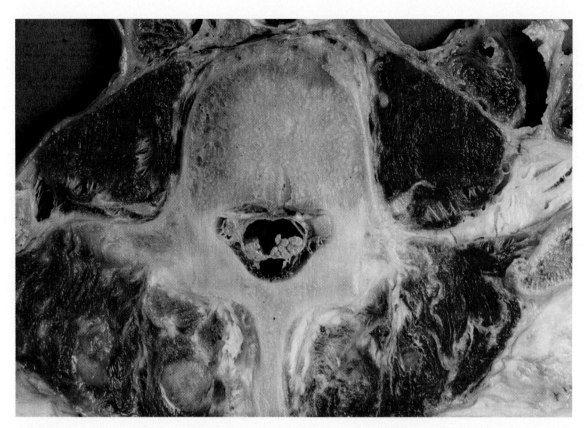

FIG. 19-1 *Transverse anatomic section through the fourth lumbar vertebra, revealing the relationship of the lumbar plexus and related structures.*

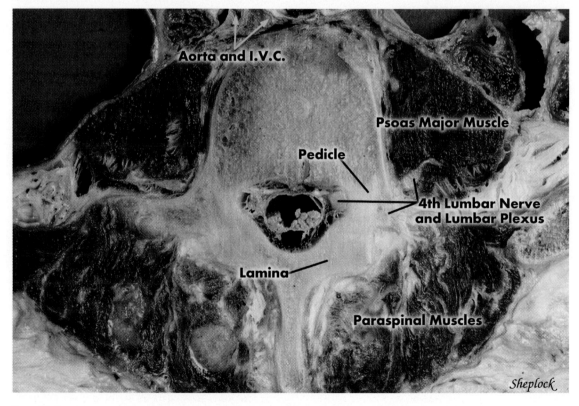

FIG. 19-2 *Corresponding computer-enhanced image of the anatomic section with annotation.*

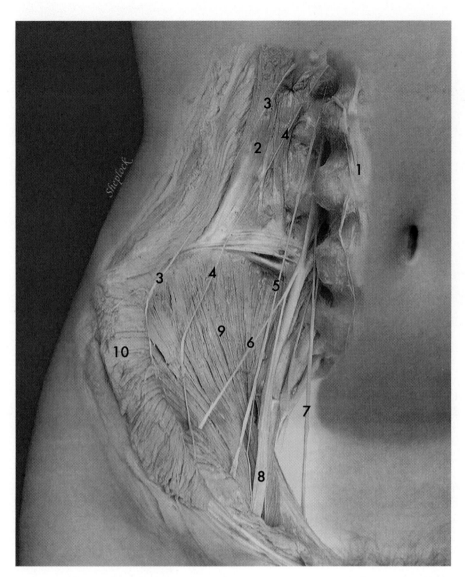

FIG. 19-3 *Dissection of the lumbar plexus with the psoas muscle removed, superimposed over the surface anatomy. Key: 1, third lumbar vertebra and anterior longitudinal ligament; 2, quadratus lumborum muscle; 3, iliohypogastric nerve; 4, ilioinguinal nerve; 5, genitofemoral nerve; 6, lateral femoral cutaneous nerve; 7, obturator nerve; 8, femoral nerve; 9, iliacus muscle; 10, internal oblique muscle.*

INDICATIONS

Blockade of the lumbar plexus in conjunction with sacral plexus blockade is used to provide anesthesia for surgery involving the lower extremity. It is also useful in pain management for the diagnosis and treatment of various pain complaints of the lower extremity.

REGIONAL ANESTHETIC TECHNIQUE

Blockade of the lumbar plexus as a unit can be accomplished by injecting local anesthetic into the fascial sheath surrounding the plexus. This can be done with either of two techniques, the psoas compartment technique or the inguinal paravascular technique.

Psoas Compartment Block

Immediately after emerging from the intervertebral foramina, the nerve roots form the lumbar plexus. This approach attempts to block the plexus as it lies in the fascial plane bordered medially by the vertebral column, dorsally by the quadratus lumborum muscle, and ventrally by the psoas major muscle.

The patient is placed in either the lateral or prone position. If the patient is placed in the lateral position, the patient should be in a relaxed but curled position similar to that used for spinal or epidural anesthesia, with the operative side uppermost.

From the spinous process of L4, a 3-cm line is drawn caudally in the interspinal line. From the end of this line, a 5-cm line is

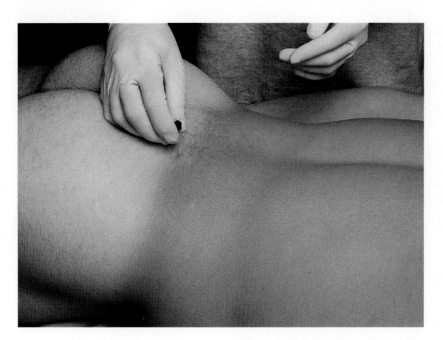

FIG. 19-4 *Blockade of the lumbar plexus via the posterior approach to the psoas compartment.*

drawn perpendicular and laterally toward the side to be blocked, usually ending at the medial edge of the iliac crest. This spot identifies the point of needle insertion. A 10- to 15-cm, 20- or 22-gauge spinal or epidural needle or a 15-cm insulated block needle may be used. A skin wheal is raised and the needle is inserted perpendicular to all planes and advanced until contact with bone is made, which identifies the transverse process of L5 and usually occurs at a depth of 5 to 10 cm.

The needle is then withdrawn, redirected slightly cephalad, and advanced until it slides over the transverse process of L5. Using the loss-of-resistance technique, the psoas compartment is usually encountered at a depth of 8 to 12 cm. The tip of the needle now lies in the psoas compartment (Fig. 19-4). The needle has passed through the quadratus lumborum muscle but not so far as to be in the substance of the psoas muscle. Needle placement can be confirmed with the aid of a nerve stimulator, checking for stimulation of the quadriceps muscles, eliciting paresthesias into the thigh, or advancing the needle slightly into the psoas muscle and reconfirming a loss of resistance while withdrawing the needle slightly into the psoas compartment (Fig.

19-5). A continuous technique is possible when using a Tuohy needle by passing a standard epidural catheter into the psoas compartment and injecting through it as would be done for epidural anesthesia.

After the needle or catheter is placed, and after careful aspiration, 30 to 40 ml of local anesthetic is injected in divided doses. It is often helpful to have the patient remain in the lateral position for a few minutes after injection to limit lateral spread of the drug.

Inguinal Paravascular Block
This technique, described by Winnie, is also known as the three-in-one block of the lower extremity. The lumbar plexus is "sandwiched" between the psoas major, quadratus lumborum, and iliacus muscles and is enclosed by the fascia of these three muscles.

This technique is based on the supposition that injecting local anesthetic in sufficient amount at the level of the inguinal ligament will force the anesthetic to track proximally along fascial planes to anesthetize the lumbar plexus. On the basis of the distribution of the local anesthetic, this technique may be considered a ventral approach to the psoas compartment.

The patient is placed in the supine position, with the leg to be anesthetized slightly abducted. A right-handed operator will stand at the patient's right side, whereas a left-handed operator may find it more convenient to stand at the patient's left side, regardless of the side being anesthetized. A 3- to 4-cm, 22-gauge block needle is inserted through a skin wheal raised approximately 1 cm lateral to the femoral artery and slightly below the inguinal ligament. The needle is directed slightly cephalad and advanced until either a femoral nerve paresthesia is elicited or, if using a nerve stimulator, contraction of the quadriceps muscles is elicited. After careful aspiration, 30 to 40 ml of local anesthetic is injected in divided doses (Fig. 19-6).

A continuous technique is possible with this approach by substituting a Tuohy or Crawford-tip needle for the regional block needle. It is often easier to pass the catheter after at least a portion of the initial dose of local anesthetic is administered through the needle before introducing the catheter into the perivascular fascial sheath. Alternatively, the fascial sheath may be initially cannulated with an 18-gauge intravenous catheter using the technique described previously. Then, using the Seldinger (over-the-wire) technique, a 12- to 15-cm catheter can be advanced into the sheath.

SIDE EFFECTS AND COMPLICATIONS

Complications of the psoas compartment block are rare when careful attention to technique is observed. Intrathecal, epidural, or intravascular injections are possible, and the patient should be monitored accordingly. Complications of the inguinal paravascular block are also rare. Intravascular injection may occur if careful aspiration has not been performed. Inadvertent puncture of the femoral artery may lead to the formation of a hematoma in the inguinal region. Rarely, nerve injury may occur if the injection is intraneural.

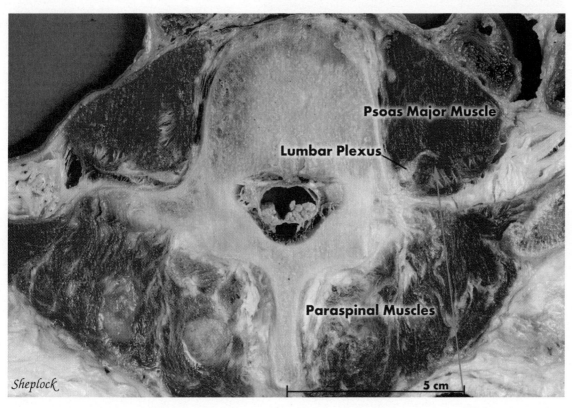

Psoas Major Muscle

Lumbar Plexus

Paraspinal Muscles

Sheplock

5 cm

FIG. 19-5 *Transverse anatomic section through the fifth lumbar vertebra, with computer-enhanced image of needle (arrow) placement required for blockade of the lumbar plexus in the psoas compartment.*

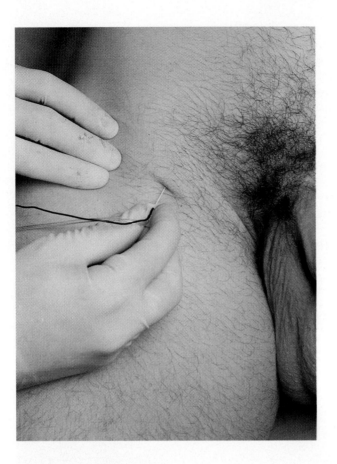

FIG. 19-6 *Blockade of the lumbar plexus via the inguinal perivascular (Winnie 3-in-1) approach.*

SUGGESTED READINGS

Adriani J, editor: *Labat's regional anesthesia: techniques and clinical applications*, ed. 4, St. Louis, 1984, Warren H. Green.

Anderson JE, editor: The lower limb. In *Grant's atlas of anatomy*, ed. 7, Baltimore, 1982, Williams and Wilkins.

Chayen D, Nathan H, Chayen M: The psoas compartment block, *Anesthesiology* 15:95-99, 1976.

Hoerster W, Nessler R: Blocks of the lumbosacral plexus. In Zenz M, editor: *Regional anesthesia*, ed. 2, St. Louis, 1990, Mosby.

Winnie AP, Ramamurthy S, Durrani Z: The inguinal paravascular technique of lumbar plexus anesthesia: "the 3-in-1 block", *Anesthesia and Analgesia* 52:989, 1963.

Woodburne RT, editor: The lower limb. In *Essentials of human anatomy*, ed. 7, New York, 1983, Oxford University Press.

CHAPTER 20

Femoral Nerve

Patrick M. McQuillan

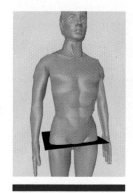

Introduction The femoral nerve is both a sensory and motor nerve. Blockade produces anesthesia of the anterior portion of the upper leg and medial calf and results in inability to abduct the leg or extend the lower leg. This block is easily performed with a high degree of success and minimal side effects. It can be a useful adjunct for postoperative pain relief in adults and children.

ANATOMIC RELATIONSHIPS

The femoral nerve is the largest branch of the lumbar plexus. It is formed by the posterior branches of the second, third, and fourth lumbar nerves. The nerve emerges through the fibers of the psoas muscle at its lower lateral border and descends in the interval between the psoas and iliacus muscles. It passes under the inguinal ligament in the groove formed by these muscles in a position immediately lateral to the femoral artery (Figs. 20-1 and 20-2). On entering the femoral triangle of the upper thigh, the femoral nerve divides into numerous articular, muscular, and cutaneous branches. It is important to remember that, at the level of the inguinal ligament, the femoral nerve divides into an anterior or more superficial bundle and a posterior or deeper bundle of nerve fibers (Fig. 20-3). The branches of the posterior bundle are primarily motor, which innervate the quadriceps muscle. Sensory fibers supply the knee joint with its terminal branch, the saphenous nerve, providing cutaneous innervation over the medial portion of the lower extremity as far distal as the medial malleolus. The anterior bundle, which is primarily sensory, supplies nerve fibers that innervate the skin of the anterior thigh and a motor branch to the sartorius muscle.

INDICATIONS

Surgical indications include soft tissue exploration, biopsy, and repair of lacerations of the anterior thigh. When used in conjunction with other nerve blocks, complete anesthesia of the leg may be effected. Complete or partial analgesia may be produced to provide relief for painful conditions of the upper leg, including femoral shaft and neck fractures, as well as knee surgery.

REGIONAL ANESTHETIC TECHNIQUE

This technique is known as the classic approach of Labat. The patient is placed in the supine position, with the right-handed operator positioned to the patient's right side. A left-handed operator may find it more comfortable to perform this block from the patient's left side. The patient's leg should be slightly abducted to allow for easy palpation of landmarks.

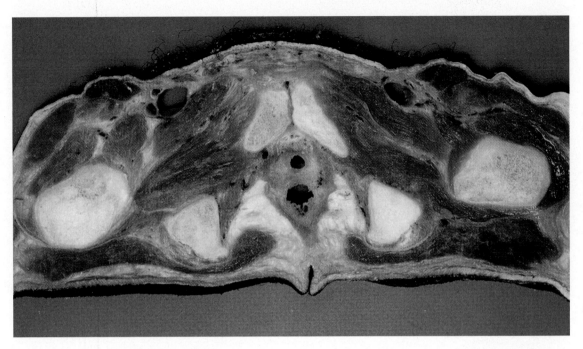

FIG. 20-1 *Transverse anatomic section through the upper leg, revealing the relationship of the femoral nerve, artery, vein, and related structures.*

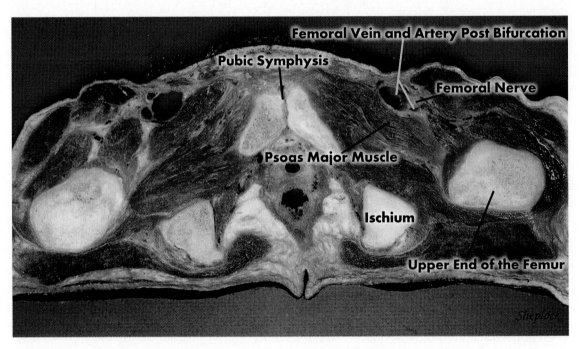

FIG. 20-2 *Corresponding computer-enhanced image of the anatomic section with annotation.*

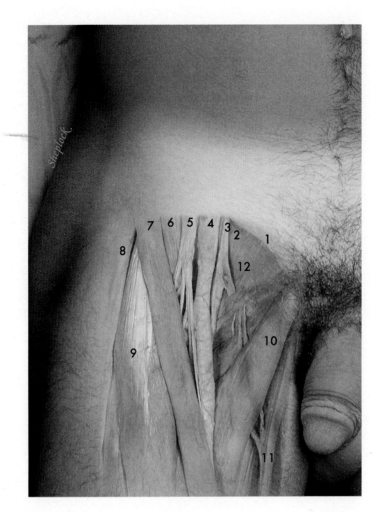

FIG. 20-3 *Dissection of the femoral nerve with the superficial vessels and nerves and the fascia lata removed, superimposed over the surface anatomy. Key: 1, inguinal ligament; 2, position of femoral canal; 3, femoral vein; 4, femoral artery; 5, femoral nerve; 6, Iliacus muscle; 7, sartorius muscle; 8, fascia lata overlying tensor fascia lata; 9, rectus femoris muscle; 10, adductor longus muscle; 11, gracilis muscle; 12, pectineus muscle.*

The point just lateral to the femoral artery, and inferior to the inguinal ligament along a line drawn from the anterior superior iliac spine to the pubic tubercle, locates the site of needle insertion (Fig. 20-4). A 3- to 4-cm needle is inserted perpendicular to the skin through the fascial plane (iliacus fascia), and approximately 20 ml of local anesthetic is injected after careful aspiration to reduce the risk of intravascular injection. Eliciting paresthesias or the use of a nerve stimulator may be helpful in performing this block. The volume of local anesthetic may be administered in divided doses in a medial-to-lateral injection sequence, but lateral to the artery, so as to distribute the local anesthetic over the branches of the femoral nerve at that level.

Assessment of the block is performed by testing sensation over the anterior thigh and demonstrating paresis of the lower leg extensors.

SIDE EFFECTS AND COMPLICATIONS

Complications may include intravascular injection and hematoma. Intravascular injections may occur in either the femoral artery or vein. This may be avoided by careful needle positioning and aspiration before injection. Direct nerve injury is highly unlikely, although it is a theoretic possibility.

An occasional side effect of this block is associated blockade of the obturator and lateral femoral cutaneous nerves. Blockade of the sympathetic fibers that course with the femoral nerve is of no clinical significance.

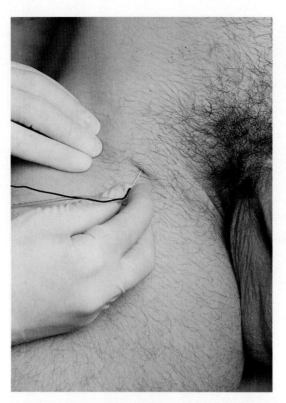

Fig. 20-4 *Blockade of the femoral nerve inferior to the inguinal ligament.*

SUGGESTED READINGS

Bridenbaugh PO: The lower extremity: somatic blockade. In Cousins M, Bridenbaugh PO, editors: *Neural blockade*, ed. 2, Philadelphia, 1988, JB Lippincott.

Labat G: *Regional anesthesia: its technic and clinical application*, Philadelphia, 1924, WB Saunders.

Woodburne RT, editor: The lower limb, In *Essentials of human anatomy*, ed. 7, New York, 1983, Oxford University Press.

CHAPTER 21

Lateral Femoral Cutaneous Nerve

Patrick M. McQuillan

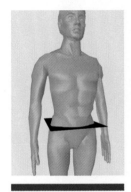

Introduction The lateral femoral cutaneous nerve is a pure sensory nerve of the lateral aspect of the thigh. Blockade of this nerve is performed with ease and a high degree of success. It is useful in providing anesthesia over the lateral aspect of the thigh.

ANATOMIC RELATIONSHIPS

The lateral femoral cutaneous nerve is a direct branch of the lumbar plexus with contributions from the second and third lumbar nerve roots. It courses through the pelvis along the lateral border of the psoas muscle, deep to the iliac fascia and anterior to the iliacus muscle (Figs. 21-1 and 21-2). It penetrates the fascia immediately inferior and medial to the anterior superior iliac spine and divides into anterior and posterior branches that become subcutaneous about 10 cm caudad to the anterior superior iliac spine. The larger anterior branch distributes over the lateral aspect of the front of the thigh as far caudal as the knee. Its terminal fibers form part of the patellar plexus, which needs to be included in blockade of the leg for surgical procedures involving the knee. The smaller posterior branch supplies the skin over the lateral portion of the buttock distal to the greater trochanter to about the middle of the thigh (Fig. 21-3).

INDICATIONS

Blockade of the lateral femoral cutaneous nerve is usually used in conjunction with blockade of other nerves to provide anesthesia for surgical procedures involving the leg. Its primary contribution is in providing analgesia for tourniquet pain. Alone, it is used to provide anesthesia for superficial procedures on the lateral thigh, such as skin grafting. It is also used in the diagnosis and treatment of meralgia paresthetica, a pain syndrome involving the lateral femoral cutaneous nerve.

REGIONAL ANESTHETIC TECHNIQUE

The patient is placed in the supine position, with the right-handed operator positioned to the patient's right side. A left-handed operator may find it more convenient to stand at the patient's left side. The injection site is identified at a point 2 cm medial and 2 cm inferior to the anterior superior iliac

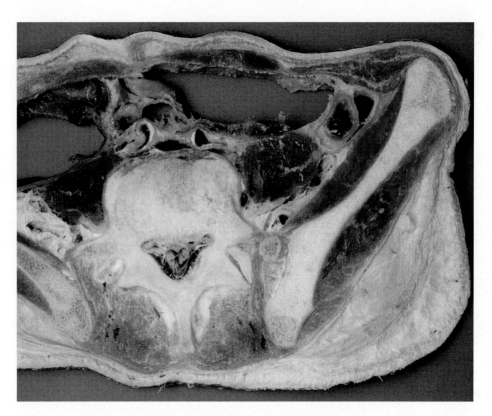

FIG. 21-1 *Transverse anatomic section through the pelvis, revealing the relationship of the lateral femoral cutaneous nerve and related structure.*

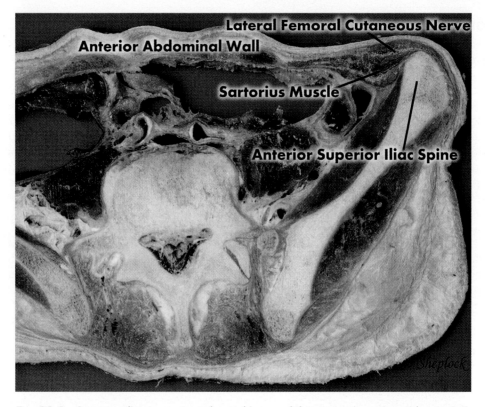

FIG. 21-2 *Corresponding computer-enhanced image of the anatomic section with annotation.*

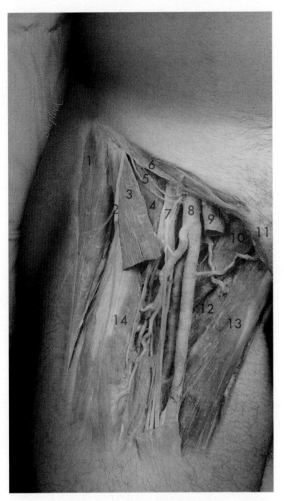

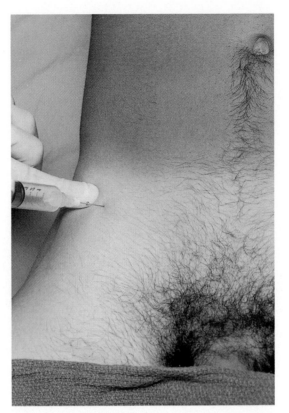

Fig. 21-4 *Blockade of the lateral femoral cutaneous nerve.*

Fig. 21-3 *Dissection of the lateral femoral cutaneous nerve, with all veins (except the upper femoral vein) and the sartorius muscle removed and superimposed over the surface anatomy. The distribution of the lateral femoral cutaneous nerve is represented in yellow. Key: 1, tensor fascia lata muscle; 2, lateral femoral cutaneous nerve; 3, sartorius muscle; 4, iliacus muscle; 5, superficial circumflex iliac artery; 6, inguinal ligament; 7, femoral nerve; 8, femoral artery; 9, femoral vein; 10, pectineus muscle; 11, spermatic cord; 12, adductor brevis muscle; 13, adductor longus muscle; 14, rectus femoris muscle.*

spine. A 3- to 4-cm needle is inserted through a skin wheal and advanced perpendicular to the skin through the fascia lata (Fig. 21-4). This fascia is identified by a "release" or a "pop" as a needle passes through it. After careful aspiration, 10 to 15 ml of local anesthetic are injected above and below the fascia

lata in a medial-to-lateral fanlike distribution to ensure "painting" the nerve branches at this level. An alternate technique is to direct the needle through a skin wheal in a lateral and cephalad direction until the needle encounters the iliac bone just medial and caudal to the anterior superior iliac spine. Local anesthetic is then injected in a medially-directed, fanlike fashion to assure blockade of the nerve.

SIDE EFFECTS AND COMPLICATIONS

In theory, direct nerve injury is possible, but in clinical practice this is one of the few nerve blocks with no side effects or complications.

SUGGESTED READINGS

Bridenbaugh PO: The lower extremity: somatic blockade. In Cousins M, Bridenbaugh PO, editors: *Neural blockade,* ed. 2, Philadelphia, 1988, JB Lippincott.

Labat G: *Regional anesthesia: its technic and clinical application,* Philadelphia, 1924, WB Saunders.

Woodburne RT, editor: The lower limb. In *Essentials of human anatomy,* ed. 7, New York. 1983, Oxford University Press.

CHAPTER 22

Obturator Nerve

Patrick M. McQuillan

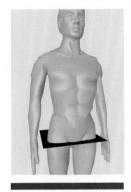

Introduction The obturator nerve is both a motor and a sensory nerve. Blockade produces anesthesia over the medial aspect of the distal thigh and paresis of the leg adductors. The obturator nerve is rarely blocked alone, but frequently blocked in conjunction with the femoral, sciatic, and lateral femoral cutaneous nerves to provide anesthesia for the lower extremity.

ANATOMIC RELATIONSHIPS

The obturator nerve arises from the anterior branches of the second, third, and fourth lumbar nerves and descends through the pelvis along the medial border of the psoas muscle. It accompanies the obturator artery and vein to the obturator foramen and through the obturator canal into the thigh (Figs. 22-1 and 22-2). In the thigh it divides into anterior and posterior branches. The anterior branch supplies an articular branch to the hip joint, motor branches to the superficial adductors, and a cutaneous branch to the medial aspect of the distal thigh. The posterior branch supplies the deep adductors and an articular branch to the posterior knee joint (Fig. 22-3).

INDICATIONS

The obturator nerve is usually blocked in conjunction with the lateral femoral cutaneous, femoral, and sciatic nerves for surgical procedures on the leg. The block used

alone is useful in aiding in the diagnosis and treatment of pain syndromes involving the hip joint, as well as relieving adductor spasms of the hip.

REGIONAL ANESTHETIC TECHNIQUE

The patient is placed in the supine position with the leg slightly abducted. The right-handed operator is positioned to the patient's right side. It is often more convenient for a left-handed operator to be positioned at the left side of the patient. Special attention should be paid, as in all clinical care, to the modesty of the patient when performing this block.

The landmark to identify is the tip of the pubic tubercle. The injection sight is identified at a point 1 to 2 cm lateral and 1 to 2 cm caudad to the pubic tubercle (Fig. 22-4). A skin wheal is raised and a 7- to 8-cm block needle is inserted perpendicular to the skin until the horizontal ramus of the pelvis is encountered, at a depth of 1.5 to 4 cm. The needle is then withdrawn and redirected lat-

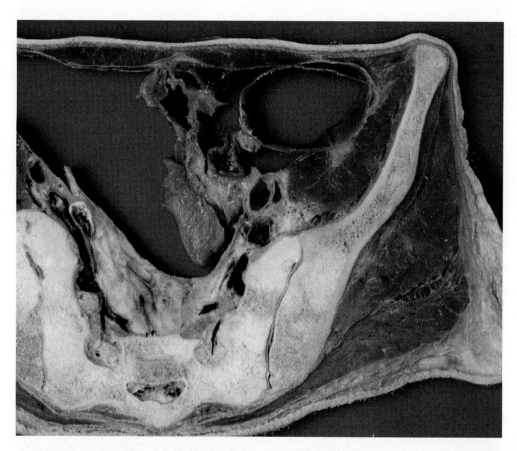

FIG. 22-1 *Transverse anatomic section through the pelvis, revealing the relationship of the obturator nerve and related structures.*

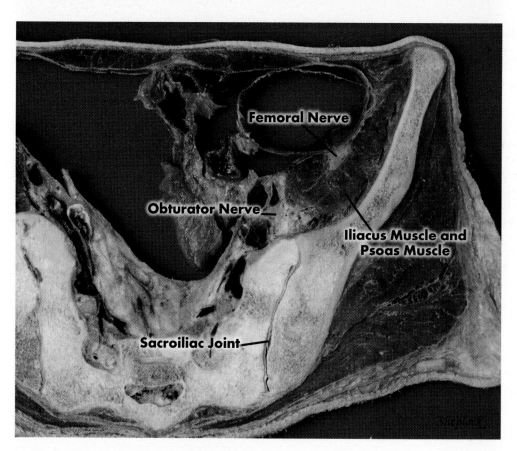

FIG. 22-2 *Corresponding computer-enhanced image of the anatomic section with annotation.*

erally 2 to 3 cm deeper than the pelvic ramus. The needle now lies in close proximity to the obturator canal. After careful aspiration, 10 to 15 ml of local anesthetic are injected in a fan-like fashion to distribute the local anesthetic in the area of the obturator nerve. The success of this block most often depends on the volume of local anesthetic.

An alternative technique is to abduct the leg on the operative side and insert the block needle at a point just posterior to the most proximal (tendenous) portion of the adductor longus muscle, advancing in the direction of the femoral pulse (Fig. 22-3). At a depth of 3 to 6 cm the obturator nerve is encountered, eliciting a paresthesia or adduction of the leg if a nerve stimulator is used. After careful aspiration, 10 to 15 ml of local anesthetic is injected. This technique avoids both directional change of the needle and the possibility of the needle contacting the periosteum.

Assessment of the block is performed by testing sensation over the lower medial thigh and demonstrating paresis of the leg adductors.

SIDE EFFECTS AND COMPLICATIONS

Intravascular injection may rarely occur into either the obturator artery or vein. Careful aspiration before injection nearly eliminates this potential complication. Careful attention to the bony landmarks and the depth of needle insertion reduces the chance of needle placement into surrounding structures such as the bladder, rectum, vagina, or spermatic cord.

SUGGESTED READINGS

Bridenbaugh PO: The lower extremity: somatic blockade. In Cousins, M, Bridenbaugh PO, editors: *Neural blockade*, ed. 2, Philadelphia, 1988, JB Lippincott.

Labat G: *Regional anesthesia: its technic and clinical application*, Philadelphia, 1924, WB Saunders.

Woodburne RT, editor: The lower limb. In *Essentials of human anatomy*, ed. 7, New York, 1983, Oxford University Press.

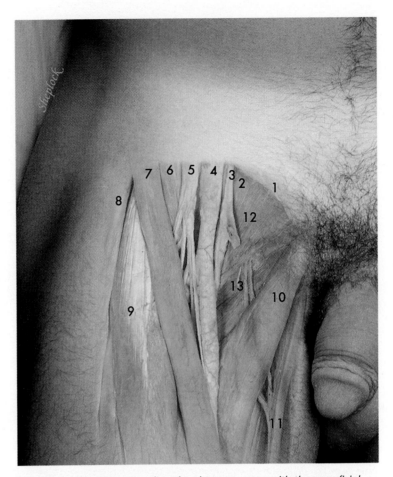

FIG. 22-3 *Dissection revealing the obturator nerve with the superficial vessels, nerves, and the fascia lata removed, superimposed over the surface anatomy. Key: 1, inguinal ligament; 2, femoral canal; 3, femoral vein; 4, femoral artery; 5, femoral nerve; 6, iliacus muscle; 7, sartorius muscle; 8, fascia lata overlying tensor fascia lata muscle; 9, rectus femoris muscle; 10, adductor longus muscle; 11, gracilis muscle; 12, pectineus muscle; 13, branches of the obturator nerve.*

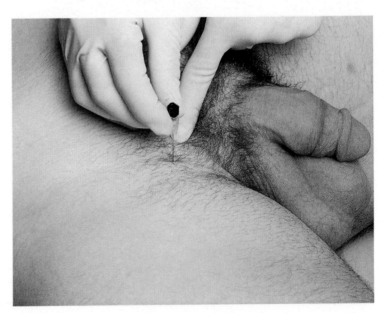

FIG. 22-4 *Blockade of the obturator nerve.*

CHAPTER 23

Peripheral Nerves at the Knee

John C. Keifer
Patrick M. McQuillan

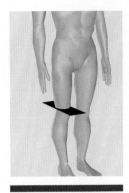

Introduction Three nerves can be blocked at the level of the knee. Two mixed nerves, the tibial and common peroneal, are branches of the sciatic nerve. The saphenous nerve, a sensory nerve, is the terminal extension of the femoral nerve. The success of neural blockade at the knee requires an appreciation of the anatomy of the popliteal fossa.

ANATOMIC RELATIONSHIPS

The popliteal fossa is a diamond-shaped area bounded inferiorly by the medial and lateral heads of the gastrocnemius muscle and superiorly by the long head of the biceps femoris laterally, and the tendons of the semitendinous and semimembranous muscles medially. It contains the posterior tibial and common peroneal nerves, an abundance of fat and connective tissue, and the popliteal vessels (Figs 23-1 and 23-2).

The sciatic nerve bifurcates in the distal thigh into a larger tibial nerve that is made up of nerve roots from L4-5 and S1-3, and a smaller common peroneal nerve made up of nerve roots from L4-5 and S1-2. After bifurcation, the tibial and common peroneal nerves maintain their anatomic relationships as they course down the leg, with the posterior tibial nerve being more medial and the common peroneal nerve being more lateral. In the popliteal fossa the common peroneal nerve separates and exits at the fossa's lateral margin, following the course of the biceps femoris tendon; the common peroneal nerve courses around the head of the fibula and lies directly on the bone under the fascia. It subsequently divides into a superficial and deep branch. The tibial and common peroneal nerves are located superficial to the popliteal vessels and about midway between the skin and posterior surface of the femur, usually at a depth of 1.5 to 2 cm in an adult. As a result of this proximity in the popliteal fossa, these nerves are blocked simultaneously with one injection (Fig. 23-3).

The posterior tibial nerve provides motor innervation to the back of the lower leg and cutaneous innervation from the popliteal fossa to the ankle. The common peroneal nerve provides articular innervation to the knee joint, cutaneous innervation to the lateral side of the leg, heel, and ankle, and motor innervation to the muscles of the anterior lateral compartment of the lower leg.

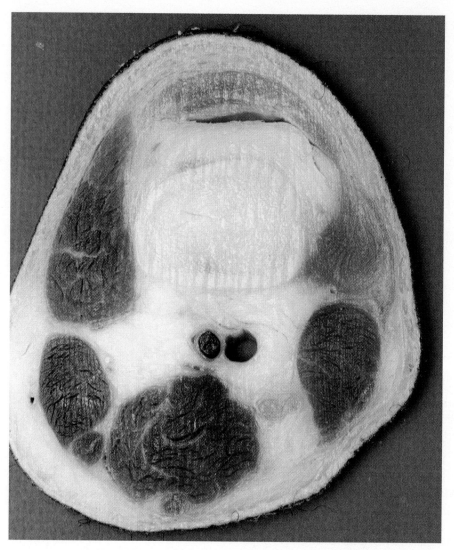

FIG. 23-1 *Transverse anatomic section through the leg at the popliteal fossa, revealing the relationship of the posterior tibial and common peroneal nerves and related structures.*

The saphenous nerve, made up of nerve roots from L1-4, is the sensory terminal branch of the femoral nerve. The femoral nerve supplies sensation to the skin over the medial, anterior medial, and posterior medial aspects of the leg, extending from just above the knee to as far distal as the plantar surface of the great toe (Fig. 23-4).

the upper leg, groin, or buttock. They can be used to provide both anesthesia for procedures on the foot and ankle, while still allowing use of a tourniquet above the ankle. They are useful for providing postoperative pain relief in adults as well as children and in both the diagnosis and treatment of pain syndromes of the lower extremity.

INDICATIONS

The greatest advantage of nerve blocks at the knee is the ability to provide anesthesia to an entire distal lower extremity while avoiding the more problematic potential complications of centroneuraxis blockade or the relative discomfort of blockade of these nerves in

REGIONAL ANESTHETIC TECHNIQUE

The patient is placed in the prone position and asked to flex the leg to aide in identifying the margins of the popliteal fossa. The operator is positioned at the patient's side with the margins of the popliteal fossa identified. The fossa itself is divided into equal medial and

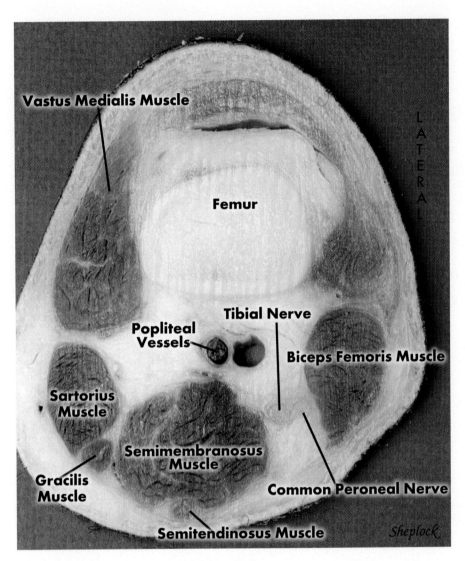

Vastus Medialis Muscle

L
A
T
E
R
A
L

Femur

Tibial Nerve

Popliteal
Vessels

Biceps Femoris Muscle

Sartorius
Muscle

Semimembranosus
Muscle

Gracilis
Muscle

Common Peroneal Nerve

Semitendinosus Muscle

Sheplock

FIG. 23-2 *Corresponding computer-enhanced image of the anatomic section with annotation.*

lateral triangles, with the base of the two triangles being the skin crease behind the knee joint. The base of both triangles forms a line between the medial and lateral epicondyles of the femur. A skin wheal is raised 5 cm proximal to the skin crease and 1 cm lateral to the midline of the triangle. A 3- to 6-cm, 22-gauge regional block needle is inserted in a 45º to 60º anterosuperior direction and advanced until a paresthesia is obtained, usually at a depth of 1.5 to 2 cm in an adult. Alternately, a nerve stimulator may be used and needle proximity to the nerves identified by eliciting either plantar flexion, stimulating the posterior tibial nerve, or plantar dorsiflexion with stimulation of the common peroneal nerve. After careful aspiration, 35 to 40

ml of a local anesthetic is injected (Fig. 23-5). The tibial nerve may be blocked in isolation through a skin wheal raised at the midpoint of the interepicondylar line, advancing the block needle perpendicular to the skin to a depth of 1.5 to 3 cm until either a paresthesia or motor stimulation is elicited. Ten ml of a local anesthetic is then injected after careful aspiration. The common peroneal nerve may be blocked in isolation through a skin wheal raised 1 to 2 cm posterior to the head of the fibula. The needle is advanced perpendicular to the skin until it just releases through the fascial plane or encounters the substance of the fibula. If the fibula is encountered, the needle is withdrawn 2 to 3 mm and 5 ml of a local anesthetic is injected. The saphenous

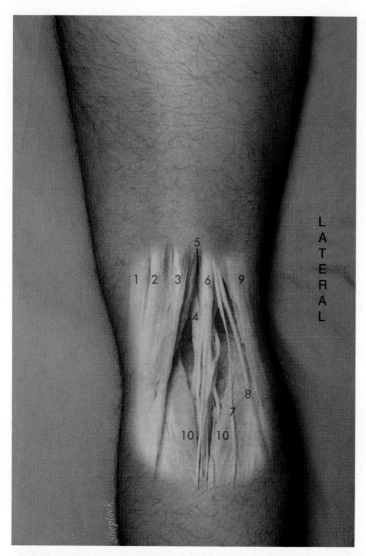

FIG. 23-3 *Dissection of the popliteal fossa superimposed over the surface anatomy. Key: 1, gracialis muscle; 2, semimembranosus muscle; 3, semitendinosus muscle; 4, popliteal artery; 5, popliteal vein; 6, tibial nerve; 7, lateral cutaneous nerve of the calf; 8, common peroneal nerve; 9, biceps femoris muscle; 10, gastrocnemius muscle.*

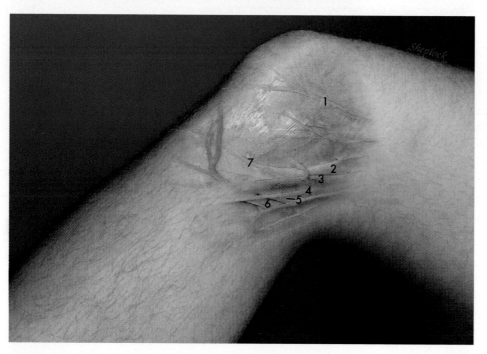

FIG. 23-4 *Dissection of the saphenous nerve of the medial right knee superimposed over the surface anatomy. Key: 1, medial femoral cutaneous nerve branches; 2, sartorius muscle; 3, saphenous vein; 4, saphenous nerve; 5, gracialis muscle; 6, semitendinosus muscle; 7, infrapatellar branch of the saphenous nerve.*

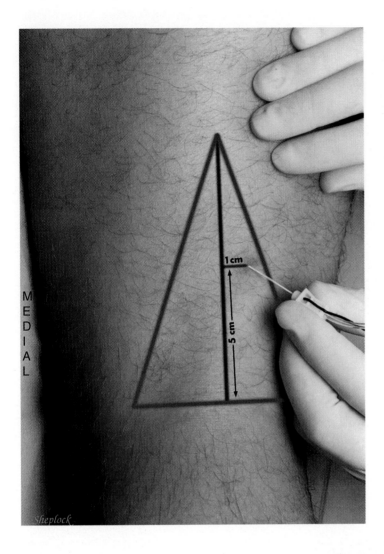

FIG. 23-5 *Blockade of the posterior tibial and common peroneal nerves in the popliteal fossa.*

nerve may be blocked by injecting 5 ml of local anesthetic in a subcutaneous ring from the medial aspect of the tibia to the border of the patellar tendon (Fig. 23-6).

SIDE EFFECTS AND COMPLICATIONS

Complications of these nerve blocks are extremely rare. Careful aspiration should be performed before each injection to avoid the potential for intravascular injection of local anesthetic.

SUGGESTED READINGS

Bridenbaugh PO: The lower extremity: somatic blockade. In Cousins M, Bridenbaugh PO, editors: *Neural blockade*, ed. 2, Philadelphia, 1988, JB Lippincott.

Haerster W: Blocks in the area of the knee joint. In Wolfe, editor: *Regional anesthesia*, ed. 2, St. Louis, 1990, Mosby.

Rorie DK, Beyer DE, Nelson DO et al: Assessment of block of the sciatic nerve in the popliteal fossa, *Anesth Analg* 59:371-376, 1980.

Woodburne RT, editor: The lower limb. In *Essentials of human anatomy*, ed. 7, New York, 1983, Oxford University Press.

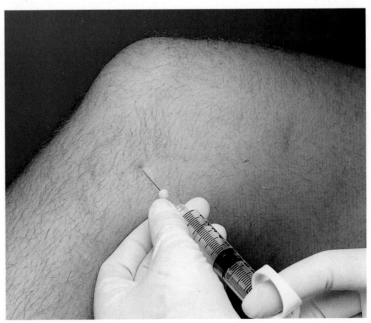

FIG. 23-6 *Blockade of the saphenous nerve at the antero-medial aspect of the lower leg.*

CHAPTER 24

Peripheral Nerves at the Ankle

John C. Keifer
Patrick M. McQuillan

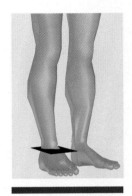

Introduction The principal nerve trunks innervating the leg divide into five terminal nerves that include the posterior tibial, sural, superficial peroneal, saphenous and deep peroneal nerves. Each nerve must be blocked individually. Blockade of the nerves at the ankle have a very high success rate even in inexperienced hands.

ANATOMIC RELATIONSHIPS
Posterior Tibial Nerve

The posterior tibial nerve (L4-L5, S1-S3) is the larger of the two branches of the sciatic nerve coursing through the lower leg in conjunction with the posterior tibial artery and vein. At the level of the ankle it lies just posterior to the medial malleolus. This nerve provides sensory innervation to the ankle and foot (Figs. 24-1 and 24-2).

Sural Nerve

The sural nerve is a pure sensory nerve formed from branches of the tibial and common peroneal nerve. It becomes subcutaneous just distal to the midlower leg and provides sensory innervation to the ankle and foot (Figs 24-1 and 24-2).

Superficial Peroneal Nerve

The superficial peroneal nerve (L4-L5, S1-S2) perforates the deep fascia on the anterior aspect of the distal lower extremity and provides sensory innervation to the dorsum of the feet and toes (Figs. 24-1 and 24-2).

Deep Peroneal Nerve

The deep peroneal nerve (L4-L5, S1-S2) courses through the lower extremity, down the anterior aspect of the interosseous membrane between the malleoli of the ankle, and onto the dorsum of the foot just lateral to the dorsalis pedis (anterior tibial) artery and the tendon of the extensor hallucis longus (Figs. 24-1 and 24-2).

Saphenous Nerve

This nerve is the terminal sensory branch of the femoral nerve. It becomes subcutaneous on the medial side of the knee joint, then follows the saphenous vein to the medial malleolus and onto the medial portion of the foot (Figs. 24-1 and 24-2).

INDICATIONS

An ankle block or isolated nerve blocks at the ankle are indicated for nearly all procedures of the foot, including amputations, debridements, and bunionectomies, as well as for providing postoperative pain relief in both children and adult (Fig. 24-3). The usefulness of this block is limited if a tourniquet is required.

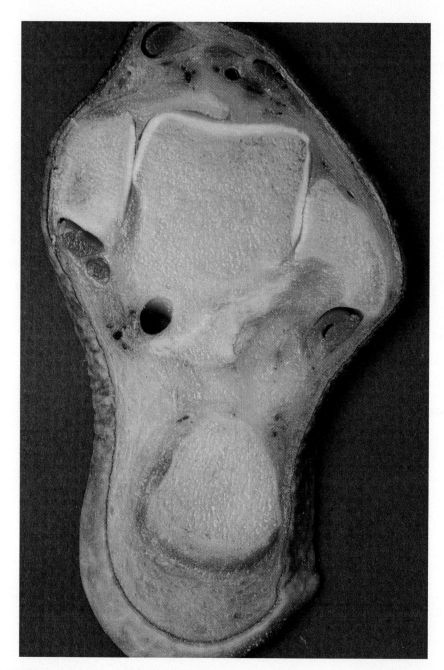

FIG. 24-1 *Transverse anatomic section through the lower leg at the ankle, revealing the relationship of the posterior tibial, sural, superficial peroneal, deep peroneal, and saphenous nerves, as well as related structures.*

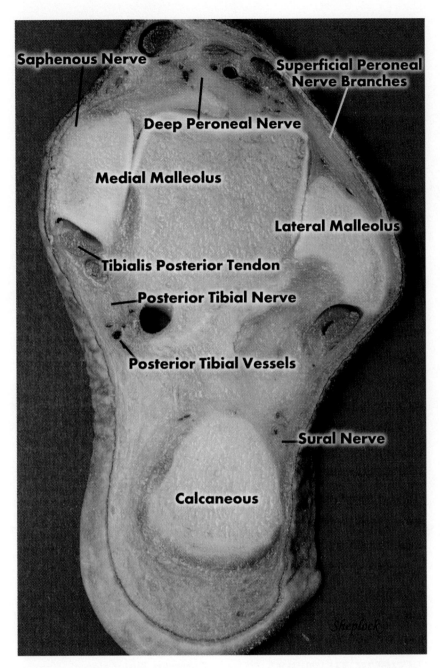

FIG. 24-2 *Corresponding computer-enhanced image of the anatomic section with annotation.*

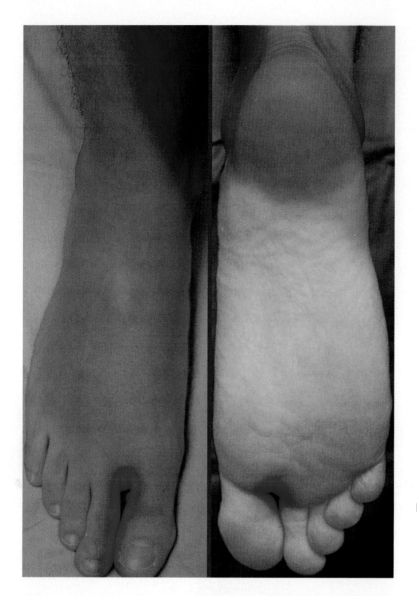

FIG. 24-3 *Sensory nerve distribution of the foot. Key:* blue, *sural nerve;* green, *superficial peroneal nerve;* purple, *saphenous nerve;* red, *deep peroneal nerve;* yellow, *plantar (posterior tibial) nerve;* brown, *calcaneal (posterior tibial) nerve.*

REGIONAL ANESTHETIC TECHNIQUES

To provide complete anesthesia to the foot, all five nerves must be blocked. The patient is placed in the supine position, with the ankle propped up on folded sheets or towels. Because of the subcutaneous infiltration in a relatively sensitive area, intravenous sedation and/or analgesia is a useful adjunct. All the nerves can be blocked at the level of the malleoli of the ankle. A skin wheal is raised at the site of each injection. In general, these blocks are field blocks, and eliciting paresthesias or using a nerve stimulator are not necessary for a high success rate.

Posterior Tibial Nerve

With the patient in the supine position and the leg externally rotated, the needle is inserted through a skin wheal just posterior to the posterior tibial artery on the medial side of the ankle. The insertion point can also be determined by marking a point just anterior to the achilles tendon at the level of the medial malleolus. A 2.5-cm needle is advanced perpendicular to the skin until the posterior portion of the tibia is encountered. The needle is withdrawn 2 to 3 mm and, after careful aspiration, 5 ml of local anesthetic is injected (Fig. 24-4).

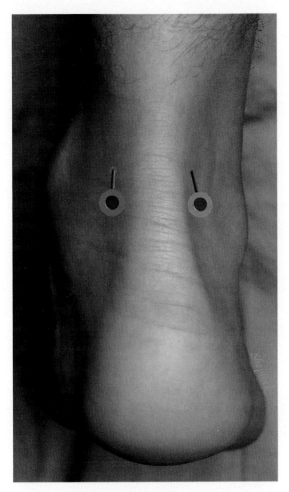

FIG. 24-4 *Needle insertion points for blockade of the posterior tibial (green) and sural (yellow) nerves at the posterior ankle.*

Sural Nerve

With the patient in the supine position and the leg internally rotated, a skin wheal is raised just anterior to the achilles tendon at the level of the lateral malleolus. A 2.5-cm needle is inserted through the skin wheal and directed subcutaneously to the lateral malleolus. Five ml of a local anesthetic are injected in a fanlike fashion while withdrawing the needle (Fig. 24-4).

Superficial Peroneal Nerve

With the patient in the supine position, this nerve is blocked by injecting 5 ml of local anesthetic subcutaneously from the anterior border of the tibia to the anterior border of the lateral malleolus (Fig. 24-5).

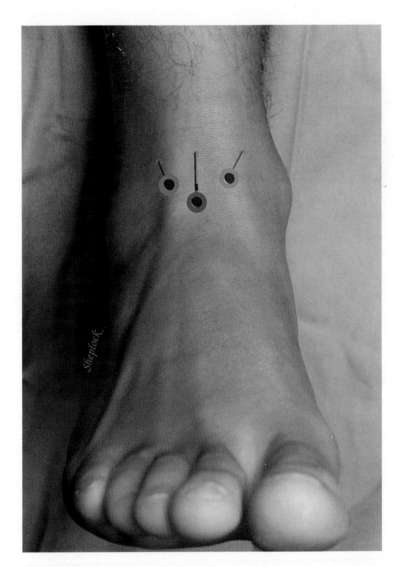

FIG. 24-5 *Needle insertion points for blockade of the superficial peroneal (green), deep peroneal (red), and saphenous (yellow) nerves at the anterior ankle.*

Deep Peroneal Nerve

With the patient in the supine position, the ankle is dorsiflexed, then relaxed to identify the extensor hallucis longus tendon. The dorsalis pedis artery is then identified just lateral to the tendon, and 2 to 3 ml of local anesthetic is injected through a skin wheal deep to the fascia on either side of the artery, to the extensor retinaculum (Fig. 24-5).

Saphenous Nerve

With the patient in the supine position, a skin wheal is raised just proximal and anterior to the medial malleolus. Three to five ml of local anesthetic is injected in a fanlike fashion in the area of the saphenous vein, with care being taken to avoid piercing the vein (Fig. 24-5).

SIDE EFFECTS AND COMPLICATIONS

Complications of this block are rare. If a large volume of local anesthetic is used, creating a ring around the ankle, vascular compromise could potentially occur, especially if the local anesthetic solution contains epinephrine.

SUGGESTED READINGS

Bridenbaugh PO: The lower extremity: somatic blockade. In Cousins M, Bridenbaugh PO, editors: *Neural blockade*, ed. 2, Philadelphia, 1988, JB Lippincott.

Haerster W: Blocks of the peripheral nerves in the area of the ankle. In Wolfe, editor: *Regional anesthesia*, ed. 2, St. Louis, 1990, Mosby.

Woodburne RT, editor: The lower limb. In *Essentials of human anatomy*, ed. 7, New York, 1983, Oxford University Press.

CHAPTER 25

Digital Nerves of the Foot

■

John C. Keifer
Patrick M. McQuillan

■

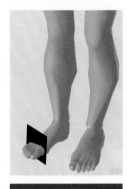

Introduction The individual nerves of the digits of the foot may be blocked at the level of the metatarsals or at the base of the phalanges. These blocks are easy to perform even in inexperienced hands.

ANATOMIC RELATIONSHIPS

The digital nerves of the foot follow a similar pattern as those described for the hand. Each nerve passes through the intermetatarsal space alongside each toe (Figs. 25-1 and 25-2). The sole of the foot is innervated primarily by the posterior tibial nerve. After passing behind the medial malleolus, the posterior tibial nerve divides into the plantar digital nerves. The plantar digital nerves are larger than the dorsal digital nerves and terminally send twigs onto the dorsum of the phalanx. The digital branch of the lateral plantar nerve supplies the lateral 1½ toes. The digital branch of the medial plantar nerve supplies the medial 3½ toes. The dorsum of the foot is innervated by the superficial and deep peroneal nerves. The deep peroneal nerve divides at the extensor retinaculum into medial and lateral branches. The medial branch divides into two dorsal digital branches that inner-vate adjacent sides of the first and second digits. The superficial peroneal nerve innervates the dorsum of the rest of the toes.

INDICATIONS

This block is useful primarily for limited procedures involving one or two digits, or as an adjunct for postoperative pain relief in both children and adults.

REGIONAL ANESTHETIC TECHNIQUES

Blockade at the Level of the Metatarsals

The patient is placed in a supine position, and skin wheals are raised over the distal intermetatarsal space. A total of 2 to 3 ml of a non–epinephrine-containing local anesthetic solution is injected in a fanlike fashion subcutaneously, as well as deep to the metatarsals to ensure blockade of both dorsal and plantar digital nerves (Fig. 25-3).

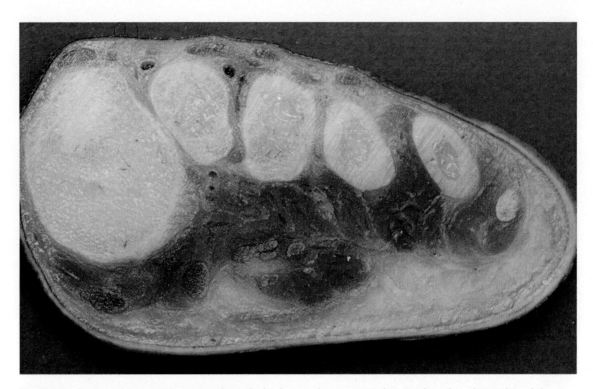

FIG. 25-1 *Transverse anatomic section through the foot at the metatarsals, revealing the relationship of the digital nerves and related structures.*

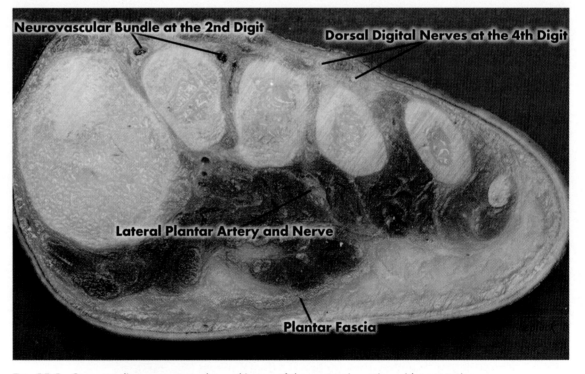

FIG. 25-2 *Corresponding computer-enhanced image of the anatomic section with annotation.*

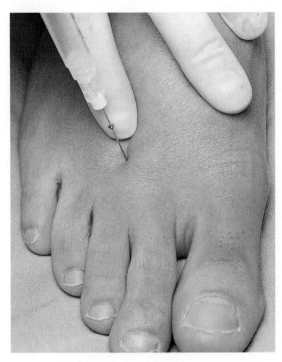

Fig. 25-3 *Needle insertion points for blockade of the digital nerves at the metatarsals.*

Blockade at the Level of the Digits

With the patient in the supine position, 2 to 3 ml of a non–epinephrine-containing local anesthetic solution is injected through skin wheals into the web space of the dorsal surface on either side of the digit to be blocked (Fig. 25-4).

SIDE EFFECTS AND COMPLICATIONS

Complications are extremely rare. Large volumes of a local anesthetic and epinephrine-containing solutions should not be used to avoid the risk of vascular compromise to the digits.

SUGGESTED READINGS

Bridenbaugh PO: The lower extremity: somatic blockade. In Cousins M, Bridenbaugh PO, editors: *Neural blockade,* ed. 2, Philadelphia, 1988, JB Lippincott.

Haerster W: Blocks in the area of the knee joint. In Wolfe, editor: *Regional anesthesia,* ed. 2, St. Louis, 1990, Mosby.

Woodburne RT, editor: The lower limb. In *Essentials of human anatomy,* ed. 7, New York, 1983, Oxford University Press.

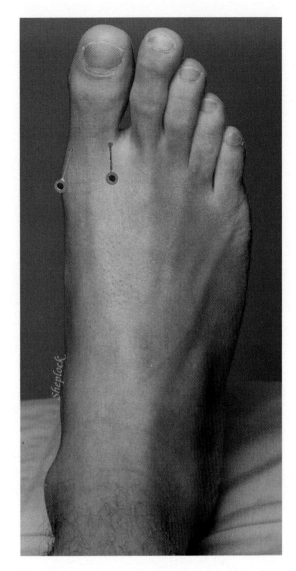

Fig. 25-4 *Needle insertion points for blockade of the digital nerves at the phalanges.*

Anatomy for Neural Blockade of the Sympathetic Nervous System

Part

6

CHAPTER 26

Stellate Ganglion

Quinn Hogan

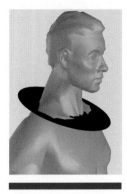

Introduction Since the stellate ganglion is formed by the embryologic fusion of the first thoracic sympathetic ganglion with the inferior cervical ganglion, a suitable alternative name is the thoracocervical ganglion. For a peripheral nervous structure, it is fairly large, typically measuring 2 cm in length, 1 cm wide, and 0.5 cm in an anterior/posterior plane. Its position at the cephalad end of the paired thoracic paravertebral sympathetic chains makes it a physiologic bottleneck: virtually all sympathetic efferent activity to the arms and head must pass through it on the way to the brachial plexus or to the cervical trunk, the continuation of the paravertebral sympathetic chain into the neck.

The basic wiring plan of the sympathetic efferent system is as follows. Signals originate from cells in the intermediolateral cell column of the spinal cord in segments T1 through L2 that give rise to lightly myelinated preganglionic B fibers. These emerge with the ventral spinal roots, pass through the white rami communicantes, and then join the paravertebral sympathetic chain. Once in the chain, the preganglionic fibers may ascend, descend, travel to prevertebral structures (celiac, mesenteric, and other plexuses) via splanchnic nerve branches from the chain, or synapse in the various paravertebral ganglia with postganglionic cells. The nonmyelinated postganglionic C fibers leave the paravertebral chains in the gray rami communicantes to travel to the segmental nerves and other structures.

There are important deviations from this basic plan. Sympathetic fibers may pass directly from the second or third intercostal nerves to the brachial plexus via the nerves of Kuntz. Many preganglionic efferents are nonmyelinated. The white and gray rami, which are indistinguishable on gross examination, are not purely preganglionic and postganglionic efferents, respectively. Gray rami often carry small myelinated cells that are visceral afferent or postganglionic efferent. Finally, synapses between preganglionic and postganglionic fibers may occur at many sites other than paravertebral ganglia, such as in the rami and peripheral nerves. These features contribute to the incomplete sympathetic denervation that may follow surgical removal or local anesthetic blockade of the stellate ganglion.

ANATOMIC RELATIONSHIPS

In vivo imaging and sections of cadavers frozen in toto show the stellate ganglion at the inferior margin of the head of the first rib (Figs 26-1 and 26-2). Dissection studies often observe the ganglion at a higher site, but this may be due to the loss of the downward traction of the lung. It is always immediately lateral to the longus colli muscle and posterior to the vertebral artery (Fig. 26-3). The par-

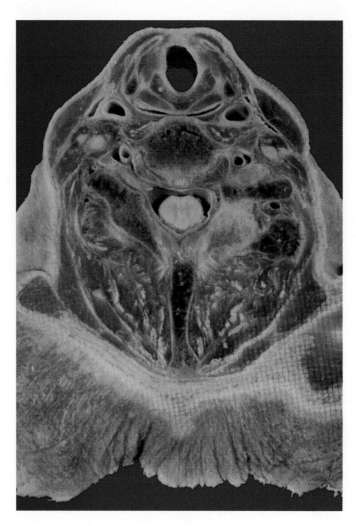

FIG. 26-1 *Transverse anatomic section through the sixth cervical vertebra, revealing the sympathetic chain and related structures.*

avertebral sympathetic chain rises from its very posterior location in the chest to a position in the neck anterior to the transverse processes, where it (in the form of the cervical trunk) lies on the anterior surface of the cervical portion of the longus colli muscle. Since the vertebral artery does the reverse—that is, goes from an anterior position at its origin from the subclavian artery to a location posterior to the cervical trunk within the foramina transversaria in the transverse processes of C6 and above—the vertebral artery penetrates the chain, usually at a position just cephalad to the stellate ganglion.

INDICATIONS

Blockade of the stellate ganglion is used for diagnosis and treatment of conditions involving autonomic dysfunction, including vascular insufficiency, hyperhidrosis, and a variety of painful syndromes. It may occasionally be used, especially on the left side, if sympathetic imbalance is thought to be contributing to ventricular arrhythmias.

REGIONAL ANESTHETIC TECHNIQUE

Injections intended to deliver solution to the stellate ganglion are often made at the level of the sixth cervical vertebra, either directly on the anterior tubercle of C6 (Chassaignac's tubercle) or medial to it. The patient is placed in the supine position, with additional support under the shoulders to extend the neck. Pressure from the operator's fingers laterally displaces the sternocleidomastoid muscle and the carotid sheath, containing the carotid artery, jugular vein, and the vagus nerve. A 22-gauge needle is inserted perpendicular to the horizontal plane until contact is made with the anterior tubercle of

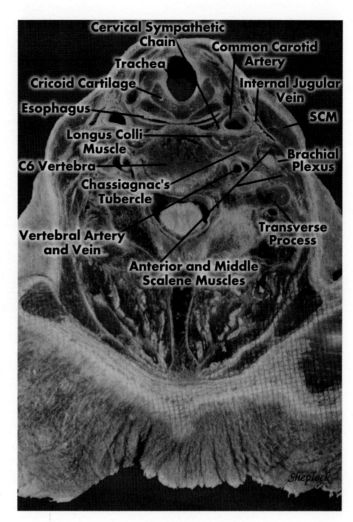

Cervical Sympathetic Chain
Common Carotid Artery
Trachea
Cricoid Cartilage
Internal Jugular Vein
Esophagus
SCM
Longus Colli Muscle
C6 Vertebra
Brachial Plexus
Chassiagnac's Tubercle
Vertebral Artery and Vein
Transverse Process
Anterior and Middle Scalene Muscles

Sheplock

FIG. 26-2 *Corresponding computer-enhanced image of the anatomic section with annotation.*

C6, usually at a depth of only about 1 cm. Injection of 5 to 12 ml of local anesthetic should follow slight withdrawal so the needle tip is not within the periosteum (Fig. 26-4). The cervical trunk at this level is within the superficial layers of the prevertebral fascia that extends from the anterior tubercle to cover the anterior scalene muscle laterally and the longus colli muscle medially. Local anesthetic injected just superficial to the tubercle or longus colli muscle will therefore reliably block the cervical trunk, producing sympathetic denervation of the head with enophthalmos, miosis, anhidrosis, nasal mucosal hyperemia, and facial and conjunctival flushing. Contralateral cervical trunk block is possible because of the free passage of fluid across the midline in this tissue plane.

Blockade of the cervical and brachial sympathetic fibers is also sought using blocks at the C7 level. These block are problematic for two reasons. First, the vertebral artery is anterior to the C7 transverse process, exposing it to puncture and anesthetic injection, which is toxic in minute (<1 ml) amounts because of direct arterial delivery to the brain stem. Although the vertebral artery may also occasionally be anterior to the transverse processes at higher levels, it is most often protected within the foramen transversarium. After aspiration, injections should always be initiated by a small test dose (0.5 ml or less). Second, because the seventh cervical vertebra has a transitional design and lacks an anterior tubercle, injections directed by bony contact with the transverse process will be into the compartment containing the brachial plexus, lessening the degree to which the block is selective for sympathetic fibers. This may also be why injections at the C7 level are somewhat more thorough in producing sympathetic blockade of the arm.

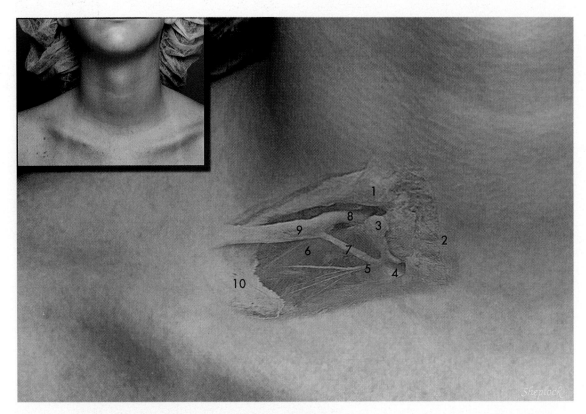

FIG. 26-3 *Dissection of the stellate ganglion and brachial plexus as they relate to the first and second ribs, superimposed over the surface anatomy. Key: 1, head of the first rib; 2, anterior longitudinal ligament; 3, sympathetic trunk and ganglion; 4, ventral ramus of the second thoracic nerve; 5, second intercostal nerve; 6, second rib; 7, communication with the first thoracic nerve; 8, ventral ramus of the first thoracic nerve; 9, lower trunk of the brachial plexus; 10, first rib.*

SIDE EFFECTS AND COMPLICATIONS

Inadequate stellate ganglion blockade is apparent if signs of sympathetic interruption fail to develop in the upper extremity. Although Horner's syndrome may ensue, this does not indicate stellate ganglion block since it will also follow cervical trunk block. The spread of solution after injection at the C6 anterior tubercle may be anterior to the ganglion and flows into the mediastinum, resulting in incomplete block.

The stellate ganglion lies less than 1 cm anterior to the inferior roots (C8 and T1) of the brachial plexus, separated only by nonfibrous adipose tissue. Even with small-volume injections at the T1 level, directed by CT scanner, obvious block of the brachial plexus may occur. Any block that delivers enough anesthetic to the ganglion to block it may also subtly alter function in the adjacent somatic roots (Figure 26-5). In addition, only the medial insertion of the anterior scalene muscle separates the site of injection for stellate block from the brachial plexus. For these reasons, it is important to search for evidence of somatic (motor, sensory) block if selective sympathetic block is being used to discern the role of the sympathetic nervous system in the pathogenesis of a condition.

Injection of less than 1 ml of local anesthetic into the vertebral artery may result in loss of consciousness or seizure, since the drug arrives undiluted in the brain stem. Proximity to the nerve roots of the brachial plexus requires caution to avoid injection into nerve root sleeves that may be in continuity with the subarachnoid space. Solution injected into the proximal segmental nerve dissects proximally to emerge in the cerebrospinal fluid. To avoid these complications, cerebrospinal fluid or blood must be sought by aspiration before injection, a small test dose must precede the full dose, and the patient must not be so sedate as to obscure a paresthesia from needle contact with a somatic nerve. Full resuscitation equipment should be available.

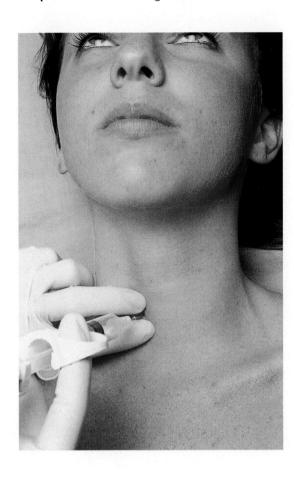

SUGGESTED READINGS

Carron H, Litwiller R: Stellate ganglion block, *Anesth Analg* 54:567-570, 1975.

Erickson SJ, Hogan Q: CT-guided injection of the stellate ganglion: description of technique and efficacy of sympathetic blockade, *Radiology* 188:707-709, 1993.

Hogan QH, Erickson SJ: Magnetic resonance imaging of the stellate ganglion, *Am J Roentg* 158:655-659, 1992.

Hogan Q, Erickson S, Haddox J et al: The spread of solutions during "stellate ganglion" blockade, *Reg Anesth* 17:78-83, 1992.

Kirgis H, Kuntz A: Inconstant sympathetic neural pathways, *Arch Surg* 44:95-102, 1942.

Malmqvist E, Bengtsson M, Sorensen J: Efficacy of stellate ganglion block: a clinical study with bupivacaine, *Reg Anesth* 17:340-347, 1992.

Moore DC: *Stellate ganglion block*, Springfield, IL, 1954, Thomas.

FIG. 26-4 *Blockade of the stellate ganglion at Chassaignac's tubercle of the sixth cervical vertebrae.*

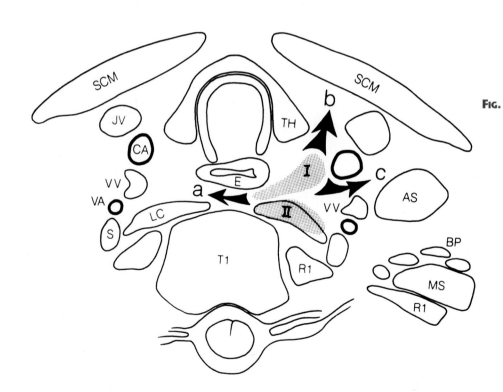

FIG. 26-5 *Patterns of fluid spread from paratracheal injections at the C6 or C7 level. The most common pattern (I) is anterior to the prevertebral fascia with extension medially/contralaterally (a), anteriorly between the trachea and carotid (b), or laterally (c). A less common pattern (II) is deep to the prevertebral fascia in or around the longus colli muscle. AS, anterior scalene muscle; BP, brachial plexus; CA, carotid artery; E, esophagus; JV, jugular vein; LC, longus colli muscle; MS, middle scalene muscle; R1, first rib; S, stellate; TH, thyroid; T1, thoracic vertebral body; VA, vertebral artery; VV, vertebral vein.*

CHAPTER 27

Celiac Plexus

Marshall D. Bedder

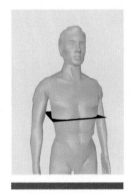

Introduction The structure of the celiac plexus has been described differently by numerous authors in the anatomic literature. There appears to be great anatomic variation and little consensus of opinion regarding shape, location, and afferent nerve supply. Celiac plexus blockade with subsequent neurolysis has been advocated for pain secondary to pancreatic cancer, other visceral malignancies, and pain secondary to pancreatitis. Multiple techniques and visualization protocols have been developed for blockade of the celiac plexus.

ANATOMIC RELATIONSHIPS

The celiac plexus is the largest of the major autonomic plexuses. It is located anterior to the superior aspect of the first lumbar vertebral body (Figs. 27-1 and 27-2). The celiac plexus is made up of two major celiac ganglion, right and left, as well as associated ganglia, secondary plexi, and nerve fibers representing the greater, lesser, and least splanchnic, vagus, and phrenic nerves. Associated ganglia with the celiac ganglia are the aorticorenal ganglion and the superior mesenteric ganglion. Secondary plexuses arising from or connected with the celiac plexus include the phrenic, splenic, hepatic, left gastric intermesenteric, suprarenal, renal, testicular or ovarian, superior mesenteric, and inferior mesenteric.

The celiac ganglia have classically been described as irregular masses, oval or semilunar in shape. Recent studies indicate a triangular shape on both sides as the most common. This retroperitoneal structure, which lies between the adrenal glands, has anterior relationships including the lesser sac and stomach. The pancreas usually overlies the origin of the superior mesenteric artery and may overlie the celiac plexus. Posterior to the plexus are the celiac artery, superior mesenteric artery (SMA), aorta, and the crura of the diaphragm. It appears the ganglia are related to both the celiac trunk and the SMA and postsynaptic fibers arising from the celiac ganglia and enveloping both vessels. The base of the triangular ganglia is almost parallel to the abdominal aorta (Fig. 27-3).

Preganglionic sympathetic fibers are carried via the greater and lesser splanchnic nerves, while postganglionic branches accompany the branches of the celiac artery along the parasympathetic vagal fibers. The splanchnic nerves enter the lateral pole of the ganglia; the posterior vagus supplies a small branch to the upper pole, while the inferior pole is connected to the aortorenal ganglion. Sensory afferent fibers from the viscera enter the medial margin of the celiac ganglia.

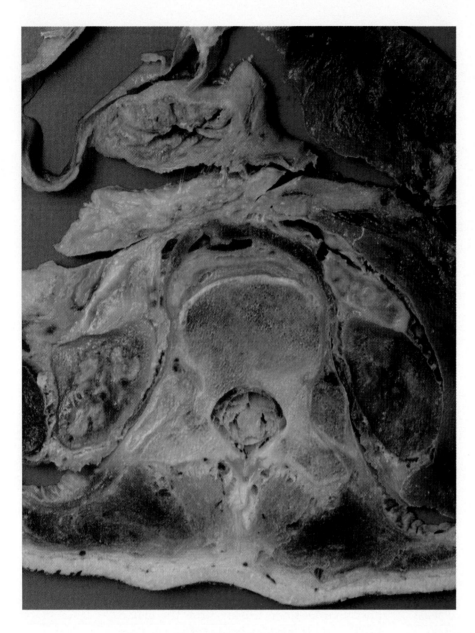

FIG. 27-1 *Transverse anatomic section at the level of the first lumbar vertebra, revealing the location of the celiac plexus and related structures.*

INDICATIONS

The major indication for neurolytic celiac plexus block (NCPB) has been pancreatic cancer. NCPB has also been reported to be effective in a variety of nonpancreatic intraabdominal malignancies. Although advocated by some for pain secondary to chronic pancreatitis, the literature is most inconclusive for this indication.

REGIONAL ANESTHETIC TECHNIQUE

Celiac plexus blockade has been described by both posterior and anterior approaches. Multiple posterior approach techniques have been advocated, and various imaging techniques with fluoroscopy or computer tomography (CT) have been used to confirm needle placement.

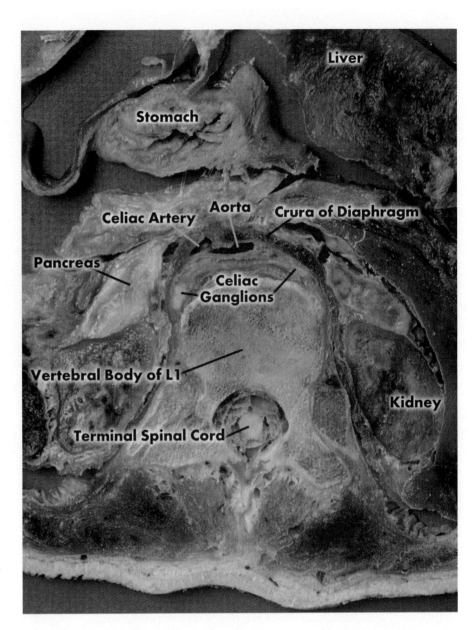

FIG. 27-2 *Corresponding computer-enhanced image of the anatomic section with annotation.*

Celiac plexus blockade by the retrocrural approach remains the standard approach to the celiac plexus. The patient should have intravenous access and have standard monitoring. The patient is positioned prone on the procedure table, with a bolster or pillow under the abdomen to reverse the normal lumbar lordosis. The patient's head is turned to the side for comfort and the arms are abducted. Attention to sterile preparation and wide draping of the field should be emphasized. Bilateral skin wheals of local anesthetic are made approximately 7 to 8 cm lateral from the midline at the L1 vertebral body. The local anesthetic infiltration should be inferior to the twelfth rib and extend deep for patient comfort.

A 10- to 15-cm suitable block needle, 20- or 22-gauge, is used, depending on patient body habitus. The needle is initially advanced

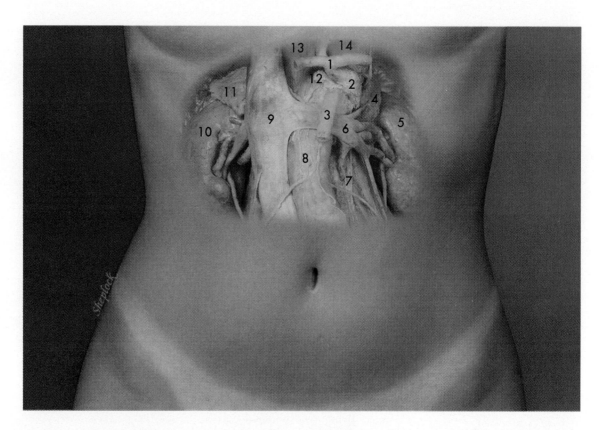

FIG. 27-3 *Dissection of the celiac plexus, with related structures superimposed over the surface anatomy. Key: 1, celiac artery trunk; 2, left celiac ganglion; 3, superior mesenteric artery; 4, left adrenal gland; 5, left kidney; 6, left renal vein; 7, left sympathetic trunk; 8, abdominal aorta and aortic plexus; 9, inferior vena cava; 10, right kidney; 11, right adrenal gland; 12, right celiac ganglion; 13, right crus of diaphragm; 14, left crus of diaphragm.*

from just under the twelfth rib at a 45° angle from the horizontal and can be visualized radiographically until it makes contact with the lateral border of the L1 vertebral body, usually at 7 to 9 cm (Fig. 27-4). A needle with depth markings or movable markers is useful to aid in correct placement. The needle is then withdrawn either to the subcutaneous tissue or the skin and redirected at a steeper angle to pass off the anterolateral aspect of the L1 vertebral body (Fig. 27-5). Previous depth determinations combined with radiographic imaging will help guide needle placement beyond the point of bony contact. The left-side needle is then advanced carefully 1.5 to 3 cm or until aortic pulsations are transmitted to the needle shaft. The right-side needle can then be advanced to a similar or slightly deeper position (Fig. 27-6).

Injection of contrast material under fluoroscopy or CT is used to confirm needle placement. Anteroposterior views should demonstrate contrast material in the retroperitoneal space at the L1 vertebral level, with midline spread and no extravasation (Figs. 27-7 and 27-8). Aspiration in four quadrants has been advocated to check for blood, urine, or CSF. A standard test dose will reveal additional information regarding inadvertent subarachnoid placement. Diagnostic blockade with local anesthetic is recommended before NCPB, but its effectiveness in predicting the efficacy of neurolytic blocks or in assessing analgesia has been questioned. Recommendations for diagnostic blockade vary widely; 20 to 30 ml unilaterally or bilaterally of 1% xylocaine, 0.25% bupivacaine, or other solutions may be used. NCPB is performed with 25 to 50 ml of 50% alcohol through each needle. Other recommendations have included 25 ml of 50% alcohol and 0.125% bupivacaine through each needle or 5 ml of 2% xylocaine before alcohol injection to decrease the pain of injection.

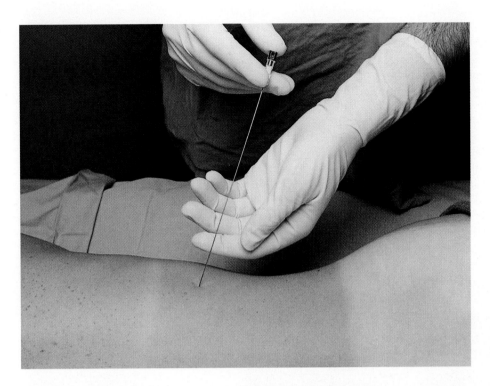

Fig. 27-4 *Initial needle placement for celiac plexus blockade.*

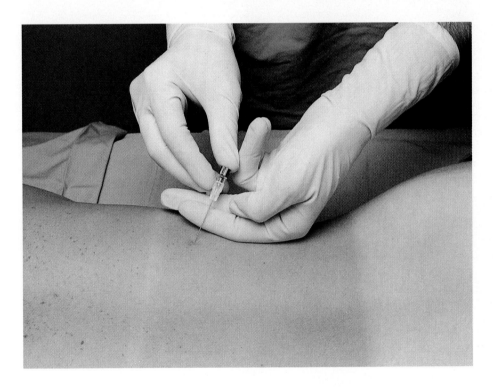

Fig. 27-5 *Final needle position for celiac plexus blockade.*

SIDE EFFECTS AND COMPLICATIONS

Orthostatic hypotension is the most frequent side effect with celiac plexus blockade due to the decrease in sympathetic tone and resulting splanchnic vessel pooling. Elderly patients, as expected, appear more prone to orthostatic hypotension, and it has been recommended that all patients be admitted for a 24-hour period of observation and treatment with intravenous hydration.

Injection of the local anesthetic test dose into the vena cava can result in cardiovascular toxicity or seizures.

Other serious side effects reported include pneumothorax, subarachnoid or epidural injection, retroperitoneal hematoma, renal necrosis or hemorrhage, paraplegia, monoparesis with loss of anal and bladder function, inability to ejaculate, diarrhea, retroperitoneal fibrosis, and aortic pseudoaneurysm.

Imaging techniques including fluoroscopy, CT scans, and ultrasound have all been used and are recommended to decrease the potential for less common but serious side effects.

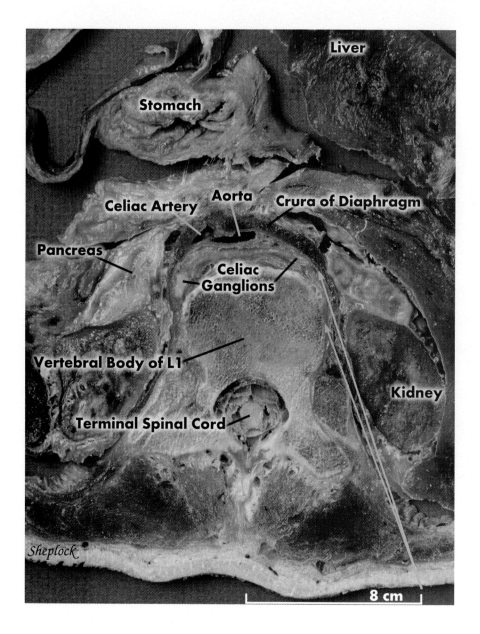

FIG. 27-6 *Transverse image at the level of the first lumbar vertebra, demonstrating both initial needle placement (yellow arrow) and final needle position (green arrow) when performing a celiac plexus blockade via the retrocrural technique.*

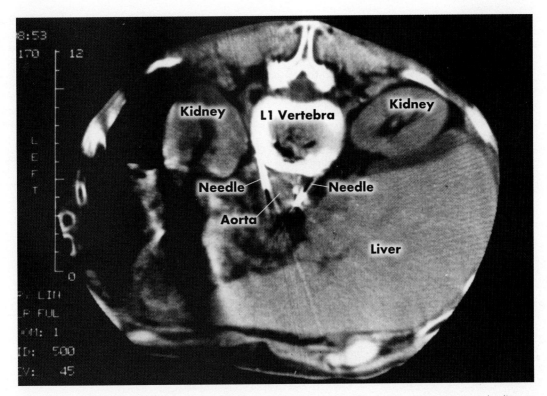

FIG. 27-7 *Computer tomography (CT) image revealing proper needle placement for retrocrural celiac plexus blockade at the L1 vertebra.*

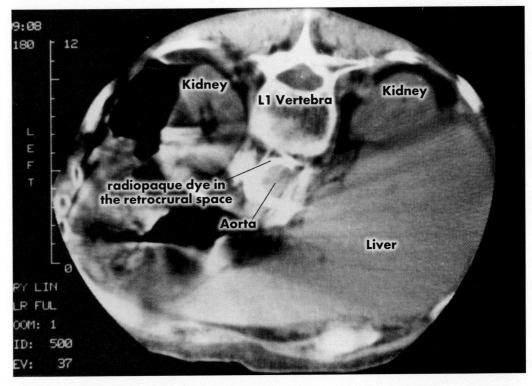

FIG. 27-8 *Computer tomography (CT) image revealing proper needle placement for retrocrural celiac plexus blockade, which is confirmed by the injection of contrast material into the retroperitoneal space anterior to the L1 vertebra.*

SUGGESTED READINGS

Brown D: A retrospective analysis of neurolytic celiac plexus block for nonpancreatic intra-abdominal cancer pain, *Reg Anesth* 14(2):63-65, 1989.

Ischia S, Ischia A, Polai E et al: Three posterior percutaneous celiac plexus block techniques: a prospective, randomized study in 61 patients with pancreatic cancer pain, *Anesthesiology* 76(4):534-540, 1992.

Mercandante S: Celiac plexus block versus analgesics in pancreatic cancer pain, *Pain* 52(2):187-192, 1993.

Moore DC, Bush WH, Burnett LL: Celiac plexus block: a roentgenographic, anatomic study of technique and spread of solution in patients and corpses, *Anesth Analg* 60:369-379, 1981.

Paz A, Rosen A: The human celiac ganglion and its splanchnic nerves, *Acta Anat* 136:129-133, 1989.

Sharfman WH, Walsh TD: Has the analgesic efficacy of neurolytic celiac plexus block been demonstrated in pancreatic cancer pain? *Pain* 41:267-271, 1990.

Thompson G, Moore DC: Celiac plexus, intercostal and minor peripheral nerve blockade. In Cousins MJ, Bridenbaugh PO, editors: *Neural blockade in clinical anesthesia and management of pain*, Philadelphia, 1988, JB Lippincott.

Williams PL, Warwick R, Dyson M et al, editors: Coeliac plexus. In *Gray's anatomy*, Edinburgh, 1989, Churchill Livingstone.

CHAPTER 28

Lumbar Sympathetic Ganglion

John C. Rowlingson

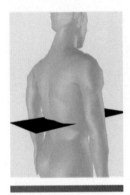

Introduction The use of lumbar sympathetic blocks (LSB) has been applied to the management of painful conditions of the pelvis and lower extremities and to labor pain. It is important to emphasize that LSB provides only interruption of sympathetic innervation and its effects are *not* confounded by additional sensory or motor blockade.

ANATOMIC RELATIONSHIPS

The lumbar sympathetic chain is a continuation of the thoracic chain. After passage through the abdomen, the sympathetic fibers course behind the common iliac vessels and enter the pelvis anterior to the ala of the sacrum. The lumbar chain descends into the abdominal cavity from the thoracic cage through the hiatus of the diaphragm. It lies in a space bounded medially by the lumbar vertebrae, posteriorly by the psoas muscle and fascia and the retroperitoneal fascia, and anterolaterally by the great vessels and abdominal contents. The aorta is anterior and slightly medial to the chain on the left side, and the vena cava almost overlies the chain on the right side (Figs. 28-1 and 28-2). In comparison to the thoracic sympathetic chain, the lumbar chain is more medial and anterior (Fig. 28-3).

The fascia and body of the psoas muscle ordinarily separate the sympathetic nerves from the lumbar spinal (somatic) nerves. The fascia attaches to the upper and lower edges of the vertebrae, as well as the intervertebral disks. Thus an arch is formed adjacent to the edge of the vertebral body through which the segmental lumbar vessels pass, and sympathetic fiber branches can course to join the lumbar somatic nerves. In general, blockade of somatic nerves does not occur when a LSB is done, though the presence of this conduit predicts the possibility that this might happen. Somatic nerve block would be most devastating if overflow of neurolytic agents were to occur.

Variation exists in the actual physical organization of the lumbar sympathetic chain even within the same patient and when comparing side to side. A clinical implication of this reality is that diagnostic blocks may need to be done at a few levels to assure an adequate trial of sympathetic interruption. Although there are typically five lumbar vertebrae, there may be only four lumbar sympathetic ganglia, due to fusion of the twelfth thoracic with the first lumbar ganglion. These ganglia may be segmentally oriented or grouped together, most commonly at the L2, L3, or L4 levels. The size of the ganglia varies from 3 to 5 mm to 10 to 15 mm in width. The lumbar sympathetic chain contains not only the preganglionic and

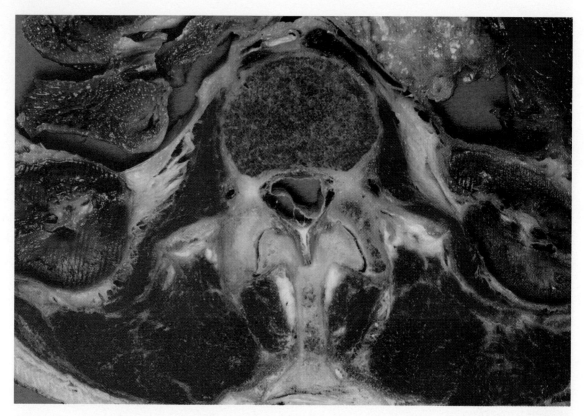

FIG. 28-1 *Transverse anatomic section through the lumbar spine at L2, revealing the sympathetic chain, vertebra, somatic nerve roots, and associated structures.*

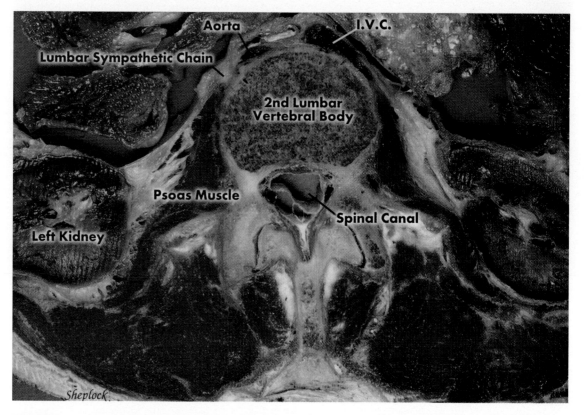

FIG. 28-2 *Corresponding computer-enhanced image of the anatomic section with annotation.*

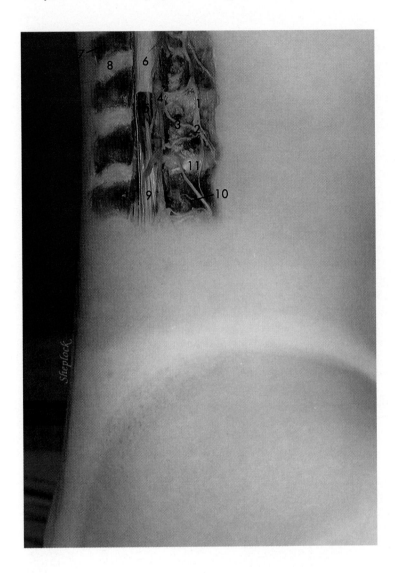

FIG. 28-3 *Dissection of the sympathetic chain and associated structures viewed from the right with parts of the vertebral arches and meninges removed, superimposed over the surface anatomy. Key: 1, sympathetic trunk; 2, sympathetic ganglion; 3, rami communicantes; 4, dorsal root ganglia of the first lumbar nerve; 5, spinal cord; 6, dura mater; 7, spinous process of the twelfth thoracic vertebra; 8, interspinous ligament; 9, cauda equina; 10, body of the third lumbar vertebra; 11, intervertebral disk.*

postganglionic fibers to the pelvis and lower extremities but also some nociceptive afferent fibers. Most of the sympathetic fibers to the lower extremities pass through the L2 or L3 ganglia, so blockade at either of these levels will provide near-complete sympathetic block of the legs (producing arterial vasodilation) as well as relief of visceral pain from the uterus, cervix, ipsilateral kidney, ureter, upper portion of the bladder, testicle, part of the transverse colon, descending colon, and the rectum.

INDICATIONS

No specific application of LSB alone in surgical anesthesia exists. The technique has been used by some for analgesia in the first stage of labor. LSBs with local anesthetics are used in a diagnostic and prognostic mode before therapeutic neurolytic blocks. The most traditional use of LSB has been in the management of painful conditions of the lower extremities or pelvic viscera. The etiology of these pathologic states may relate to: (1) altered blood flow as with reflex sympathetic dystrophy/causalgia, peripheral vascular disease, or thrombophlebitis; (2) visceral pain as with renal colic or cancer of the leg, colon, or pelvic organs; (3) neuralgic/deafferentation pain associated with peripheral nerve injury, leg trauma, infection, radiation neuritis, phantom limb pain, or postherpetic neuralgia; or (4) sympathetic nervous system problems such as hyperhidrosis.

REGIONAL ANESTHETIC TECHNIQUE

The patient is placed in the prone position, with a pillow under the iliac crests to flatten the lumbar lordosis and facilitate palpation of the necessary landmarks. A less common alternative is to have the patient in a decubitus position with the affected side uppermost. Placement of an IV is recommended, especially when neurolytic blocks are done. Sedatives and analgesics should be used judiciously, because patient cooperation is important for assessing outcome.

The spinous processes in the midline of the prone patient are identified and a line drawn over them from L1 to L5. Thereafter, various techniques advise marking a spot for needle insertion that is 5, 5 to 7.5, 7 to 10, and even 12 cm lateral to the midline at the level of the desired lumbar vertebral spinous process. Approaches beyond 8 cm risk needle injury to the kidney, whereas being less than 5 cm lateral to the midline makes the lateral aspect of the vertebral body difficult to hit. The point at which a line that is parallel and 7.5 cm lateral to the midline crosses the lowermost palpable rib is the needle insertion site for the L2 level (Fig. 28-4).

The skin of the low back area is prepped with alcohol or betadine. Drapes are placed to circumscribe the area and leave landmarks exposed. Skin wheals using local anesthetic are placed at all sites where therapeutic needles will be applied, and a 23- to 25-gauge spinal needle may be used to infiltrate the proposed tract of needle insertion. It is possible that generous infiltration in a thin patient may result in partial lumbar plexus block and a falsely positive response to LSB.

Because the distance to the lateral aspect of the vertebral body is approximately 6 to 8 cm in a normal adult but can be 10 cm in a large adult, needles that are 8 to 15 cm are needed for LSB. These vary in recommended gauge from 19 to 22. It is not apparent whether there is a distinct advantage of using *one* needle at L2 or L3 over using a needle at L2 *and* L4. (If a neurolytic block is to be done, use of a smaller volume of injectate through each of two needles is recommended.) The chosen needle is inserted through the skin wheal at a 30° to 45° angle off the perpendicular to the skin (Fig. 28-5, *A*).

The transverse process of the lumbar vertebrae may be contacted at a depth of 3 to 5 cm (Fig. 28-9, *yellow arrow*). It may be useful to

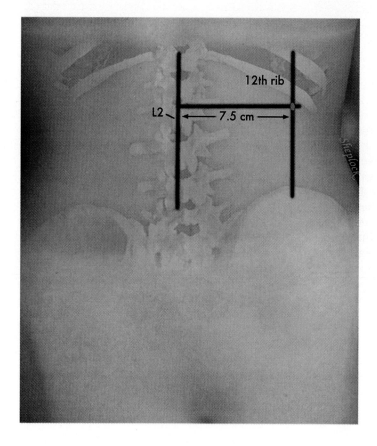

FIG. 28-4 *Computer-enhanced image of the bony landmarks and needle insertion point for performing lumbar sympathetic blockade. Key:* black line *over spinous processes of L1-L5;* brown line *over border 12th rib;* blue circle *over spinous process of L2;* red circle *over needle insertion point.*

purposefully make contact with this landmark to (1) ensure knowledge of its actual location so as to not "walk" the needle off it mistakenly and place drug adjacent to somatic nerves, and (2) make use of the fact that a marker, slid back up the shaft of the needle to two times the depth to the transverse process, is a rough guide of the depth of the targeted vertebral body. The needle must bypass the transverse process—if contacted, the needle is aimed slightly more cephalad or caudad and inserted until contact with bone is made a second time and at a greater depth (Fig. 28-5, *B*). Ideally the needle hits the upper or lower third of the vertebral body to avoid the segmental lumbar vessels that are usually in a midbody location. The bevel of the needle should face the vertebral body. With progressive steepening of the needle entry, and as the needle is withdrawn 2 to 4 cm and reinserted, contact with bone will be lost. The needle should be advanced 1 to 2 cm (Fig. 28-5, *C*) beyond this depth. Slightly more penetration may be needed to reach the L4 vertebral body than the L2 level due to the normal degree of lumbar lordosis.

The correct location of the needle tip(s) must be confirmed, and there are a number of recommended techniques (Fig. 28-9, *green arrow*).

(1) Anesthetists may use a loss-of-resistance (LOR) to air or saline technique as the needle is passed through the psoas muscle and fascia. (If LOR is used throughout placement of the needle, the anesthetist must be aware of the temporary LOR that can be felt between the quadratus lumborum and psoas muscles. Injection of drug at this location will result in lumbar plexus blockade).

(2) The needle may simply be placed percutaneously, followed by careful aspiration of the needle in at least two planes for blood, CSF, and urine.

(3) Technique number 2 is frequently combined with the subsequent administration of a dose of local anesthetic containing epinephrine, with the signs and symptoms of intrathecal or intravascular injection sought as with a classical epidural anesthesia test dose.

(4) The "feel" of the needle and its freedom of movement can be checked by looking for the "tent sign." This sign is based on the fact that, if the skin is the major tissue binding the needle, slight in-and-out movement of it will tent the skin (Fig. 28-6). However, if the skin does not tent, firm resistance to movement usually indicates the needle tip is in an intervertebral disk, viscus, or the wall of a vessel.

(5) The ultimate method to verify correct needle location is with the use of radiographic imaging. Instillation of contrast dye into properly placed needle(s) will demonstrate longitudinal spread within the space anterolateral to the lumbar vertebral bodies and outside of the psoas fascia (Figs. 28-7 and 28-8). This verification is crucial before neurolytic drugs are injected, and the pictures taken are important for the permanent record. Imaging is also recommended before diagnostic blocks are done, because no valid conclusion about the result of a diagnostic block can be made unless certainty exists that the LSB was first a technical success. If a catheter placement technique is used (as through an 18-gauge needle), documentation of accurate placement of the catheter is important because markedly smaller doses of drug will then be necessary to obtain the desired clinical effect. Ultrasonic guidance has recently been proposed as a valuable and reliable method for overseeing needle placement. A study using this technique for doing neurolytic LSBs with a phenol-glycerol mixture has noted the advantages to be excellent results, documentation of the expected spread of the injectate, far lower cost than CT or fluoroscopy, the absence of radiation exposure, and good definition of the regional anatomy before and after the procedure.

Typically, local anesthetic drugs are injected to achieve sympathetic blockade of at least a temporary nature. Most anesthetists advocate first using 5 to 15 ml of a short-acting, rapid-onset drug such as 2% 2-chloroprocaine or 1% lidocaine to verify proper needle location and expected effect. Thereafter an equal volume of 0.25% to 0.5% bupivacaine with or without epinephrine can be injected. If a single needle is placed, volumes in the 15- to 20-ml range are needed. Large volumes of local anesthetic are also advocated when therapeutic blocks are performed.

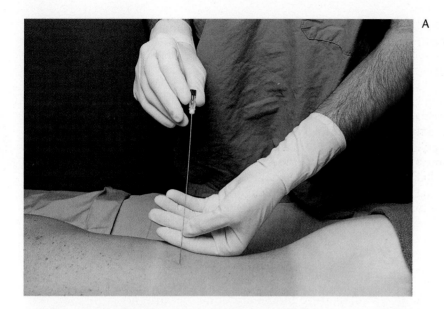

A

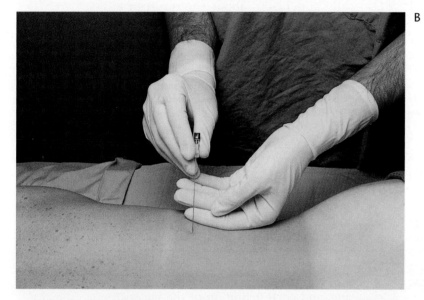

B

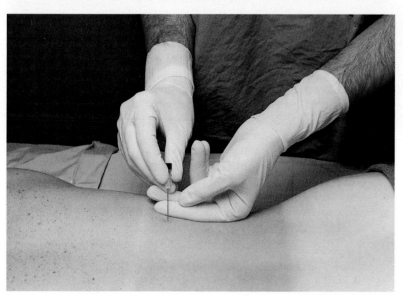

C

FIG. 28-5 *Blockade of the lumbar sympathetic chain at the second lumbar vertebra. **A**, Initial needle insertion through the skin at a 30° to 45° angle directed towards the L2 vertebra. **B**, The needle is in contact with the lateral aspect of the L2 vertebral body at a depth of 6 to 8 cm. **C**, The needle is in its final position near the sympathetic chain, 1 to 2 cm anterior to the L2 vertebral body at a depth of 9 to 14 cm.*

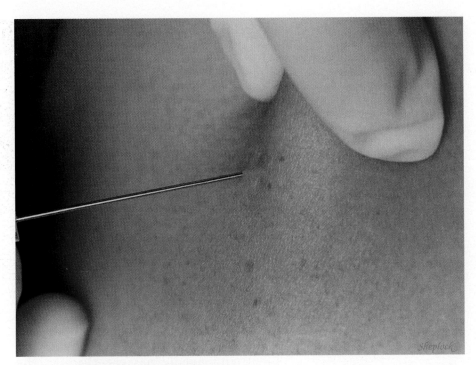

FIG. 28-6 *Tenting of the skin occurs with slight movement of the shaft only when the needle tip is free from restriction. Lack of skin tenting may indicate that the needle tip is in an intervertebral disk or viscus or vascular wall.*

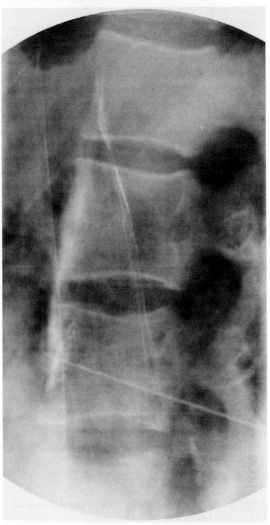

FIG. 28-7 *Lateral radiograph demonstrating proper needle placement for blockade of the lumbar sympathetic chain, confirmed by the spread of injected radioopaque contrast material along the sympathetic chain.*

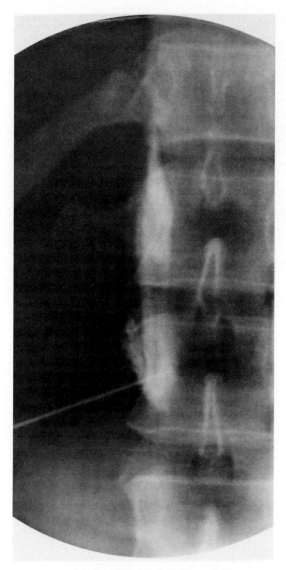

FIG. 28-8 *Anteroposterior radiograph demonstrating proper needle placement for blockade of the lumbar sympathetic chain, confirmed by the spread of injected radioopaque contrast material along the sympathetic chain.*

This technique is in contrast to using smaller volumes through two or three needles before administration of neurolytic drugs. Theoretically, a smaller volume of injectate will have less likelihood of migrating laterally along the anterior psoas fascia and causing genitofemoral neuralgia. Neurolytic agents are used only after a good to excellent response has been manifested when local anesthetic blocks have been done. Three to five ml or 45% to 95% alcohol or 5 to 8 ml of 6% to 10% phenol in water (per needle) are used. Phenol is the drug of choice due to the lower incidence of postprocedure neuritis.

The expected physiologic effects of LSB include an increase in cutaneous temperature of the ipsilateral extremity (a difference between corresponding areas of the extremity of at least 2° C is noticeable with palpation) and the lack of any sensory or motor blockade. Cutaneous temperature may be measured with thermistors taped to the skin. Loss of the sympathogalvanic reflex (SGR) is evidence of sympathectomy. The patient may volunteer that pain is decreasing or gone. The expected increase in skin blood flow can be documented by plethysmography or thermography.

SIDE EFFECTS AND COMPLICATIONS

It is very important to discriminate side effects from complications. The most common side effect of LSB is transient backache and stiffness from the positioning for the block and needle passage through the paraspinal muscles. If needed, conservative treatment with heat, ice, rest, and occasionally NSAIDs and nonspecific sedative muscle relaxants is curative. Given the intentional sympathetic blockade after LSB, orthostatic hypotension may occur though the unilateral effect of the block usually precludes a dramatic problem. Due to the proximity of large vessels, an intravascular injection of drug could occur. Lastly, the angle of approach of the needle brings it close to the roots of the lumbar plexus, and it is possible that the patient will experience a transient paresthesia into the upper ipsilateral leg. An incidence of genitofemoral neuralgia exists, which is due to poorly defined factors when local anesthetics are used but is understandable when neurolytic agents spread laterally across the anterior psoas fascia and contact the nerve. The pain can persist and may require treatment.

The regional anatomy for LSB predicts the potential complications of the technique. Most that are listed will be more devastating if neurolytic agents are used. Due to the invasive nature of the block, infection or bleeding could be created by needle passage through the skin and deeper tissues or penetration into the aorta, vena cava, or (theoretically) the lumbar vessels. Retroperitoneal hemorrhage is possible, as is bleeding into the psoas muscle sheath; the latter could result in pain being referred to the upper leg and weakness of the quadriceps. Intravascular injection that goes unrecognized

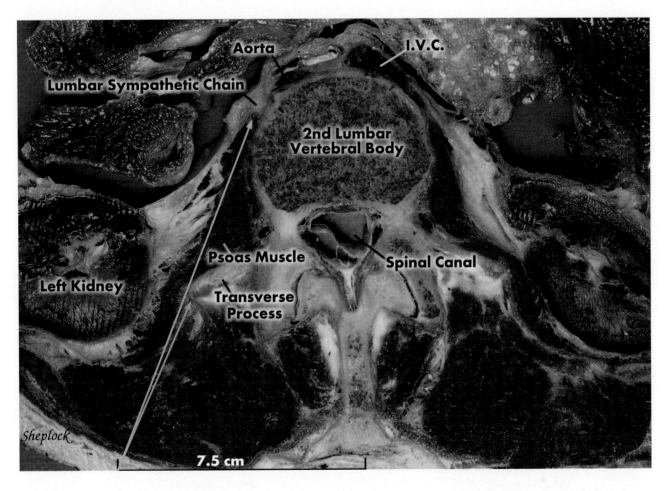

FIG. 28-9 *Transverse computer-enhanced image through the lumbar spine at L2, revealing the initial needle placement represented by the yellow arrow tip in contact with the transverse process of the vertebra and in the final position represented by the green arrow tip near the sympathetic chain.*

will lead to convulsions, hypotension, and cardiopulmonary arrest. One case has been reported of a patient sustaining permanent partial motor paralysis of the lower extremities, the cause of which may have been related to vascular injury to the anterior spinal artery or the artery of Adamkiewicz.

If the needle is not inserted past the transverse process of the lumbar vertebrae, it can be erroneously "walked off" that bony contact and placed in a position such that injection will result in an epidural or spinal block. The neurologic consequences will vary depending on the exact placement, concentration, and volume of the drug injected. Dural sleeves may extend beyond the intervertebral foramina into the paravertebral space, with the subsequent possibility that a dural cuff could be punctured during positioning of the needle for LSB and the patient could develop a post-

dural puncture headache. Intervertebral disks can be perforated, but the exact clinical implication of this is not known.

The proximity of the abdominal viscera exposes them to potential needle trauma, but the likelihood is small. The more lateral to the midline is the initial insertion of the needle, the more likely the tip is to be close to the anterolateral sympathetic chain. The closer the original insertion is to the midline, the more the needle tip goes lateral to the sympathetic chain and closer to the somatic nerves and abdominal structures. Perforation of the kidney could result in hematuria. Neurolytic agents deposited too close to the ureters can result in their stricture or occlusion. Ejaculatory failure can be a consequence of sympathetic interruption. Neurolytic agents that ascend above the diaphragm can provoke pleuritic pain.

SUGGESTED READINGS

Artuso JD, Stevens R, Lineberry PJ: Postdural puncture headache after lumbar sympathetic block: a report of two cases, *Reg Anesth* 16:288-291, 1991.

Bonica JJ, Buckley FP: Regional analgesia with local anesthetic. In Bonica JJ, editor: *The management of pain*, Philadelphia, 1990, Lea and Febiger.

Carron H, Korbon GA, Rowlingson JC: *Regional anesthesia: techniques and clinical applications*, Orlando, 1984, Grune and Stratton.

Haynsworth RF, Noe CE: Percutaneous lumbar sympathectomy: a comparison of radiofrequency denervation versus phenol neurolysis, *Anesthesiology* 74:459-463, 1991.

Jackson S, Smith D, Durkin A: Hematuria as a complication of lumbar paravertebral sympathetic block, *Reg Anesth* 11:31-33, 1986.

Jain S: Nerve blocks. In Warfield CA, editor: *Principles and practice of pain management*, New York, 1993, McGraw-Hill.

Kirvela O, Svedstrom E, Lundbom N: Ultrasonic guidance of lumbar sympathetic and celiac plexus block: a new technique, *Reg Anesth* 17:43-46, 1992.

Lofstrom JB, Cousins MJ: Sympathetic neural blockade of the upper and lower extremity. In Cousins MJ, Bridenbaugh PO, editors: *Neural blockade in clinical anesthesia and management of pain*, ed 2, Philadelphia, 1988, JB Lippincott.

Rauck R: Sympathetic nerve block. In Raj PP, editor: *Practical management of pain*, St. Louis, 1992, Mosby.

Schmidt SD, Gibbons, JJ: Postdural puncture headache after fluoroscopically guided lumbar paravertebral sympathetic block, *Anesthesiology* 78:198-200, 1993.

Sprague RS, Ramamurthy S: Identification of the anterior psoas sheath as a landmark for lumbar sympathetic block, *Reg Anesth* 15:253-255, 1990.

Wang JF, Johnson KA, Ilstrup DM: Sympathetic blocks for reflex sympathetic dystrophy, *Pain* 23:13-17, 1985.

CHAPTER 29

Superior Hypogastric Plexus and Ganglion Impar

Richard B. Patt
Ricardo Plancarte

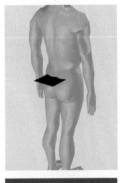

Introduction Neural blockade of selected portions of the sympathetic component of the autonomic nervous system has long been used to treat various chronic pain conditions. In addition to the classic targets of sympatholysis (stellate or cervicothoracic ganglion, thoracic ganglia, celiac plexus, and lumbar chain), new approaches to anesthetize the hypogastric plexus and ganglion impar have been recently reported. These techniques have gained rapid acceptance for the management of pelvic and perineal pain, and are described here.

ANATOMIC RELATIONSHIPS
Superior Hypogastric Plexus

The superior hypogastric plexus, alternately referred to as the plexus hypogastricus and presacral nerve, represents the pelvic extension of the abdominal sympathetic nervous system. Its (preganglionic) cells of origin are located chiefly in the lower thoracic and upper two lumbar levels of intermediolateral column of the spinal cord. Axonal fibers exit these regions as white rami communicantes to synapse in the paravertebral lumbar sympathetic chain and preaortic ganglia and plexuses. Postganglionic fibers emerge from these regions and, together with contributions from the parasympathetic sacral ganglia, form the superior hypogastric plexus.

Descriptions of the gross anatomy of the superior hypogastric plexus vary. The plexus is relatively compact at its origin (L4) and in the course of its descent into the pelvis. Broad and flat with some periaortic condensations, it occupies the midline at its proximal pole (L4-L5), where it has been referred to as the presacral nerve. Near the middle of the body of L5 it begins to divide, giving rise to the hypogastric nerves at the level of the sacral promontory. In the course of dividing and spreading laterally, the plexus takes on a more fenestrated, plexiform morphology. Moving caudad, the hypogastric nerves follow the ventral curve of the sacrum to sweep anteriorly along the side walls of the rectum bilaterally and form the inferior hypogastric plexus. They continue along the side walls of the bladder and, in the male, prostate and seminal vesicles or, in the female, cervix and vaginal fornices. Wile the orientation of the superior hypogastric plexus is predominantly longitudinal, the inferior hypogastric plexus runs transversely, extending posteroanteriorly parallel to the pelvic floor.

The superior hypogastric plexus and closely related structures (hypogastric nerves, inferior hypogastric plexuses) contribute to the innervation of most pelvic organs and vessels. Together with the inferior mesenteric ganglion (which is in continuity with the celiac plexus), it innervates the sigmoid colon and rectum. Together with branches from the renal plexus (also in continuity with the celiac plexus) it contributes to the formation of the ureteric and testicular or ovarian plexuses. In addition, filaments from the superior hypogastric plexus contribute to the plexuses surrounding the common and internal iliac arteries. The inferior hypogastric plexus further supplies the pelvic viscera and genitalia and contributes to the formation of subsidiary plexuses, for example, the superior and middle rectal, vesical, prostatic, and uterovaginal plexuses. Its branches contain visceral, glandular, vascular, and afferent fibers. Although blockade of the inferior hypogastric plexus has not been described, because the plexus is formed predominantly by fibers originating in the superior hypogastric plexus, denervation is achieved by proximal blockade.

In the sagittal (longitudinal) plane, the plexus may extend in the midline as far cephalocaudal as L4-S1. The plexus divides and continues bilaterally as the hypogastric nerves. These structures descend ventrally and, at the level of the lower portion of L5 or upper portion of S1, are the actual targets for superior hypogastric plexus block. In the transverse plane, the plexus and its major constituents are situated within the loose subserosal connective tissue of the retroperitoneum (Figs. 29-1 and 29-2).

In its proximal portion the superior hypogastric plexus lies ventral to the distal portion of the aorta, which separates it from the two lower lumbar vertebrae. Its anterior relations at this level include the parietal peritoneum and small bowel mesentery. Just distally, the aorta and inferior vena cava bifurcate, at the lower portion of L4 and upper portion of L5 respectively, while the superior hypogastric plexus continues downwards. As a result of the lateralization of the aorta and vena cava, the lower pole of the superior hypogastric plexus lies between the common iliac arteries, at first ventral to the left common iliac vein, then against the median sacral artery and vein and the L5 vertebral body. The plexus then divides into the hypogastric nerves that continue caudad and laterally at the level of L5-S1 (sacral promontory). The hypogastric nerves descend in front of the S1 vertebral body and diverge to straddle the rectum. Lateral relations include, proximally the lower paravertebral lumbar sympathetic ganglia, and distally the first sacral ganglia and internal iliac vessels.

Ganglion Impar

The peripheral portion of the sympathetic nervous system consists of paired ganglionated paravertebral chains that extend from the base of the skull to the coccyx, several major prevertebral (periaortic) plexuses (cardiac, celiac, and hypogastric), and numerous small intermediate and terminal ganglia. The paravertebral ganglia are inconstant in number due to fusion of adjacent components and anatomic variability among individuals, but the usual arrangement consists of three paired cervical ganglia, 12 paired thoracic ganglia, four paired lumbar ganglia, four paired sacral ganglia, and a single unpaired ganglion impar located near the sacrococcygeal junction. These ganglia are situated anterolateral to the vertebral column: anterior to the transverse processes in the cervical region, anterior to the heads of the ribs in the thoracic region, along the sides of the vertebral bodies in the abdomen, and in front of the sacrum in the pelvis (see Chapter 28).

The lumbar and sacral parts of the sympathetic trunks are directly contiguous at the level of the pelvic brim. The sacral sympathetic trunks and ganglia lie in the parietal pelvic fascia behind the parietal peritoneum and rectum and on the ventral surface of the sacrum, just medial to its anterior foramina

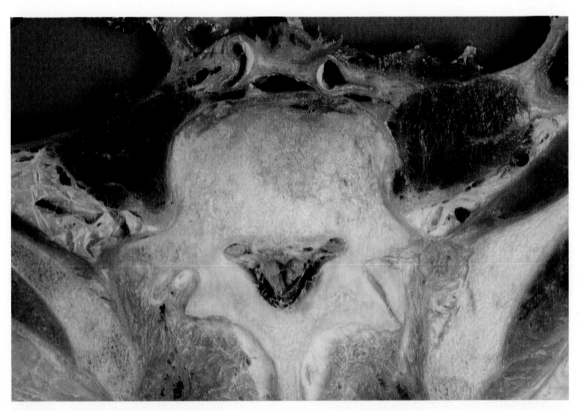

FIG. 29-1 *Transverse anatomic section through the spine at L5-S1 level, revealing the hypogastric plexus, vertebrae, and associated structures.*

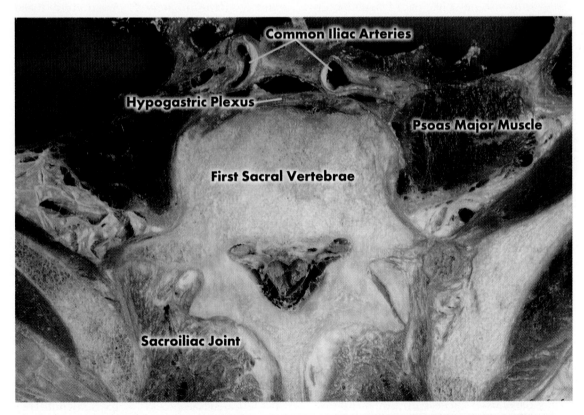

FIG. 29-2 *Corresponding computer-enhanced image of the anatomic section with annotation.*

and the exiting sacral nerves. Below, they converge and unite to form a solitary, small "ganglion impar," located anterior to the sacrococcygeal junction (Figs. 29-3 and 29-4).

The ganglion impar (also called ganglion of Walther) is a solitary retroperitoneal structure located at the level of the sacrococcygeal junction that marks the termination of the paired paravertebral sympathetic chains (Fig. 29-5). It may be prominent, delicate, or even absent. While standard anatomic texts generally provide little detail on its function, as a part of the sacral sympathetic chain it contributes to the innervation of the pelvic organs and genitalia.

INDICATIONS
Superior Hypogastric Plexus Blockade
Superior hypogastric plexus blockade may be considered for pelvic pain that has been unresponsive to more conservative interventions. Because it innervates only the pelvic viscera and vasculature, referred pain emanating from somatic structures will be unaffected. Thus, in addition to therapeutic indications, a diagnostic superior hypogastric plexus block may help distinguish between pelvic pain of visceral and somatic origin. Historic features typically associated with visceral pelvic pain (vague, poorly localized, dull, crampy, pulling, squeezing, or colicky) suggest the likelihood of a favorable response to superior hypogastric plexus block.

Most published experience with superior hypogastric plexus block have reported on the treatment of pain of oncologic origin. In addition to pain emanating directly from tumor invasion, favorable results have been obtained for pain and tenesmus due to radiation injury and rectal anastomosis. Based on beneficial results reported for presacral neurectomy, an analogous surgical procedure, superior hypogastric plexus block may be useful for patients with nononcologic pain as well. Therapeutic superior hypogastric plexus neurolysis, while an effective and minimally hazardous palliative treatment for visceral pelvic cancer pain, should be approached cautiously in patients with nonmalignant disease until further clinical studies have been performed.

Blockade of the Ganglion Impar
Blockade of the ganglion impar has thus far been reported only in abstract form, although it has been used successfully in numerous centers. Injection of the ganglion impar is indicated for perineal pain of visceral origin and sympathetically mediated genital pain that has proven unresponsive to more conservative therapy. As with superior hypogastric plexus blockade, somatic pain is unlikely to be relieved, so while ganglion impar injection can be considered as an aid to the differential diagnosis of perineal pain of undetermined etiology, it is unlikely to be therapeutic for somatically-based conditions like coccygodynia. Patients with pain in the perineal region that is vague, poorly localized, and accompanied by sensations of burning and urgency are most likely to benefit. As with superior hypogastric plexus blockade, most experience with this procedure has been with pain due to cancer, so neurolytic blockade should be performed cautiously if at all in patients with nonmalignant pain.

REGIONAL ANESTHETIC TECHNIQUE
Superior Hypogastric Plexus Blockade
Superior hypogastric block may be preceded by a single-shot L4-L5 epidural injection of 8 to 10 ml of local anesthetic to enhance patient cooperation by reducing reflex muscle spasm, ameliorating the discomfort associated with contact of needles with periosteum, and reducing movement. Alternately, these goals can be achieved with local infiltration of the intervening muscle planes.

The patient assumes the prone position with padding placed beneath the pelvis to flatten the lumbar lordosis. The lumbosacral region is cleansed aseptically. The location of the L4-L5 interspace is approximated by palpation of the iliac crests and spinous processes and is then verified by fluoroscopy. Skin wheals are raised 5 to 7 cm bilateral to the midline at the level of the L4-L5 interspace. A 17.5-cm, 22-gauge short-beveled needle is inserted through one of the skin wheals with the needle bevel directed toward the midline. A depth marker may be used to aid in needle placement. From a position perpendicular in all planes to the skin, the needle is oriented about 30º caudad and 45º mesiad so that its tip is directed toward the anterolateral aspect of the bottom of the L5 vertebral body (Fig. 29-6, *A*). The iliac crest and the transverse process of L5, which is sometimes enlarged, are potential barriers to needle passage and necessitate the use of the cephalolateral entrance site and oblique trajectory described. If the transverse process of L5 is encountered during advancement of the needle, the needle

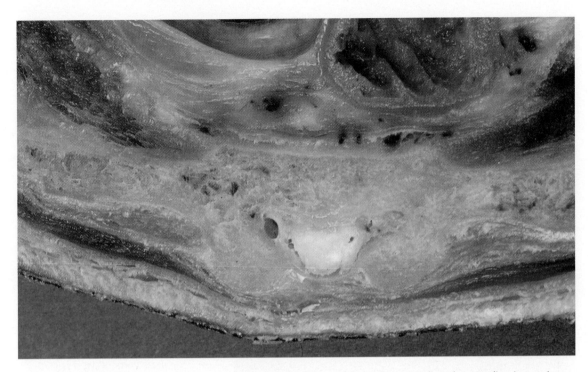

FIG. 29-3 *Transverse anatomic section through the sacrococcygeal junction, revealing the ganglion impar (ganglion of Walther) and associated structures.*

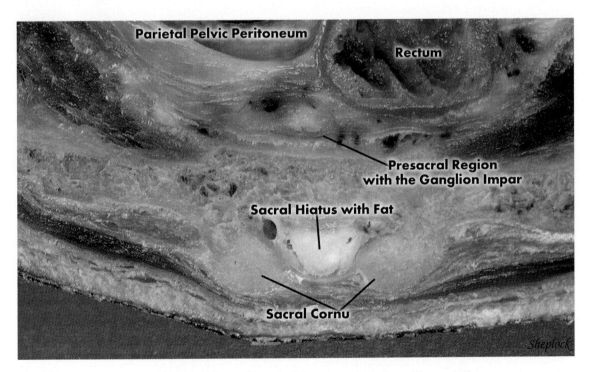

FIG. 29-4 *Corresponding computer-enhanced image of the anatomic section with annotation.*

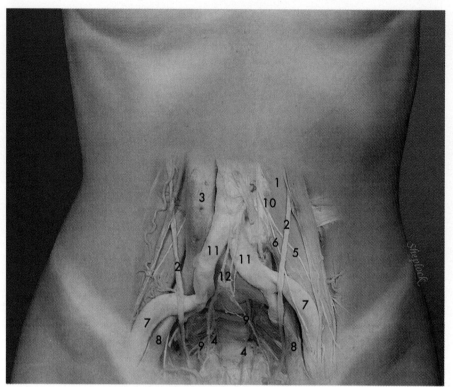

FIG. 29-5 *Dissection with much of the pelvic viscera removed, revealing the hypogastric plexus and vessels superimposed over the surface anatomy. Key: 1, psoas major muscle; 2, ureter; 3, inferior vena cava; 4, sympathetic trunk and ganglia; 5, femoral branch of the genitofemoral nerve; 6, genital branch of the genitofemoral nerve; 7, external iliac artery; 8, external iliac vein; 9, inferior hypogastric plexus and pelvic splanchnic nerves; 10, genitofemoral nerve; 11, common iliac artery; 12, superior hypogastric plexus.*

is withdrawn to the subcutaneous tissue and is redirected slightly caudad or cephalad. The needle is readvanced until the body of the L5 vertebra is encountered or until its tip is observed fluoroscopically to lie at its anterolateral aspect, at a depth of approximately 10 to 12.5 cm. If the vertebral body is encountered, gentle effort may be made to further advance the needle. If this effort is unsuccessful, the needle is withdrawn and, without altering its cephalocaudal orientation, is redirected in a slightly less mesiad plane so that its tip is "walked off" the vertebral body. The needle tip is advanced about 1 cm past the depth at which contact with the body occurred, at which point a loss resistance or "pop" may be felt, indicating that the needle tip has traversed the anterior fascial boundary of the ipsilateral psoas muscle and lies in the retroperitoneal space (Fig. 29-6, *B*). The contralateral needle is inserted in a similar manner, using the trajectory and the depth of the first needle as a rough guide.

Biplanar fluoroscopy is used during needle passage and to verify needle placement. Anteroposterior views should demonstrate the needle tips' locations at a level near the junction of the L5 and S1 vertebral bodies, and lat-eral views confirm placement of the needle tip just beyond the vertebral body's anterolateral margin. The injection of 3 to 4 ml of water-soluble contrast medium through each needle is recommended to further verify accuracy of placement and an absence of spread in the vertebral column. In the AP view, the spread of the contrast media should be confined to the midline region, and in the lateral view, a smooth posterior contour corresponding to the anterior psoas fascia indicates that needle depth is appropriate (Figs. 29-7 and 29-8). Alternately, computerized axial tomography may be used, permitting visualization of vascular structures. Additional precautions include careful aspiration for blood or cerebrospinal fluid before injection and the use of test doses of local anesthetic.

Hypogastric plexus blockade can be used for diagnostic or prognostic and therapeutic purposes. In the former case, a volume of 6 to 8 ml of local anesthetic through each needle is recommended. For neurolytic blocks, a total of 6 to 8 ml of 10% aqueous phenol injected through each needle has been used successfully. To keep the phenol in solution, a small amount of glycerine is added during its manufacture.

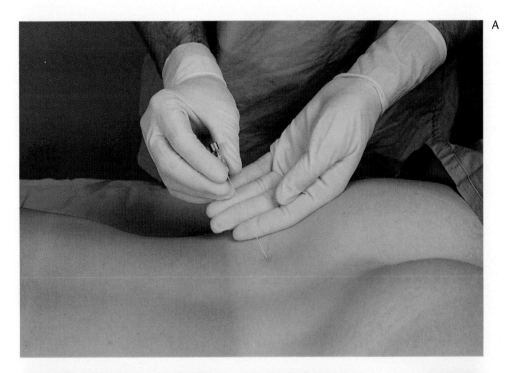

A

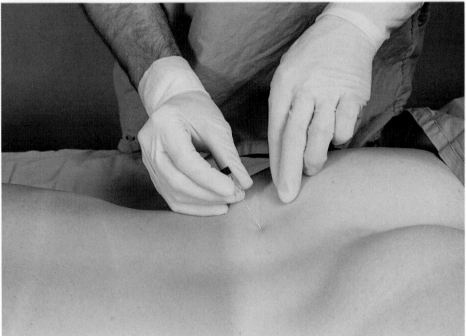

B

Fig. 29-6 *Blockade of the superior hypogastric plexus at the level of the fourth and fifth lumbar vertebral interspace. **A,** Initial needle insertion through the skin at a 45° mesiad angle and a 30° caudad angle directed towards the inferior, anterolateral aspect of the L5 vertebra. **B,** The needle in its final position near the sympathetic chain, 1 cm anterior to the L5 vertebral body at a depth of 8 to 10 cm.*

Blockade of the Ganglion Impar

The patient is positioned in the lateral decubitus position. A skin wheal is raised in the midline at the superior aspect of the intergluteal crease, over the ancoccygeal ligament and just above the anus. The stylet is removed from a standard 8.9-cm, 22-gauge spinal needle, which is then manually bent about 2.5 cm from its hub to form a 25° to 30° angle. This maneuver facilitates positioning of the needle tip anterior to the concave curvature of the sacrum and coccyx. The needle is inserted through the skin wheal with its concavity oriented posteriorly and, under fluoroscopic guidance, directed anterior to the coccyx, closely approximating the anterior surface of the bone, until its tip is observed to have reached the sacrococ-

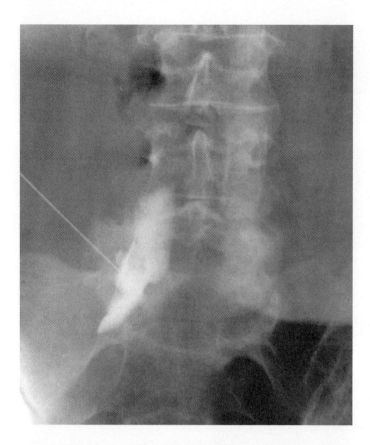

Fig. 29-7 *Anteroposterior radiograph demonstrating proper needle placement for blockade of the superior hypogastric plexus, confirmed with injected radio-opaque contrast material.*

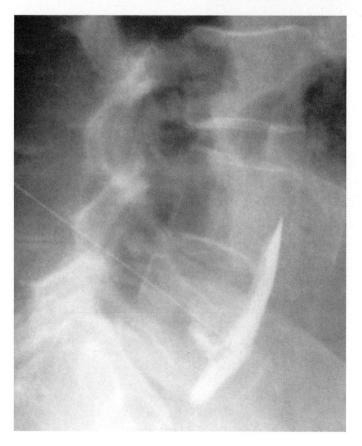

Fig. 29-8 *Lateral radiograph demonstrating proper needle placement for blockade of the superior hypogastric plexus, confirmed by the posterior spread of injected radioopaque contrast material along the anterior psoas fascia.*

cygeal junction (Fig. 29-9). Retroperitoneal location of the needle is verified by observation of the spread of 2 ml of water-soluble contrast medium, which typically assumes a smooth-margined configuration resembling an apostrophe in the lateral plane (Fig. 29-10). Placement may be difficult in individuals with exaggerated sacral curvatures, in which case a second bend may be applied to the needle shaft at the junction of its middle and distal third.

Four ml of local anesthetic is injected for diagnostic and prognostic purposes or, alternately, 4 to 6 ml of 10% phenol is injected for therapeutic neurolytic blockade.

SIDE EFFECTS AND COMPLICATIONS
Superior Hypogastric Plexus Blockade
Overall this procedure is safe, even when a neurolytic solution is used. The most likely potential problems relate to the proximity of the bifurcation of the common and internal iliac vessels. Vascular puncture is not uncommon and may theoretically lead to hemorrhage or hematoma formation, although these have not emerged as practical problems. Accidental intravascular injection may be associated with local anesthetic or phenol toxicity but can usually be avoided by immobilization of the needle, aspiration, and the use of test doses of local anesthetic and nonionic contrast medium.

Resistance to injection should be minimal, as is true generally for retroperitoneal blocks. Unexpectedly high resistance to injection may occur in cancer patients due to lymphadenopathy or local tumor growth. If an abnormally high level of resistance to injection is encountered, the needle should be repositioned to avoid unpredictable spread.

Intramuscular or intraperitoneal injection may result from an improper estimate of needle depth. These and less likely complications (subarachnoid and epidural injection, somatic nerve injury, renal or ureteral puncture) can usually be avoided by careful observation of technique.

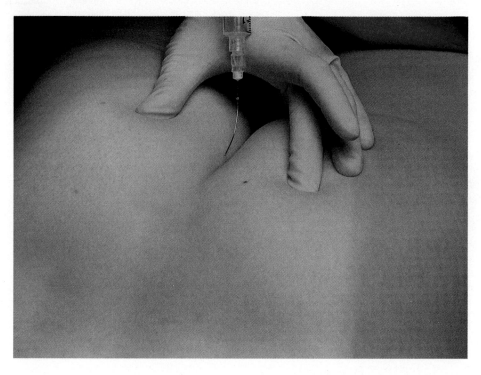

FIG. 29-9 *Blockade of the ganglion impar by passing through the anococcygeal ligament.*

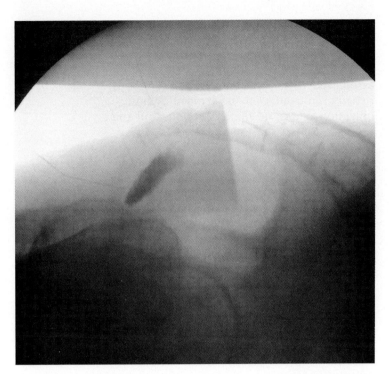

FIG. 29-10 *Lateral radiograph demonstrating proper needle placement for blockade of the ganglion impar, confirmed by the smooth-margined configuration of radioopaque contrast material resembling an apostrophe.*

Blockade of the Ganglion Impar

Under most circumstances needle placement is relatively straightforward. Local tumor invasion, particularly from rectal cancer, may prohibit the spread of injected solutions. If abnormally high resistance to injections encountered, the needle should be repositioned to avoid aberrant spread.

Due to the proximity of the sacral neural foramina and the theoretic risk of reflux into the vertebral canal, observation that the spread of contrast material is restricted to the retroperitoneum is essential. Perforation of the rectum with possible sepsis and periosteal injection may occur if the needle tip is too anterior or posterior. Toxicity due to the accidental intravascular injection of local anesthetic or phenol should be avoided by careful immobilization of the needle, aspiration, and the administration of test doses of local anesthetic and contrast medium.

SUGGESTED READINGS

Frier A. Pelvic neurectomy in gynecology, *Obstet Gyn* 1965:25-48.

Goss CM, editor: *Gray's anatomy*, Am ed. 29, Philadelphia, 1973, Lea and Febiger.

Kent E, de Leon-Cassasola OA, Lema M: Neurolytic superior hypogastric plexus block for cancer related pelvic pain, *Reg Anesth* 1992, 17 (suppl):19.

Lee RB, Stone K, Magelssen D et al: Presacral neurotomy for chronic pelvic pain, *Obstet Gynecol* 68:517-521, 1986.

Neter FH: *Atlas of human anatomy*, Summit, NJ, 1989, Ciba-Geigy.

Pitkin G: The autonomic nervous system. In Pitkin G, Southworth JL, Hingson RA, Pitkin WM, editors: *Conduction anesthesia*, ed. 2, Philadelphia, 1953, Lippincott.

Plancarte R, Amescua C, Patt R et al: Superior hypogastric plexus block for pelvic cancer pain, *Anesthesiology* 1990, 73:236.

Plancarte R, Amescua C, Patt RB: Presacral blockade of the ganglion impar (ganglion of Walther), *Anesthesiology* 1990, 73:A751.

Plancarte R, Amescua C, Patt RB: Sympathetic neurolytic blockade. In Patt RB, editor: *Cancer pain*, Philadelphia, 1993, JB Lippincott.

Snell RS, Katz J: *Clinical anatomy for anesthesiologists*, Norwalk, CT, 1988, Appleton and Lange.

Testut L, Latarjet A, Testut M: *Tratado de anatomia humana*, ed. 9, vol 4, Barcelona, Salvat Editores.

Waldman SD, Wilson WL, Kreps RD: Superior hypogastric plexus block using a single needle and computed tomography guidance: description of a modified technique, *Reg Anesth* 16:286-7, 1991.

Anatomy for Spinal Blockade

Spinal Anatomy

Quinn Hogan

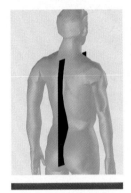

Introduction The vertebral column is the bony reference for a large variety of nerve blocks, including spinal and epidural anesthesia, blocks of paravertebral and prevertebral sympathetic structures, blocks of segmental nerves emerging from the vertebral column, and injections into the joints of the vertebral column itself. The general features pertinent to anesthesiologists are reviewed here.

ANATOMIC RELATIONSHIPS

The vertebral axis is clearly metameric in youth, with 7 cervical, 12 thoracic, 5 lumbar, 5 sacral, and 4 coccygeal vertebrae. There are 8 cervical neural segments; the eighth segmental nerve emerges between the seventh cervical and first thoracic vertebrae, while the other cervical nerves emerge above their same numbered vertebral bones and the thoracic, lumbar, and sacral nerves emerge from the vertebral column below the same-numbered bony segment (Fig. 30-1). The ability to estimate segmental level from palpable landmarks is often overestimated. The most prominent spinous process is usually the seventh cervical, and the line connecting the iliac crests (Tuffier's line) crosses the vertebral column most often at the L4-L5 disk, but there is a natural variability in anatomic parameters, and radiologic imaging is necessary to be sure of segmental level (Fig. 30-2).

Sacral vertebrae are connected in childhood by cartilage, which progresses to bony fusion after puberty. In the adult only a narrow residue of the sacral disk persists. The last lumbar or first sacral vertebra may be indeterminate in formation, with partial fusion of L5 with S1 (sacralization of L5, usually unilateral), or incomplete fusion of S1 and S2 (lumbarization of S1). The posterior roof of the sacral vertebral canal is highly variable in the midline. Fusion is typically complete down to the S5 level, where the sacral hiatus remains open. However, virtually complete closure or the entire lack of any posterior bony roof of the sacral vertebral canal are both possible. Fortunately, access to the epidural space through the sacral hiatus is consistent in children. The coccyx represents the last four vertebrae joined into a single structure.

An archetypal vertebral bone consists of elements forming a vertebral arch posteriorly and the body anteriorly. Stout pedicles that arise on the posterolateral aspects of the vertebrae fuse with the platelike laminae to enclose the vertebral foramen, which in sequence form the vertebral canal. The vertebral canal is triangular in the cervical and lumbar regions, but circular and smaller in the thoracic segments. The transverse process is based at the junction of the pedicle and lamina and extends laterally. The spinous process projects posteriorly from the midline junction of the laminae, is often bifid in the cervical column, and may not lie in the midline at other levels (Fig. 30-3).

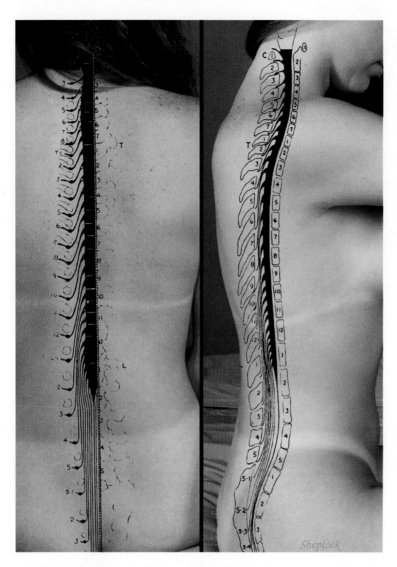

FIG. 30-1 *Posterior and lateral drawings of the relationship of the various nerves and their corresponding vertebrae.* (Overlay from Bonica JJ, editor: *The management of pain*, ed 2, Philadelphia, 1990, Lea & Febiger.)

The vertebral bodies are joined by fibrocartilaginous disks that have an avascular gelatinous core, the nucleus pulposus, surrounded by the collagenous lamellae of the annular ligament. Passage of the nuclear material through rents in the annular ligament may produce compression of the spinal cord or nerves in the vertebral canal, resulting in neurologic deficits. The intense inflammation produced by extruded disk material around segmental nerves may cause neuropathic pain (radiculopathy).

Adjacent posterior elements articulate by true diarthrodial joints, the zygapophyseal (facet) joints. The inferior articular process projecting caudally overlaps the superior articular process from the next most caudal vertebra (Fig. 30-4). In the cervical and lumbar column the facet joints are posterior to the transverse processes, while the thoracic facets are anterior to the transverse processes. The joint surfaces are halfway between the axial and coronal planes in the cervical region, in an even more coronal plane at the

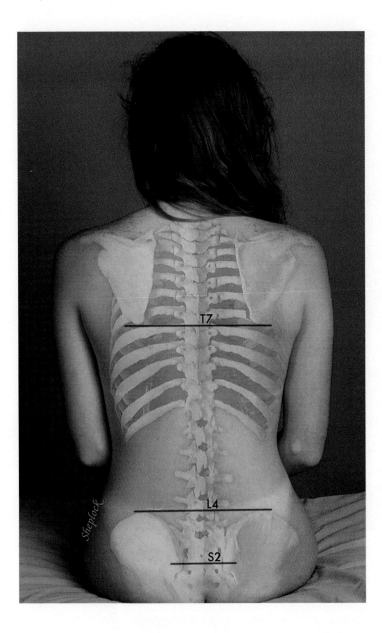

Fig. 30-2 *Computer-enhanced image of the vertebral column superimposed over the surface anatomy. T7 spine is approximately at a vertical line through the scapulae tips; L4 is approximately at a vertical line through the iliac crests; S2 is approximately at a vertical line through the posterior superior iliac spines.*

thoracic levels, and are curved in the lumbar region with the anterior portion coronal and the posterior portion sagittal. Arthritis of these joints with periarticular exostoses is also a cause of cord and nerve compression.

The anterior spinal ligament reinforces the vertebral column anterior to the vertebral bodies. The posterior longitudinal ligament does the same within the vertebral canal posterior to the vertebral bodies and may occasionally be ossified. A heavy band, the supraspinous ligament, joins the tips of the spinous processes but thins and vanishes in the lower lumbar region. The interspinous ligament is a narrow web between the spinous processes. Because these two fibrous structures are composed largely of collagen, a needle passing through them generates a characteristic snapping sensation as the fibers are parted. The ligamentum flavum, in contrast, is 80% elastin, and its dense, homogenous texture is readily appreciated as a needle

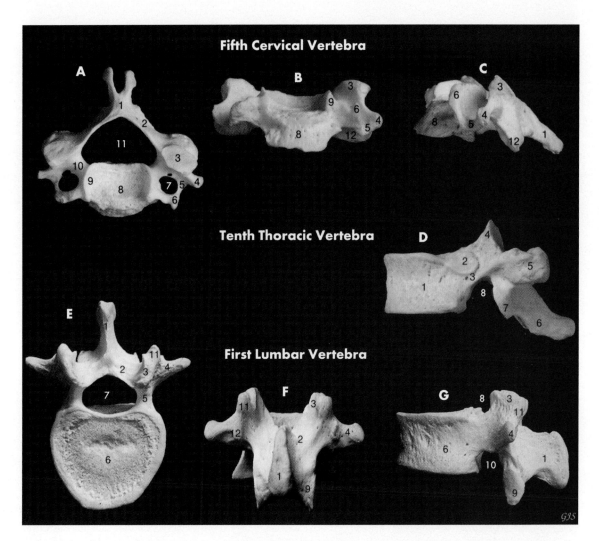

FIG. 30-3 *Comparative views of a cervical, thoracic, and lumbar vertebra demonstrating their comparative anatomy. **A**, Superior view, **B**, anterior view, and **C**, left lateral view of fifth cervical vertebra. Key: 1, Bifid spinous process; 2, lamina; 3, superior articular process; 4, posterior tubercle of transverse process; 5, intertubercular lamella of transverse process; 6, anterior tubercle of transverse process; 7, foramen of transverse process; 8, vertebral body; 9, uncus (posterolateral lip); 10, pedicle; 11, vertebral foramen; 12, inferior articular process. **D**, Left lateral view of tenth thoracic vertebra. Key: 1, body; 2, costal facet; 3, pedicle; 4, superior articular process; 5, transverse process; 6, spinous process; 7, inferior articular process; 8, inferior vertebral arch. **E**, Superior view, **F**, posterior view, and **G**, left lateral view of first lumbar vertebra. Key: 1, spinous process; 2, lamina; 3, superior articular process; 4, transverse process; 5, pedicle; 6, vertebral body; 7, vertebral foramen; 8, superior vertebral arch; 9, inferior articular process; 10, inferior vertebral notch; 11, mamillary process; 12, accessory process.*

passes through it (Figs. 30-5 and 30-6). Tension in the ligamentum flavum is evident as it retracts to half its length on sectioning. It spans from the anterior surface of the cephalad lamina of an adjacent pair of vertebrae to the posterior aspect of the lower lamina. The right and left halves meet at an angle of less than 90º, and a gap may be present in the midline. The lateral edges wrap anteriorly around the facet joints, reinforcing their joint capsule. Margins of the ligamenta flava may include bone even in young subjects.

The lateral wall of the vertebral canal is incomplete, with gaps termed intervertebral foramina between the successive pedicles (Fig. 30-7). Because the pedicles attach not to the middle of the vertebral bodies but somewhat more cephalad, the intervertebral foramina

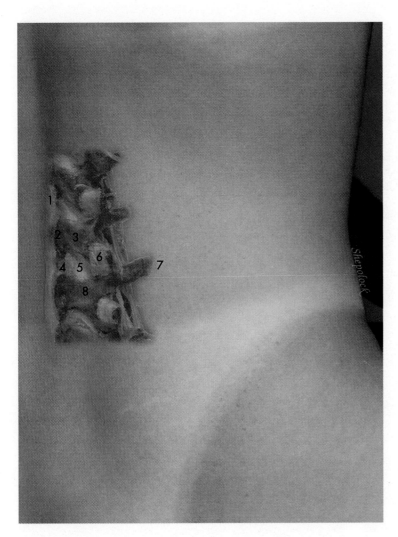

FIG. 30-4 *Dissection of the lumbar spine demonstrating the relationship of the posterior articular elements superimposed over an oblique view of the surface anatomy. Key: 1, supraspinous ligament; 2, spinous process of the fourth lumbar vertebra; 3, lamina of the fourth lumbar vertebra; 4, interspinous ligament; 5, ligamentum flavum; 6, facet (zygapophysial) joint; 7, transverse process of the fifth lumbar vertebra; 8, lamina of the fifth lumbar vertebra.*

are centered opposite the lower half of the vertebral body with the disk at the caudal end of the foramen. The borders of the intervertebral foramina are thus pedicle at the cephalad and caudal ends; anteriorly the vertebral body cephalad and the disk caudally, and a slight amount of the next vertebral body most inferiorly; and posteriorly the lamina, facet joint, and ligamentum flavum. Foraminal stenosis and radiculopathy may result from impingement on the corresponding nerve root by these structures. Disk material extrudes characteristically at a paramedian site, not in the midline that is reinforced by the posterior longitudinal ligament. Extruded material may compress the root exiting at the same level or, more commonly, the next most caudal nerve root. Loss of disk height in turn results in pathologically increased overlap of the facets

as they telescope inward, decreasing the longitudinal dimensions of the foramen. Foreshortening of the ligamentum flavum with loss of disk height causes it to buckle into the foramen, contributing to foraminal narrowing. Finally, arthritis and osteophyte formation of the facet joints may encroach on the intervertebral foramen.

The spinal cord ends with the conus medullaris, which usually lies at about the level of the L1-L2 intervertebral disk, although this is also variable (Fig. 30-8). Anterior and posterior spinal roots arise from rootlets along the cord that fuse into two or three fascicles, which are loosely bound to form each root. Segments that contribute to a plexus innervating the upper or lower extremity have roots considerably larger than at other levels. Since the cord is much shorter than the entire verte-

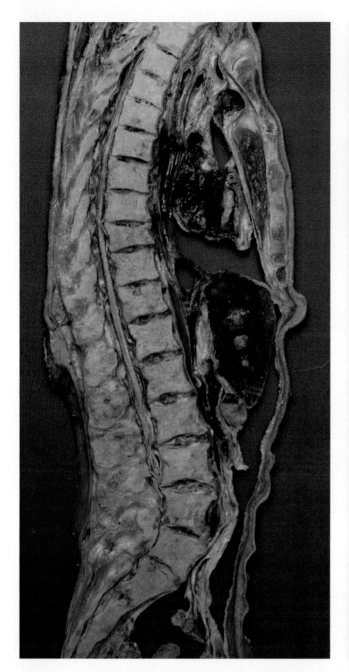

FIG. 30-5 *Sagittal anatomic section through the spine revealing the vertebral bodies, disks, spinal cord, and ligamentous and related structures.*

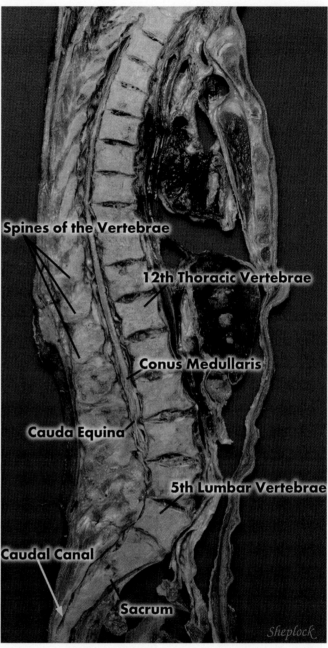

Spines of the Vertebrae

12th Thoracic Vertebrae

Conus Medullaris

Cauda Equina

5th Lumbar Vertebrae

Caudal Canal

Sacrum

FIG. 30-6 *Corresponding computer-enhanced image of the anatomic section with annotation.*

bral canal, lumbar and sacral roots are much longer; these compose the cauda equina. The roots pivot tightly around the inner and caudal aspect of the pedicle as they exit the vertebral canal (Fig. 30-7). The posterior dorsal root ganglion occurs in the foramen just after the emerging root passes the pedicle in the lum-bar region, but is further beyond the foramen in the cervical region and in the vertebral canal in the sacrum. The anterior and posterior roots divide into small fascicles lateral to the posterior root ganglion and then rearrange into anterior and posterior primary rami of the segmental nerve.

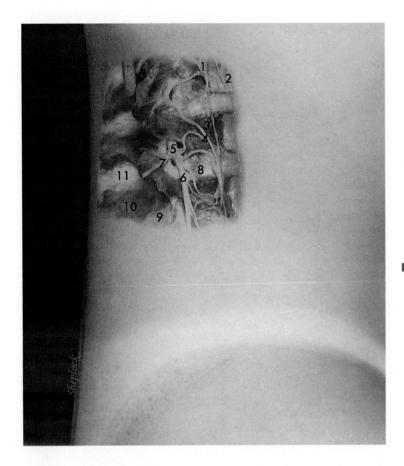

FIG. 30-7 *Dissection of the lumbar spine, revealing the intervetebral foramina, nerve roots, and related structures superimposed over a lateral view of the surface anatomy. Key: 1, sympathetic ganglion and trunk; 2, anterior longitudinal ligament; 3, first lumbar vertebra; 4, rami communicantes; 5, first lumbar nerve exiting from the intervertebral foramen; 6, ventral rami of the first lumbar nerve; 7, dorsal rami of the first lumbar nerve; 8, first lumbar intervertebral disk; 9, facet (zygapophysial) joint; 10, spinous process of the second lumbar vertebra; 11, interspinous ligament.*

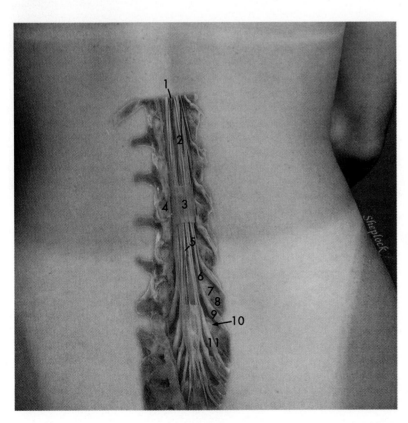

FIG. 30-8 *Computer-enhanced image of a lumbosacral spine dissection with parts of the vertebral arches and meninges removed, superimposed over the surface anatomy. Key: 1, conus medullaris of spinal cord; 2, cauda equina; 3, dura mater; 4, superior articular process of the third lumbar vertebra; 5, filum terminale; 6, roots of fifth lumbar nerve; 7, fourth lumbar intervertebral disk; 8, pedicle of fifth lumbar vertebra; 9, dorsal root ganglion of fifth lumbar nerve; 10, fifth lumbar intervertebral disk; 11, lateral part of the sacrum.*

The vertebral bodies are somewhat hour-glass-shaped. The waist is encircled by segmental vessels passing from the aorta and vena cava anteriorly to the vertebral canal and by rami communicantes following a similar route from the anterior primary ramus of the segmental nerve to the paravertebral sympathetic chain. The vessels enter the intervertebral foramina at its caudal pole.

A thorough comprehension of the vertebral column and spinal anatomy is essential for the anesthesiologist who performs any of the spinal or paraspinal nerve blocks. This understanding no doubt leads to an increase in successful blockade and a reduction of untoward complications from regional anesthetic techniques.

SUGGESTED READINGS

Cheng PA: The anatomical and clinical aspects of epidural anesthesia, *Anesth Analg* 42:398-415, 1963.

Heylings JA: Supraspinous and intraspinous ligaments of the human lumbar spine, *J Anat* 125:127-131, 1978.

Hogan Q: Tuffier's line: the normal distribution of anatomic parameters, *Anesth Analg* 78:194-195, 1993.

Kostelic J, Haughton V, Sether L: Anatomy of the lumbar spinal nerves in the neural foramen, *Clin Anat* 4:366-372, 1991.

Maigne JY, Ayral X, Guerin-Surville H: Frequency and size of ossifications in the caudal attachments of the ligamentum flavum of the thoracic spine: role of rotatory strains in their development, *Surg Radiol Anat* 14:119-124, 1992.

Miyasaka K, Kaneda K, Ito T et al: Ossification of spinal ligaments causing thoracic radiculomyelopathy, *Radiology* 143:463-468, 1982.

Trotter M: Variations of the sacral canal: their significance in the administration of caudal analgesia, *Anesth Analg* 26:192-202, 1947.

Willis TA: An analysis of vertebral anomalies, *Am J Surg* 6:163-168, 1929.

Zarzur E: Anatomic studies of the human ligamentum flavum, *Anesth Analg* 63:499-502, 1984.

CHAPTER 31

Epidural

Quinn Hogan

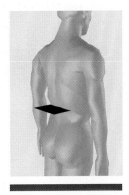

Introduction Injection into the epidural space allows the delivery of analgesic, anesthetic, or neurolytic substances to the nerve roots, spinal cord, and perhaps the segmental nerves. The use of different sites of injection and different volumes and concentrations of local anesthetic makes the epidural route a highly versatile anesthetic method. Dissection is an inadequate method to define the anatomy of the spinal canal since the contents are liquid (cerebrospinal or CSF fluid), flexible (dura), or semifluid (epidural fat), and exposure of the region by removal of the dense bony and fibrous walls destroys the native arrangement of tissue. The result is typical portrayals that are ambiguous or contradictory. The anatomy of the epidural space is becoming clarified using modern methods, particularly sectional imaging by cryomicrotome section, computerized tomography (CT) and magnetic resonance imaging (MRI), and by epiduroscopy.

ANATOMIC RELATIONSHIPS

The epidural space is the area outside the dural sac but inside the vertebral canal. The walls of the vertebral canal include the vertebral bodies and disks anteriorly, the pedicles laterally, and the laminae and ligamenta flava posteriorly. The contents of the epidural space include nerves and vessels, but the majority is fat (Figs 31-1 and 31-2). Whereas the brain is protected by a rigid case, the spinal cord must exist in the flexible vertebral column. A biomechanic accommodation is provided by a padding of epidural fat that is nearly fluid in texture and has nonadherent surfaces that permit gliding movement of the neural structures.

The epidural contents are distributed in compartments that are discontinuous circumferentially and longitudinally, separated by zones in which the dura is in contact with the vertebral canal wall and therefore is an empty space. The posterior compartment of the epidural space is filled by a fat pad that is triangular in axial section. It lies between the dura and ligamenta flava but extends slightly under the caudalmost portion of the lamina above. Since it is not adherent to these structures, catheters or fluid may pass between the surfaces of the fat, canal wall, and dura. The fat pad is attached to a posterior pedicle that enters through the gap between the right and left ligamenta flava in the midline; it may be seen as a midline filling defect in radiologic contrast studies, and as an incomplete membrane during epiduroscopy (Fig. 31-3). This epidural fat is unique in the body in having virtually no fibrous content.

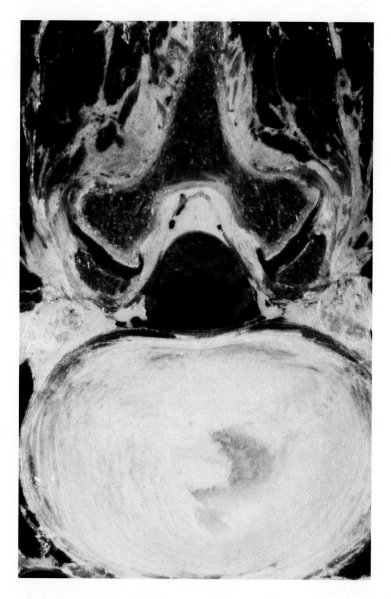

Fig. 31-1 *Transverse anatomic (cryomicrotome) section through the lumbar region, revealing the epidural space and related structures.*

Segmental nerves, vessels, and fat fill the lateral epidural compartment that forms just medial to each intervertebral foramen. Except in advanced degenerative disease, the intervertebral foramina are widely open and allow the free egress of solution injected within the vertebral canal. Historic reports of barriers in the foramina were due to tissue preparation using desiccation and barriers cannot be identified in recent studies.

Stretching laterally from the posterior longitudinal ligament is a fine membrane that completely separates the anterior epidural compartment from the rest of the vertebral canal. This anterior space is occupied almost entirely by a nearly confluent internal vertebral venous plexus, from which emerges the basivertebral vein as it penetrates into the vertebral body. Above the L4-L5 disk, the anterior epidural compartment is obliterated at the level of each disk by attachment of the posterior longitudinal ligament to the disk. Caudal to this level, especially in the caudal canal, the anterior epidural space widens to a capacious fat-filled cavity. This may contribute to difficulty in delivering local anesthetic to the L5 and S1 nerve roots during epidural anesthesia.

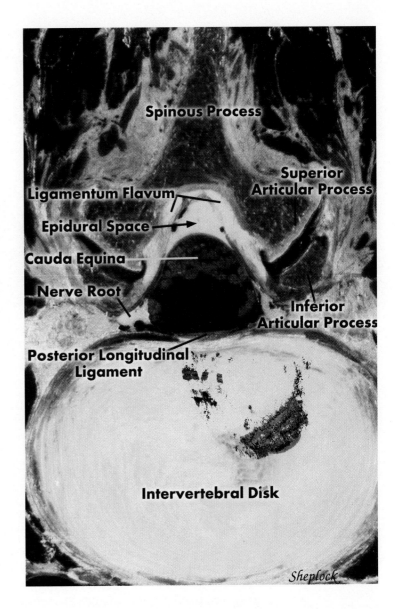

Spinous Process

Superior
Articular Process

Ligamentum Flavum

Epidural Space

Cauda Equina

Nerve Root

Inferior
Articular Process

Posterior Longitudinal
Ligament

Intervertebral Disk

Sheplock

FIG. 31-2 *Corresponding computer-enhanced image of the anatomic section with annotation.*

INDICATIONS

Epidural anesthesia can be performed for virtually any surgical procedure other than those on the head. Unlike spinal anesthesia, epidural anesthesia produces a segmental block with a lower and an upper limit of sensory blockade. It is best to place the injectate at the segmental level of the surgical procedure. This results in the maximum block at the level of maximum nociceptive stimulation, a more limited extent of block, smaller local anesthetic doses, and diminished physiologic consequences of the block. Lumbar insertion is most popular for surgery below the waist, including orthopedic procedures on the leg and hip, as well as for lower abdominal and pelvic surgery. Cesarian section is also an indication for lumbar epidural anesthesia. Thoracic placement of epidural local anesthetic is commonly used for abdominal and thoracic surgery, and is usually combined with general anesthesia to reduce vagal responses and eliminate nociception unblocked by epidural anesthesia. Cervical or cervicothoracic epidural anesthesia is less often used but is suitable for bilateral upper extremity procedures and neck surgery.

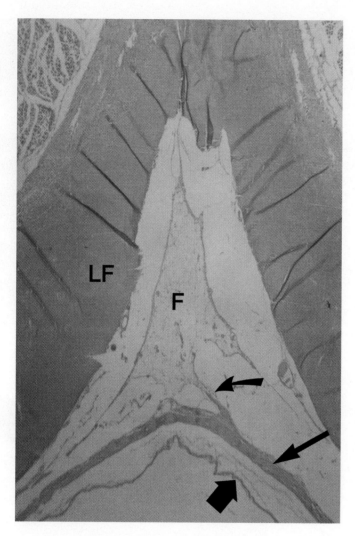

FIG. 31-3 *Posterior epidural fat (F), enclosed by dura (narrow straight arrow) and ligamentum flavum (LF). It is adherent only at its posterior midline surface and occasionally to the dura in the midline (curved arrow). The arachnoid is also evident (heavy arrow).*

Limiting the volume and concentration of local anesthetic minimizes motor block, making epidural injections an analgesic option for medical conditions (uretolithiasis, pancreatitis, angina), labor, and postoperative pain. Epidural opiates alone or in combination with dilute local anesthetics produce analgesia with minimal sensory, motor, or sympathetic block and have proved useful in treating postoperative and malignant pain. Steroid injections at various levels may be used to treat radiculopathy.

REGIONAL ANESTHETIC TECHNIQUE

Epidural needle and catheter insertion may be performed with the patient in the sitting or lateral position. Identifications of the midline, a key to success in performing epidural anesthesia, is more easily achieved with the patient sitting, particularly in a stout subject.

However, many patients with fractures, endotracheal tubes, or advanced systemic disease are unable to sit. Also, sedation is difficult with the patient upright, the vertebral column is less stable when exerting pressure with the needle (especially for thoracic and cervical procedures), and vagal responses are more likely in a sitting patient. Excessive sedation should be avoided, since an obtunded patient may fail to respond to the contact of a needle or catheter with a nerve or spinal cord so that further needle advancement or injection may worsen the injury. Adequate local anesthetic in the skin and deeper fascial and ligamentous structures permits perfection in needle placement without the anguish that repeat insertions may cause. Also, insertion of the large epidural needle is easier after identification of the spinous processes (and therefore the midline) using the smaller-gauge 3.37 cm needle for exploration and anesthetic injection.

The midline approach to the epidural space passes successively through the skin, subcutaneous tissue, supraspinous and interspinous ligaments, and hence into the ligamentum flavum. Because of the perpendicular orientation of the lumbar and cervical spinous processes, a midline needle must enter at an angle nearly perpendicular to the axis of the dural sack. The steeply overlapping thoracic spinous processes require a comparable needle angle (Fig. 31-4). The depth of the vertebral canal from the skin is highly variable, depending on level in the vertebral column, amount of subcutaneous fat, body size, and needle angle, so that no safe rule of thumb can be applied. Because the ligamenta flava are steeply arched, the vertebral canal will be entered about 1 cm more superficially in the midline than laterally, adjacent to the facet joint.

On passing anterior to the ligamentum flavum, injected air or saline readily passes into the plane between the nonadherent dorsal fat pad and canal wall. This is the "loss-of-resistance" noted when the syringe plunger suddenly yields to pressure exerted during

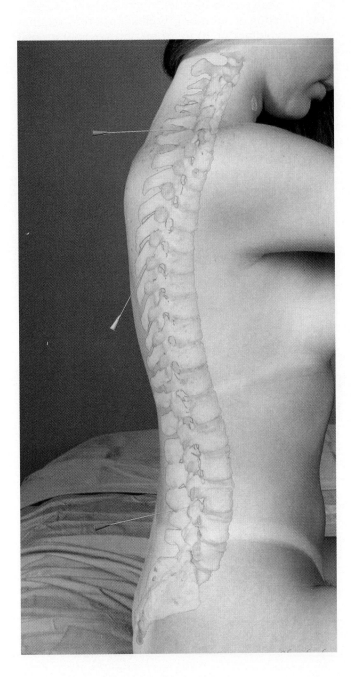

Fig. 31-4 *Computer-enhanced lateral image of the vertebral column superimposed over the surface anatomy, demonstrating the angle needed for needle placement at the cervical, thoracic, and lumbar regions.*

needle advancement (Fig. 31-5). Solution or air injected into the epidural space readily distributes between the surfaces of the various structures and encircles the dura, with only occasional impediment in the dorsal midline, where the dura may adhere to the lamina or fat. Less commonly the needle might pass into the substance of the dorsal fat pad, making catheter passage difficult. If the needle enters the spinal canal lateral to the midline, it may encounter the dura with no further advancement since the dorsal epidural fat pad may be very thin at its lateral attenuations. For this reason, rotation of the needle should be avoided because it increases the chance of the point penetrating the dura.

As the catheter is passed through the needle, a brief resistance to advancement may occur as the tip impinges on the dura (Fig. 31-6). When inserted 3 cm into the vertebral canal, the catheter tip most commonly lies laterally at the internal aspect of an intervertebral foramen, but solution will surrounds the dura circumferentially (Fig. 31-7). Even when the catheter tip lies exterior to the intervertebral foramen in the paravertebral space, distribution of the injectate is preferentially back into the vertebral canal. Catheters that pass anteriorly through the membrane that isolates the anterior epidural space are most likely to enter a vein, often with a perceptible sudden yield or "pop" as the catheter is advanced. Catheters inserted using a more cephalad needle angle, as is done with thoracic epidural catheterization or using a paramedian approach, are less apt to advance anteriorly to where the majority of large epidural veins exist.

Local anesthetic dosing depends on the site of insertion and desired extent of block. Whereas cervical or thoracic epidural injection of 4 to 8 ml of anesthetic produces a band of analgesia or anesthesia (with higher concentrations of solution), lumbar insertion requires volumes of 10 to 20 ml and possibly more if extension of the block into the thoracic segments is desired In general, doses may be reduced with increased age, obesity, and pregnancy, but these are highly variable influences.

With age, loss of disk height causes spinous processes to contact one another. Arthritic changes in the facets further complicate entry into the vertebral canal as the space between the laminae of adjacent vertebrae is narrowed. Even in younger individuals bone may grow into the margins of the ligamenta flava, which may also make needle placement difficult.

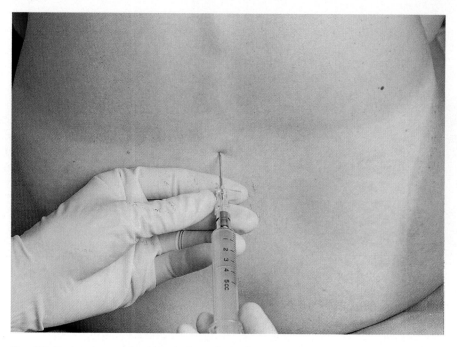

Fig. 31-5 *Lumbar epidural blockade performed via a midline approach in the sitting position. Needle placement is accomplished through the loss of resistance to air technique.*

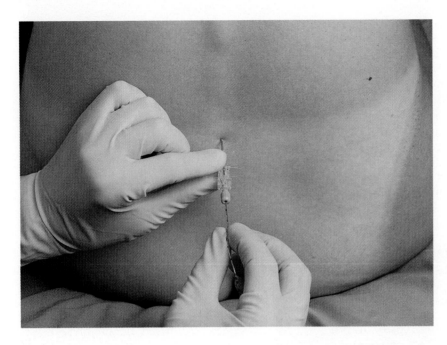

FIG. 31-6 *Lumbar epidural catheter is placed 3 to 4 cm into the epidural space through the needle. The needle is then removed with constant forward pressure on the catheter to avoid its withdrawal.*

SIDE EFFECTS AND COMPLICATIONS

Block failure is almost always due to placement of the needle tip or catheter outside the spinal canal. Incomplete block of L5 and S1 during lumbar epidural anesthesia is probably due to the large size of the roots and the greatly enlarged spinal canal at those levels; injected solution is not compelled to remain in close apposition to the nerves. In contrast, doses must be greatly reduced in the thoracic levels, where the canal and roots are small. Unilateral block probably represents passage of solution along only one side of the canal due to the catheter tip lodging on that side. No evidence of an impenetrable midline fibrous barrier exists, and unilateral distribution is more likely the result of the lateral channel being the least resistant path. Aberrant distribution is less probable after injection through the needle, which is almost certain to lie in the posterior epidural space and therefore not far from the midline.

Compared to spinal anesthesia, a large local anesthetic dose is used, especially for lumbar epidural anesthesia. Such doses, if inadvertently administered intrathecally, will result in extensive block with hypotension and ventilatory compromise. Blood pressure and ECG monitoring is desirable during the procedure, as is supplemental oxygen. Epidural anesthesia must be performed only when intubation and support of the circulation may be promptly initiated. Injection of all or part of the anesthetic solution between the arachnoid and dura mater (i.e., into the subdural space) may result from the needle lacerating the dura but not the more velamentous arachnoid. Peculiar and unanticipated evens may ensue, such as extensive but unilateral blocks if the solution remains in the subdural space, or sudden extensive spinal block with respiratory arrest if the arachnoid finally ruptures and spills the accumulated injectate into the CSF.

Injection of the local anesthetic intravascularly may lead to central nervous system symptoms (loss of consciousness and seizures) or cardiovascular complications (hypotension, arrhythmias, cardiovascular collapse). Local anesthetic must be injected in increments of 3 to 5 ml, with adequate intervals between doses to examine for change in blood pressure and heart rhythm. Epinephrine 5 μg/ml in the solution alerts the operator to this problem early by provoking a tachycardia. Incremental injection is also a key safety strategy to avoid massive intrathecal injection. If extensive block is identified, further injection and excessive block can be avoided.

Needle or catheter trauma very rarely results in nerve irritation or cord damage. More common is a postdural puncture headache if the epidural needle inadvertently enters the subarachnoid space. Epidural hematoma is uncommon but must be considered if backache or neural deficit persists after epidural block. The advisability of combining epidural puncture with various forms of anticoagulation is an unresolved issue. Epidural abscess is rare except when catheters remain in place for an extended period or if the subject has bacteremia, in which case antibiotics are necessary. Diagnostic imaging and surgical evaluation are urgent issues if an abscess is suspected.

SUGGESTED READINGS

Blomberg R, Olsson SS: The lumbar epidural space in patients examined with epiduroscopy, *Anesth Analg* 68:157-160, 1989.

Hatten HP: Lumbar epidurography with metrizamide, *Radiology* 137:129-136, 1980.

Hogan Q: Lumbar epidural anatomy: a new look by cryomicrotome section, *Anesthesiology* 75:767-775, 1991.

Quint DJ, Boulos RS, Sanders WP et al: Epidural lipomatosis, *Radiology* 169:485-490, 1988.

Ramsey HG: Comparative morphology of fat in the epidural space, *Am J Anat* 105:219-232, 1959.

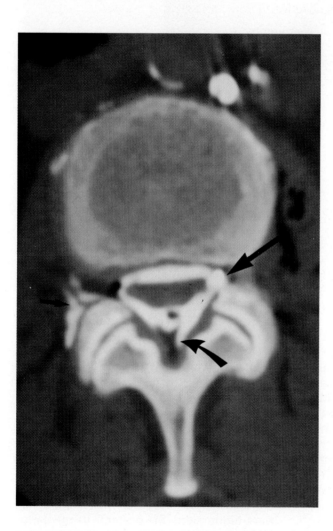

FIG. 31-7 *Radiographic view of the lumbar spine demonstrating anterolateral catheter position (large straight arrow) in the lateral epidural space following midline placement. This is the most commonly observed placement for a lumbar catheter threaded 3 to 4 cm. Nonetheless, fluid distribution is usually uniform, even out the contralateral foramen in this case (small straight arrow). The* curved arrow *demonstrates a filling defect from the posterior epidural fat.*

CHAPTER 32

Subarachnoid

■

Kenneth Drasner

■

Introduction In 1885, to treat a patient suffering from "spinal weakness and seminal incontinence," J. Leonard Corning attempted to inject approximately 4 ml of 3% cocaine between the spinous processes of the eleventh and twelfth vertebrae. Dr. Corning believed that drugs applied directly to the spinal cord acted entirely through the intermediation of the blood vessels, and he postulated that anesthetic injected into this area would be rapidly taken up by the numerous small veins and be transported to the substance of the spinal cord. Within minutes of injection, analgesia of the lower extremities and lumbosacral region ensued, which appeared to confirm his theory. Dr. Corning's early "success" notwithstanding, a thorough understanding of the underlying anatomic and physiologic principles should be considered a prerequisite to central neuraxial blockade. This chapter will discuss the anatomy of the subarachnoid space. It is not intended to be exhaustive, but rather to focus on the anatomic principles most germane to the safety and efficacy of the spinal technique.

ANATOMIC RELATIONSHIPS

The spinal cord begins at the rostral border of the medulla and, in the adult, extends approximately 45 cm to occupy the upper two thirds of the subarachnoid space. In the fetus, the spinal cord extends the entire length of the canal, but because of disproportionate growth of the neural tissue and the vertebral canal, the caudal termination comes to lie approximately at the level of the third lumbar vertebra at birth and at the lower border of the first lumbar vertebra in adulthood. To avoid possible trauma to the cord, lumbar puncture is thus not routinely performed above L4 in the infant or above L2 in the adult. It should, however, be appreciated that lumbar puncture at the L2 level is not completely devoid of risk of direct cord trauma— in approximately 2% of individuals, termination of the spinal cord occurs caudal to this level (Table 32-1).

Attached to the spinal cord are 31 pairs of nerves: 8 cervical, 12 thoracic, 5 lumbar, 5 sacral, and 1 coccygeal (see Chapter 30, Fig. 30-1). Each nerve is formed from the union of a dorsal and ventral root, composed of afferent and efferent fibers, respectively. The roots are, in turn, formed by coalitions of rootlets that emerge in nonsegmented fashion along the ventrolateral and dorsolateral aspect of the cord. The dorsal and ventral roots remain separated within the subarachnoid space, joining to form a mixed nerve only after becoming ensheathed by the dura/arachnoid distal to the dorsal root ganglia. Because the sensory fibers traverse the posterior aspect of the subarachnoid space, they tend to lie dependent—a location particularly accessible to hyperbaric solutions—when the patient is placed in the supine horizontal position.

There are eight cervical nerves, but only seven cervical vertebrae. The first seven cervical nerves exit through the intervertebral foramen above the corresponding vertebra, and the eighth through the foramen below the seventh cervical and above the first thoracic vertebra. The remaining nerves all exit below the corresponding vertebra. Because of the differential growth of the spinal cord and vertebral column, the spinal nerves become progressively longer and assume a more vertical path with caudal progression. Below the caudal termination of the cord, the remaining roots run parallel to the longitudinal axis of the subarachnoid space, resembling a horse's tail, or cauda equina. The roots move relatively freely within the cerebrospinal fluid

(CSF) and, thus, are resistant to direct trauma from a needle or catheter (Fig. 32-1).

The spinal cord is surrounded and protected by three layers of connective tissue (the meninges) and by the CSF. The outermost connective tissue layer, the dura mater, originates at the foramen magnum as an extension of the inner, or meningeal layer of cranial dura and extends caudally to terminate between the S1 and S4 level (Table 32-1).

The dura is a tough fibroelastic membrane that, although easily penetrated by a needle, provides a formidable barrier to a catheter positioned in the epidural space. Indeed, it has been demonstrated that "epidural" catheters are incapable of penetrating sections of postmortem dura, even when maximum pressure is applied while the dura is held taut. Thus true "migration" of an epidural catheter—i.e., from the epidural to the intrathecal space through an intact dura—probably rarely, if ever, occurs.

On the inner surface of the dura, separated only by a thin film of serous fluid, lies the arachnoid membrane. It is avascular and, although far more delicate than the dura, provides the major barrier to diffusion of drug from the epidural to the intrathecal space. Because the dura and arachnoid are adjacent, penetration of the dura by a spinal needle is usually accompanied by passage of the tip through the arachnoid membrane (Fig. 32-2). However, injection of drug (or passage of a catheter) into the subdural space can, and does, occur. Subdural injection of all or part of an intended intrathecal dose of anesthetic may result in complete or partial failure of the technique due to the relative impermeability of the arachnoid membrane. Of note, the side hole position of a pencil-point needle might increase the likelihood of injection into the subdural space; this possibility can be minimized or eliminated if, after obtaining free flow of CSF, the needle is advanced slightly further before injection.

The innermost layer of spinal meninges, the pia, is a highly vascular structure closely applied to the cord. Along the lateral surface between the dorsal and ventral roots, an extension of this membrane forms a dense serrated longitudinal shelf, the denticulate ligament, which attaches to the dura, providing lateral suspension. At the caudal end, the spinal cord tapers to form the conus medullaris and the pia continues interiorly as a thin filament, the filum terminale. At the

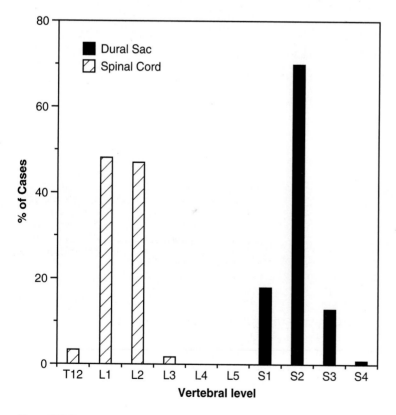

TABLE 32-1

The vertebral level of termination of the spinal cord and dural sac. Data for spinal cord termination are adapted from Reimann and Anson's pooled data of 801 cases from four studies. Sacral termination histogram is derived from the data for 160 cases reported by Evison et al.

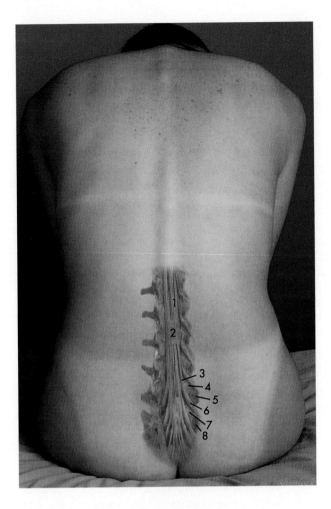

FIG. 32-1   *Dissection of lumbosacral spine with parts of the vertebral arches and meninges removed, superimposed over the surface anatomy. Key: 1, cauda equina; 2, dura mater; 3, roots of fifth lumbar nerve; 4, fourth lumbar intervertebral disk; 5, pedicle of fifth lumbar vertebra; 6, dorsal root ganglion of fifth lumbar nerve; 7, fifth lumbar intervertebral disk; 8, lateral part of the sacrum.*

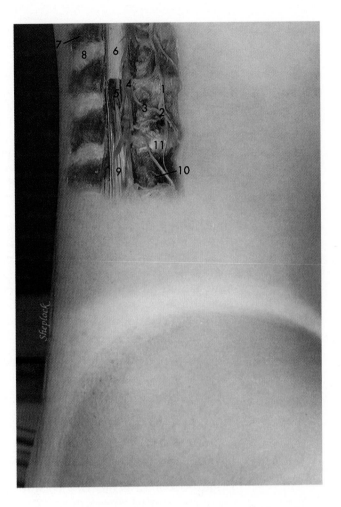

FIG. 32-2   *Dissection of the lumbar region viewed from the right with parts of the vertebral arches and meninges removed, demonstrating the spinal cord, cauda equina, meninges, and related structures superimposed over the surface anatomy. Key: 1, sympathetic trunk; 2, sympathetic ganglion; 3, rami communicantes; 4, dorsal root ganglia of the first lumbar nerve; 5, spinal cord; 6, dura mater; 7, spinous process of the twelfth thoracic vertebra; 8, interspinous ligament; 9, cauda equina; 10, body of the third lumbar vertebra; 11, intervertebral disk.*

caudal termination of the dural sac, this filament becomes enveloped by the dura and extends inferiorly to attach to the posterior wall of the coccyx.

INDICATIONS

Spinal anesthesia is the preferred technique for many surgical procedures involving the lower abdomen, perineum, or lower extremities. Some advocate its use in select cases involving the upper abdomen and thorax; others argue that, because of the potential for patient discomfort and the significant respiratory and hemodynamic effects associated with the extensive anesthesia required for such procedures, spinal anesthesia is less preferable to a well-conducted general anesthetic. Spinal anesthesia has, in fact, been used successfully for cases involving the head and neck, but this application has never achieved widespread popularity.

Spinal anesthesia is useful for obstetric procedures such as vaginal delivery and cesarean section. Differential spinal blockade has also been used in the diagnosis of various pain syndromes.

Few absolute contraindications to spinal anesthesia exist. Certainly, few clinicians would consider the technique in the presence of a bleeding diathesis, full anticoagulation, elevated intracranial pressure, infection at the site of puncture, or patient refusal. Other conditions, such as preexisting neurologic disease, abnormal anatomy, and mitral or aortic stenosis, represent relative contraindications that must be balanced against potential advantages. In some cases, due to medicolegal considerations or a perceived relationships to an underlying ailment (e.g., back pain), it may be wise to forego the procedure even though no true medical contraindication exists.

REGIONAL ANESTHETIC TECHNIQUES
Single Injection vs Continuous Spinal Anesthesia

Spinal anesthesia is most commonly achieved by injection of a single dose of a local anesthetic through a needle. The duration of block can be manipulated by the choice of anesthetic agent, selection of dose, and the addition of vasoconstrictors. Alternately, a catheter can be threaded into the subarachnoid space and anesthesia can be achieved and maintained through repetitive administration of local anesthetic (continuous spinal anesthesia or CSA). The single-injection technique is easier, faster, and avoids the potential for catheter-induced trauma to neural tissue. However, CSA does have potential advantages: local anesthetic can be titrated to effect; anesthesia can be maintained for long cases, yet permit rapid recovery following completion of surgery; and extent of blockade can be better controlled, potentially reducing the incidence of hypotension.

Patient Position

Spinal anesthesia can be readily performed with the patient in the lateral decubitus, sitting, or prone position. The lateral decubitus position affords the greatest patient comfort and is obviously well-suited for the sedated patient.

The sitting position encourages flexion and facilitates recognition of the midline, a particularly important consideration in the obese patient. CSF pressure is elevated and the lumbar dural sac distended, facilitating placement and recognition of the needle tip within the subarachnoid space. However, the relatively high CSF pressure can, at times, be a disadvantage. If a continuous spinal technique is performed with an epidural catheter, considerable fluid may be lost while attempting to thread the catheter through a large-bore needle.

The prone position is rarely used except for perineal procedures performed in the "jackknife" position. Performance of spinal anesthesia in this position is technically more demanding, due to limited flexion, low CSF pressure, and a contracted dural sac. The relative difficulty encountered in obtaining CSF before and after injection attests to the importance of the latter two factors.

Approach

Spinal anesthesia can be accomplished using a midline or a lateral (paramedian) approach. The midline approach is technically easier and more frequently chosen if adequate flexion can be achieved. Because the needle passes through less sensitive structures, this approach produces less discomfort and, thus, requires less local infiltration. However, the paramedian approach is more useful in challenging circumstances such as significant narrowing of the interspinous space, calcification of the ligaments, or inability to flex—the area available for passage through the interlaminar foramen is significantly larger for a needle advanced from an inferolateral position (particularly when the lumbosacral spine is not flexed). The paramedian approach also permits orientation of the needle closer to the longitudinal axis of the subarachnoid space, promoting cephalad spread; this may contribute to the higher success rate associated this approach. In addition, a more cephalad needle orientation confers the advantage for passage of a catheter for continuous spinal anesthesia, particularly if a large-bore catheter is used.

Because of the orientation of the L5 spinous process, the L5-S1 interspace cannot be readily accessed from the midline, so a paramedian approach is required. Most often this is accomplished using the technique of Taylor. As originally described, an intradermal wheal is placed 1 cm below and 1 cm medial to the lowermost prominence of the posterior-superior iliac spine. To reach midline at the lumbosacral interspace, the needle is advanced with an upward angle of 55° and a medial angle determined by the width of the sacrum. Because L5-S1 is the largest interspace and remains accessible in the absence of flexion, it is somewhat surprising that the Taylor approach is rarely used (Fig. 32-3).

Interspace

When selecting the interspace to be used for needle insertion, one must consider the position of the needle or catheter relative to the caudal termination of the spinal cord, the perceived ease of needle insertion, and the influence of interspace on distribution of local anesthetic within the subarachnoid space. The importance of the latter factor is often overlooked, but is demonstrated by the data from two prospective studies investigating the etiologies of failed spinal anesthetics (Table 32-2). In both studies the incidence of failure increased as the injection was performed at progressively more caudal site. A notable

exception, however, is the low failure rate associated with the Taylor approach, which may reflect the prevalent use of this technique for more caudal procedures or promotion of cephalad spread of anesthetic by the cephalad needle orientation.

Table 32-2 Rate of failed spinal anesthetics relative to the level of lumbar puncture.

SITE OF PUNCTURE	MUNHALL ET AL FAILED		TARKKILA FAILED	
	TOTAL	%	TOTAL	%
T12-L2	0/0	NA	1/41	2.4
L2-3	0/56	0	7/541	1/3
L3-4	5/85	5.9	43/1197	3.7
L4-5	3/44	7.3	7/94	7.4
L5-S1	0/15	0	0/3	0

Modified from Munhill R, Sukhani R, Winnie A: Incidence and etiology of failed spinal anesthetics in a university hospital: a prospective study, Anesth Analg 67:843-848, 1988; Tarkkila P: Incidence and causes of failed spinal anesthetics in a university hospital: a prospective study, Reg Anesth 16:48-51, 1991.

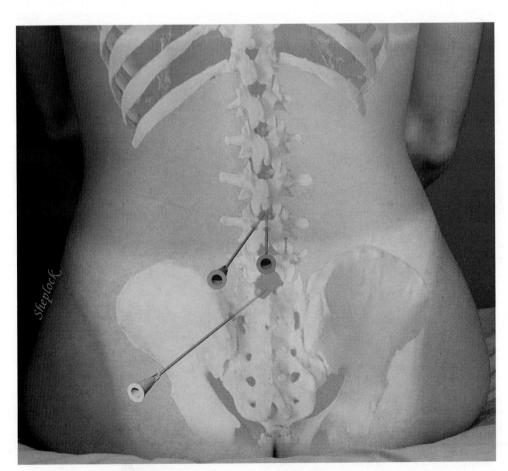

FIG. 32-3 *Computer-enhanced image of the spine and bony landmarks superimposed over the surface anatomy to demonstrate the point of needle insertion for a midline (red), paramedian (green), and Taylor's (yellow) approach to the subarachnoid space.*

Technique

Following identification of the interspinous space and appropriate cleansing of the skin, local anesthetic is infiltrated at the anticipated site of puncture. For the midline approach, anesthetic is injected into the skin and subcutaneous tissue just cephalad to the lower spinous process. In adults, an 8.75 cm spinal needle is inserted and progressively advanced, with a slight cephalad orientation, through the supraspinous ligament, interspinous ligament, ligamentum flavum, and epidural space to reach the dura (Fig. 32-4). However, the use of a 26-gauge or smaller spinal needle is facilitated by placing an introducer into the interspinous ligament before needle insertion to prevent needle deflection or distortion. (With larger needles, use of an introducer rests more on personal preference.) If a cutting needle, such as a Quincke, is used, orienting the bevel parallel to the longitudinal axis may promote spreading of the dural fibers and reduce the risk of postdural puncture headache. In addition, it should be appreciated that the path of a cutting needle tends to veer away from the bevel. Thus the practitioner may choose to direct the needle slightly toward the bevel to compensate; the amount of compensation required is less if a larger needle is chosen or an introducer is used. Following penetration of the dura, the needle should be advanced slightly to ensure that the bevel or side port rests entirely within the subarachnoid space. Once within the subarachnoid space, needles having side ports can be rotated to take advantage of the directional flow of the local anesthetic stream; bevel direction of an open-tipped cutting needle has no effect on the stream trajectory. After demonstrating good flow of CSF, local anesthetic is injected (Table 32-3).

Using the paramedian approach, the needle is generally inserted at a point slightly more caudad and 1 to 2 cm lateral to the midline (Fig. 32-5). Success rests on understanding the anatomy and appropriate angulation of the needle rather than on a specific point of insertion. The most common mistake is to underestimate the distance to the dura and, consequently, angle the needle so that it crosses the midline.

SIDE EFFECTS AND COMPLICATIONS

The immediate adverse effects of spinal anesthesia occur as a direct consequence of the physiology of neural blockade and commonly include nausea, vomiting, hypotension, and bradycardia. For example, in a recent prospective study of 1008 spinal anesthetics,

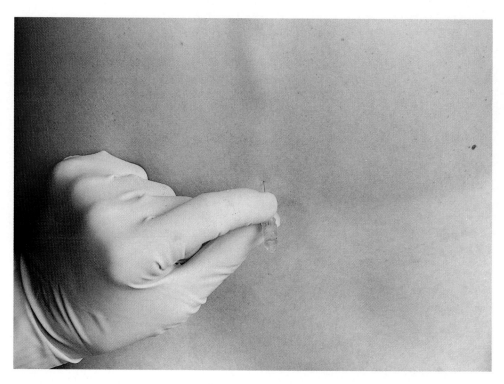

FIG. 32-4 *Spinal anesthesia performed via a midline approach in the sitting position.*

Table 32-3   Dosing for Subarachnoid Blockade (Adult)

		Dose (mg) to Achieve			Duration (min)	
		L4	T10	T4	With Epi	Without Epi
Lidocaine	Hyperbaric	40-50	50-75	75+	60-90	60-90+
	Isobaric		40-50		60-90	60-90
Bupivacaine	Hyperbaric	7.5	10-12	15	90-150	90-150
	Isobaric		10		90-150	90-150
Tetracaine	Hyperbaric	5	6-10	12-15	180-270	120-180
	Isobaric		10-12		180-270	120-180
	Hypobaric	5-10			180-270	120-180

Epi=epinephrine.

bradycardia. For example, in a recent prospective study of 1008 spinal anesthetics, hypotension and bradycardia occurred in 33% and 13% of patients, respectively. In the same study, multivariant analysis revealed several variables associated with the risk of developing one or more side effects. Most significantly, a peak block height >T5 was associated with increased risk for all four of these side effects. In addition to limiting block height, the study identified other modifications in technique that might reduce risk, including the use of plain solutions of local anesthetic (to reduce the risk of hypotension, nausea, or vomiting); performance of spinal puncture at or below the L3-L4 interspace (hypotension); combined spinal and general anesthesia (hypotension); and use of procaine (nausea or vomiting). Although limiting block height and using a lower interspace may reduce the risk of side effects, it is important to note that these strategies also increase the possibility of inadequate anesthesia.

Although immediate adverse effects are generally not serious and easily treated, profound bradycardia and cardiac arrest can occur. As of 1988, analysis of the closed-claims database had identified 14 cases of cardiac arrest in healthy patients undergoing spinal anesthesia for relatively minor surgical procedures. Analysis of these cases suggested that early recognition of the severity of the problem and prompt treatment of asystole with a full resuscitation dose of epinephrine may be critical factors affecting favorable outcome.

Delayed adverse effects or complications of spinal anesthesia range from relatively minor common problems such as headache and backache to rare but severe complications such as arachnoiditis and paralysis. Many factors have been identified or suggested to affect the incidence of postdural puncture headache, including age, sex, needle size, angle of approach and tip configuration, early ambulation, solutions used for skin preparation, and the type of drugs administered.

The potential causes of major neurologic sequelae are numerous and include infection, trauma, ischemia and neurotoxic reactions. Such sequelae are rarely associated with modern techniques. However, the recent occurrence of several cases of cauda equina syndrome after continuous spinal anesthesia has renewed concern regarding the potential for neural injury following spinal anesthesia. Substantial evidence suggests that these injuries resulted from a direct neurotoxic effect of the local anesthetic. The manner in which neurotoxicity may occur can be appreciated by understanding the factors affecting toxicity and how the anatomy of the subarachnoid space affects the distribution of local anesthetic.

The analysis of four cases of cauda equina syndrome following continuous spinal anesthesia revealed two common factors: the development of a restricted block, indicating limited distribution of the local anesthetic within the subarachnoid space, followed by administration of a dose of local anesthetic greater than that usually used with a single-injection technique. It appeared that the combination of maldistribution and a relatively high dose of local anesthetic exposed neural tissue to a toxic concentration of anesthetic. Subsequent cases suggested the same etiology.

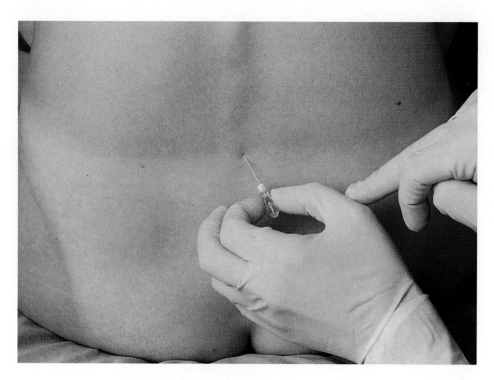

FIG. 32-5 *Spinal anesthesia performed via a paramedian approach in the sitting position.*

Studies performed with models of the subarachnoid space further support this etiology for injury: administration of hyperbaric local anesthetic through a sacrally-directed catheter produces a restricted distribution, and potentially neurotoxic concentrations may be achieved with clinically administered dosages. Several factors appear to affect distribution, including catheter size, tip configuration, tip position, injection rate, and injection velocity.

Although injury associated with microcatheters has received much attention, the tip of any sacrally-directed catheter will likely rest caudal to the peak of the lumbosacral curve. Thus hyperbaric local anesthetic may accumulate in the sacral sac, resulting in a relatively restricted block and high peak anesthetic concentration. Moreover, maldistribution can occur with any spinal technique; it is, perhaps, the most common cause for a "failed" single-injection spinal anesthetic. If a repeat injection is performed after a failed spinal, the potential exists for anesthetic to distribute in the same restricted fashion, resulting in neurotoxic concentrations.

Based on these considerations, preliminary guidelines for both continuous and single-inject spinal anesthesia have been proposed. These guidelines include administration of anesthetic at the lowest effective concentration; placement of a limit on the amount of local anesthetic used to establish a block; administration of a "test dose" followed by assessment of the extent of blockade; the use of maneuvers to increase the spread of local anesthetic should maldistribution occur (e.g., alteration of the lumbosacral curvature or use of a local anesthetic with a different baricity); and abandonment of the technique if well-distributed sensory anesthesia is not achieved before the limit is reached.

With the single-injection technique, aspiration of CSF should be attempted immediately before and after injection of local anesthetic. If CSF is aspirated following anesthetic injection, it should be assumed that local anesthetic has been delivered into the subarachnoid space—total anesthetic dosage should be limited to the maximum dose a clinician would consider reasonable to administer in a single injection. If an injection is repeated, the technique should be modified to avoid reinforcing the same restricted distribution. If CSF cannot be aspirated after injection, repeat injection of a "full" dose of local anesthetic should not be considered unless careful sensory examination (including sacral dermatomes) reveals no evidence of blockade. Recent events would also suggest that relatively high doses of anesthetic should be avoided when a restricted distribution is deliberately sought (i.e., saddle block).

Four cases of transient radicular irritation following spinal anesthesia have been recently reported. These cases suggest an additional mechanism by which anatomy might affect local anesthetic toxicity. In addition to dependent pooling of local anesthetic, it is suggested that transient neurologic toxicity may have resulted, in part, from increased vulnerability from stretching of the sacral roots produced by the lithotomy position. The significance of this complication has yet to be determined, but it does suggest that local anesthetic toxicity may be responsible for less severe, but more common, complications of spinal anesthesia, such as backache.

It should be apparent that the efficacy of spinal anesthesia depends on an understanding of the anatomy of the subarachnoid space. Although recent injuries have renewed concern about the potential for neural injury following spinal anesthesia, understanding and appreciating the factors that predispose to injury should permit continued safe use of this valuable technique.

SUGGESTED READINGS

Caplan R. Ward R, Posner K Et al: Unexpected cardiac arrest during spinal anesthesia: a closed claims analysis of predisposing factors 68:5-11, 1988.

Carpenter R, Caplan R, Brown D et al: Incidence and risk factors for side effects of spinal anesthesia, *Anesthesiology* 76:906-916, 1992.

Corning J: Spinal anesthesia and local medication of the cord, *NY Med J* XLII:483-485, 1885.

Crone L, Vogel W: Failed spinal anesthesia with the Sprotte needle (letter), *Anesthesiology* 75:717-8, 1991.

Drasner K, Rigler M: Repeat injection after a "failed spinal": at times, a potentially unsafe practice, letter; *Anesthesiology* 75:713-14; 1991.

Drummond GB, Scott DHT: Deflection of spinal needles by the bevel, *Anesthesia* 35:854, 1980.

Evison G, Windsor P, Duck F: Myelographic features of the normal sacral sac, *Brit J Radiol* 52:777-780, 1979.

FDA Safety Alert: Cauda equina syndrome associated with the use of small-bore catheters in continuous spinal anesthesia, May 29, 1992.

Hardy P: Can epidural catheters penetrate dura mater? an anatomical study, *Anaesthesia* 41:1146-1147, 1986.

Jonnesco T: Remarks on general spinal analgesia, *Brit Med J* 1396-1401, 1909.

Lambert D, Hurley R: Cauda equina syndrome and continuous spinal anesthesia, *Anesth Analg* 72:817-819, 1991.

Munhall R, Sukhani R, Winnie A: Incidence and etiology of failed spinal anesthetics in a university hospital: a prospective study, *Anesth Analg* 67:843-848, 1988.

Reimann A, Anson B: Vertebral level of termination of the spinal cord, with report of a case of sacral cord, *Anatomic Rec* 88:127-137, 1944.

Rigler M. Drasner K: Distribution of catheter-injected local anesthetic in a model of the subarachnoid space, *Anesthesiology* 75:684-692, 1991.

Rigler M, Drasner K. Krejcie T et al: Cauda equina syndrome after continuous spinal anesthesia, *Anesth Analg* 72:27-281, 1991.

Ross B, Coda B, Heath C: Local anesthetic distribution in a spinal model: a possible mechanism of neurologic injury after continuous spinal anesthesia, *Reg Anesth* 17:69-77, 1992.

Schneider M, Ettlin T, Kaufmann M et al: Transient neurologic toxicity after hyperbaric subarachnoid anesthesia with 5% lidocaine, *Anesth Analg* 76:1154-7, 1993.

Sechzer P: Subdural space in spinal anesthesia, *Anesthesiology* 24:869-870, 1963.

Swisher J. Drasner K. Rigler M et al: Does port orientation of side-port spinal needles affect the segmental concentration of local anesthetic injected into a model of the subarachnoid space? *Anesthesiology* 77:A881, 1992.

Tarkkila P: Incidence and causes of failed spinal anesthetics in a university hospital: a prospective study, *Reg Anesth* 16:48-51, 1991.

Taylor J: Lumbosacral subarachnoid tap, *J Urol* 43:561, 1940.

CHAPTER 33

Caudal

Linda Jo Rice

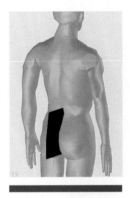

Introduction The sacral approach to the epidural space produces a more reliable and effective block of the sacral nerves than does the lumbar route. This caudal approach is probably the most popular regional technique performed in pediatric patients. Its versatility stems from the technical ease of performance on young children, who have not yet developed the pubertal fat pad or the fused sacra that make this block technically more difficult in adults. Caudal block is, therefore, much more popular in pediatric patients than in adults.

The caudal approach is, however, frequently employed in the treatment of chronic pain in adults. It is particularly useful when the epidural space has been interrupted by previous surgery.

ANATOMIC RELATIONSHIPS

The sacral hiatus, situated at the lower end of the sacrum, is very easy to identify in infants and young children. The triangular sacrum is formed by the fusion of the five sacral vertebrae. Its ossification is incomplete at birth. The vertebral arches become completely ossified and unite with one another and with the vertebral bodies by age 8. The hiatus is due to the nonfusion of the fifth sacral vertebral arch immediately cephalad to the coccyx, and is covered by the sacrococcygeal membrane (Figs. 33-1 and 33-2). The large bony processes on each side are the cornua. In infants and young children these landmarks are easily palpable or even visible through the skin because of the absence of the large sacral pad of fat that usually develops at puberty (Fig. 33-3). Unfortunately, considerable anatomic variations exist in this area in adults, resulting in differences in size and shape of the hiatus that make its identifica-tion difficult (Fig. 33-4). In some instances, even the insertion of a needle into the sacral canal may be impossible.

The sacral canal is triangular in cross section. In addition to the dural and arachnoid sacs, it contains sacral nerves, blood vessels, lymphatics, and areolar fat. The dural and arachnoid sacs usually terminate at the level of the second sacral vertebra in adults but may extend to the S3 or S4 levels in infants. The sacral hiatus is relatively more cephalad in infants, so the distance between the sacral hiatus and the end of the dural sac is relatively short.

The epidural fat in the newborn and small child has a gelatinous, spongy appearance with distinct spaces between the fat lobules. In the adult epidural space the lobules are more densely packed and surrounded by fibrous strands. Thus the infant's epidural space offers less resistance to the cephalad advancement of catheters than does that of the adult.

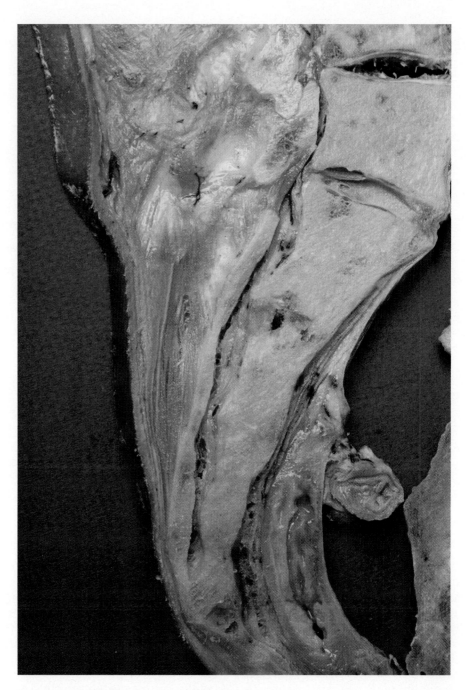

FIG. 33-1 *Sagittal anatomic section through the sacrum.*

INDICATIONS

Single-shot caudal blockade can be used to provide analgesia for most outpatient surgical procedures below the level of the umbilicus or even higher. "Sacral segment" surgeries such as clubfoot repair, circumcision, hypospadias repair, or rectal surgery are ideal for the caudal approach. The caudal block is ideal for pediatric patients because it is technically easier to perform than other approaches to the central neuraxis. In addition, the use of dilute local anesthetics such as 0.125% of 0.25% bupivacaine provide prolonged analgesia without motor blockade. This lack of motor blockade is a distinct advantage for pediatric outpatient surgery. The single-shot approach is most frequently used in adult patients for injection of

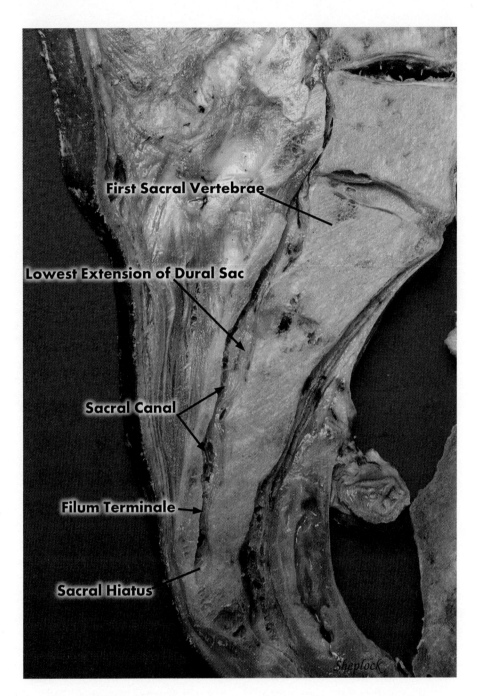

First Sacral Vertebrae

Lowest Extension of Dural Sac

Sacral Canal

Filum Terminale

Sacral Hiatus

Sheplock

Fig. 33-2   *Corresponding computer-enhanced image of the anatomic section with annotation.*

a steroid-local anesthetic mixture for the treatment of various chronic pain syndromes.

Continuous caudal blockade has been used successfully for upper abdominal and even thoracic surgery in pediatric patients, in addition to surgical sites below the umbilicus. In pediatric patients, because of the loose areolar fat, catheters can be placed in the epidural space via the caudal canal and reliably threaded as far as the high thoracic region. Low-dose opioids, in conjunction with low concentrations of local anesthetics, are often infused via these catheters for profound postoperative analgesia. Continuous caudal blockade is rarely employed in adult patients.

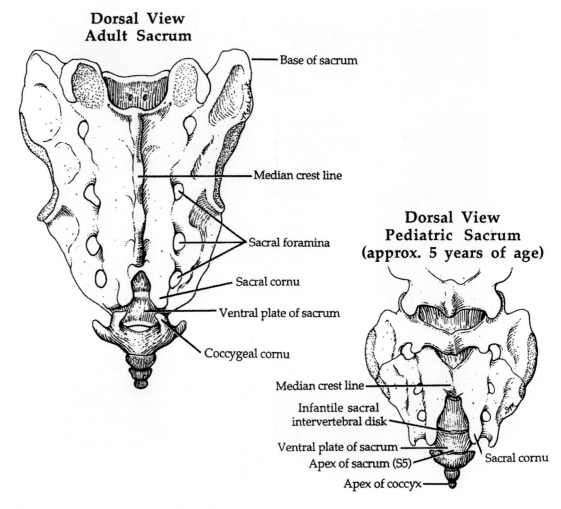

**Dorsal View
Adult Sacrum**

— Base of sacrum

— Median crest line

— Sacral foramina

— Sacral cornu

— Ventral plate of sacrum

— Coccygeal cornu

**Dorsal View
Pediatric Sacrum
(approx. 5 years of age)**

Median crest line —

Infantile sacral
intervertebral disk —

Ventral plate of sacrum —

Apex of sacrum (S5) —   — Sacral cornu

Apex of coccyx —

Fig. 33-3 *Posterior views of adult and pediatric sacrums for comparison.*

REGIONAL ANESTHETIC TECHNIQUES

With the patient in the prone or lateral position, the sacral hiatus is identified (Fig. 33-5). Apply firm pressure to identify the coccyx with the nondominant index finger, then palpate in a cephalad direction, moving the finger gently from side to side. The first pair of bony protuberances encountered are the two cornua of the sacrum that surrounds the sacral hiatus. The cornua should be marked.

Following careful skin preparation, the sacral hiatus is again identified, using firm pressure by the nondominant index finger. Asepsis must be maintained either by wearing sterile gloves or, less ideally, by palpating the skin through a sterile alcohol swab.

Once the sacral hiatus has been identified, the caudal space is entered using a short (2.5 cm), 23-gauge needle (Fig. 33-6). The needle must be placed exactly in the midline and inserted at a 60° angle to the coronal plane, perpendicular to all other planes. The bevel of the needle should be facing anteriorly to minimize the chance of piercing the anterior sacral wall (the most common reason for aspirating blood). The needle is advanced, and a distinct loss-resistance ("pop") is felt as the sacrococcygeal membrane is pierced. The needle is then lowered to an angle of 20° and advanced an additional 2 to 3 mm to make sure that all of the bevel surface is in the caudal space (Fig. 33-7). Further advancement of the needle is not necessary and will *increase* the chances of dural puncture. After the absence of blood or CSF has been demonstrated following attempted aspiration, the appropriate amount of local anesthetic is injected slowly in an incremental fashion.

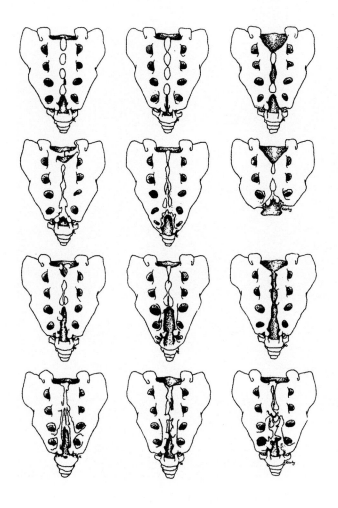

FIG. 33-4 *Posterior views of adult sacrums demonstrating distinct variations.* From Cousins MJ, Bridenbaugh PO, editors: *Neural blockade in clinical anesthesia and management of pain,* ed 2, Philadelphia, 1988, JP Lippincott.

Alternative methods of performing this block include the use of a butterfly needle or a needle and extension tube combination. The block is performed in a similar fashion in adults, frequently employing an 18-gauge intravenous needle and catheter. Following placement of the needle, the catheter is easily advanced into the caudal space, allowing the injection of local anesthetic to be fractionated.

Three important variables determine the quality, duration, and extent of any block: volume, total dose, and concentration of the drug. Using the desired local anesthetic solution, a volume of 0.5 ml/kg will result in an adequate sacral block. One ml/kg is used to block the lower thoracic nerves, and 1.25 ml/kg to reach the midthoracic region. These large volumes are difficult to administer to adults. The total milligram per kilogram dose should always be checked to ensure that it is within the acceptable safe dose of the drug.

Caudal block is most often employed in adults for rectal procedures, for which a total volume of 15 to 20 ml of local anesthetic is required. This approach is also useful for reaching the lower lumbar epidural space, particularly if the patient has had previous lumbar spinal surgeries.

Continuous caudal blockade is becoming the state-of-the-art for postoperative pain management in pediatric patients undergoing intraabdominal or lower extremity surgery. In contrast to the single-shot caudal block, in which the bevel of the needle should be pointed anteriorly, the bevel of the Tuohy or Crawford needle should be pointed posteriorly so that the catheter will advance more easily.

In infants and children it is possible to advance a caudal catheter to the thoracic level, obviating the need for a thoracic epidural catheter. This technique requires careful attention to catheter placement,

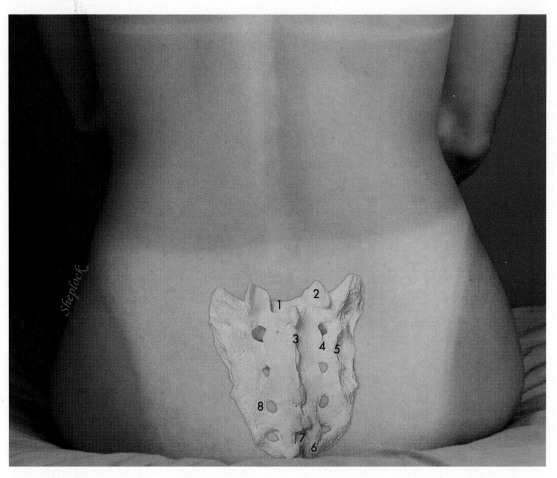

FIG. 33-5 *Image of the sacrum superimposed over the surface anatomy. Key: 1, sacral canal; 2, superior articular process; 3, median sacral crest; 4, intermediate sacral crest; 5, lateral sacral crest; 6, sacral cornu; 7, sacral hiatus; 8, third dorsal sacral foramen.*

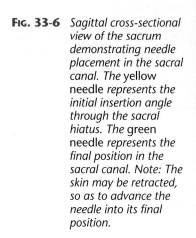

FIG. 33-6 *Sagittal cross-sectional view of the sacrum demonstrating needle placement in the sacral canal. The yellow needle represents the initial insertion angle through the sacral hiatus. The green needle represents the final position in the sacral canal. Note: The skin may be retracted, so as to advance the needle into its final position.*

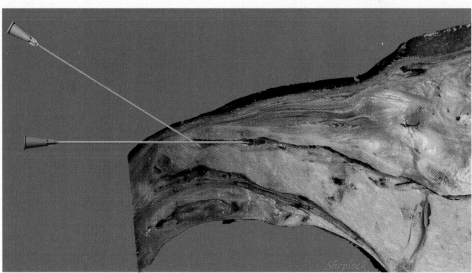

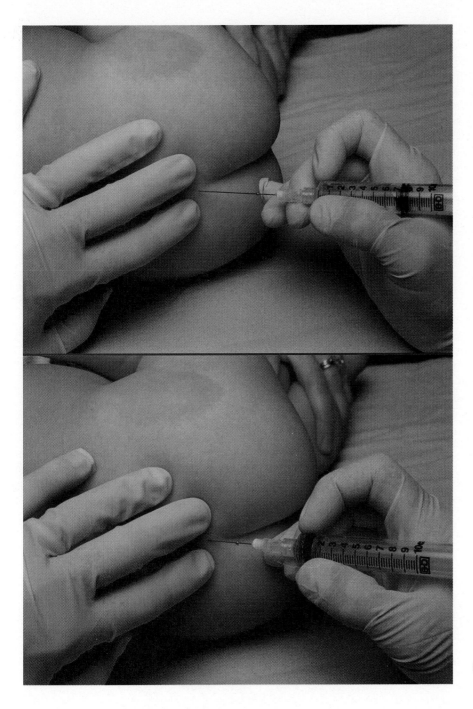

Fig. 33-7 *Caudal blockade of a pediatric patient in the lateral position.*

especially by refraining from forcing the catheter. It is suggested that catheter tip placement be confirmed radiographically before its use. Caudal catheter kits are commercially available. Although there have been no reports of postcatheter infection, daily inspection of the catheter insertion site is imperative.

SIDE EFFECTS AND COMPLICATIONS

Although infection is frequently listed among the complications of caudal block, it generally is not noted in clinical practice. However, careful attention to asepsis continues to be critical. The possibility of intraosseous injection must always be considered when caudal blocks are performed in children. The cancellous mass of sacral bone is covered by a wafer-thin, brittle layer of cortex that can easily be penetrated. Intraosseous penetration is suggested by the appearance during aspiration of a gritty aspirate in a small volume of apparently pure blood. This complication is best avoided by inserting the needle in the line of the sacral canal, avoiding excessive force, and keeping the bevel of the needle directed toward the anterior surface so that it slides over, rather than penetrates, the anterior plate of the sacrum.

Intravenous injection can be prevented by repeated gentle aspiration after each needle movement. Unfortunately, the use of epinephrine in a test dose to assist in identification of intravascular injection is unreliable in pediatric patients undergoing halothane anesthesia. Test doses should be performed in adult patients similar to the way they are performed in other approaches to the epidural space.

Venous air embolisms may occur when the "loss-of-resistance" (to air) technique is used. Thus this technique should be avoided in pediatric patients.

SUGGESTED READINGS

Berde CB: Convulsions associated with pediatric regional anesthesia, *Anesth Analg* 75:164-166, 1992.

Fisher QA, McComiskey CM, Hill JL et al: Postoperative voiding interval and duration of analgesia following peripheral or caudal nerve blocks in children, *Anesth Analg* 17:173-177, 1993.

Gunter JB, Eng C: Thoracic epidural anesthesia via the caudal approach in children, *Anesthesiology* 76:935-938, 1992.

McClain BC: *Pediatric caudal anesthesia: an illustrated handbook*, Augusta, Georgia, 1990, Medical College of Georgia.

Rice LJ, Britton JB: Pediatric regional anesthesia, *Adv Anesth* 11:237-284, 1993.

Sethna NF, Berde CB: Venous air embolism during identification of the epidural space in children, *Anesth Analg* 76:925-927, 1993.

Willis RJ: Caudal epidural blockade. In Cousins MJ, Bridenbauth PO, editors: *Neural blockade in clinical anesthesia and management of pain*, Philadelphia, 1988, JB Lippincott.

Anatomy for Neural Blockade of Axial Nerves

Part

8

CHAPTER 34

Intercostal Nerve

Marc B. Hahn

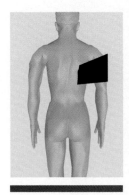

Introduction Blockade of the intercostal nerves produces anesthesia or analgesia in a thoracic dermatomal distribution. The blockade of intercostal nerves is a useful technique for the treatment of postoperative or posttraumatic pain, as well as various chronic pain maladies. This block may be performed at multiple levels or bilaterally.

ANATOMIC RELATIONSHIPS

The intercostal nerves arise from the anterior rami of the first through twelfth paired thoracic nerve roots (Figs. 34-1 and 34-2). Fibers from the first thoracic nerve join with fibers of C8 to become the lowest trunk of the brachial plexus.

The intercostal nerves pass at the inferior border of the corresponding rib between the external and internal intercostal muscles, which are superficial, and the innermost intercostal muscle. The nerve travels inferior to the intercostal artery and vein in the costal groove (Fig. 34-3). At the midaxillary line the intercostal nerve gives off the lateral cutaneous branch, which supplies cutaneous sensation to the lateral thorax and abdomen. The lateral cutaneous branch of the first intercostal nerve supplies sensation to the skin of the axilla. The lateral cutaneous branch of the second intercostal nerve is the intercostalbrachial nerve, which supplies sensation to the skin of the

medial aspect of the arm. Just before the midline, the intercostal nerve gives off the anterior cutaneous branch, which supplies cutaneous sensation to the anterior thorax and abdomen (Fig. 34-4). Motor branches of the first six pairs of intercostal nerves supply the corresponding intercostal, subcostal, serratus posterior superior, and transverse thoracic muscles. The lower five pairs supply the intercostal, subcostal, serratus posterior inferior, transverse, oblique, and rectus abdominal muscles.

The twelfth thoracic nerve is not considered an intercostal nerve because it travels in a subcostal course. Fibers of the twelfth thoracic nerve join with fibers from L1 to become the ilioinguinal and iliohypogastric nerves.

INDICATIONS

Blockade of one or more intercostal nerves can provide profound anesthesia or analgesia in a dermatomal distribution (see Fig. 1 in the Preface).

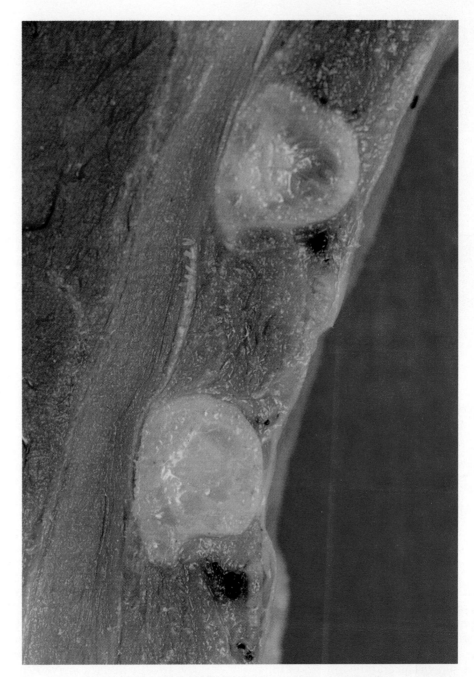

FIG. 34-1 *Parasagittal anatomic section of the chest wall, demonstrating the relationship of the ribs, musculature, thoracic cavity, and intercostal neurovascular bundle.*

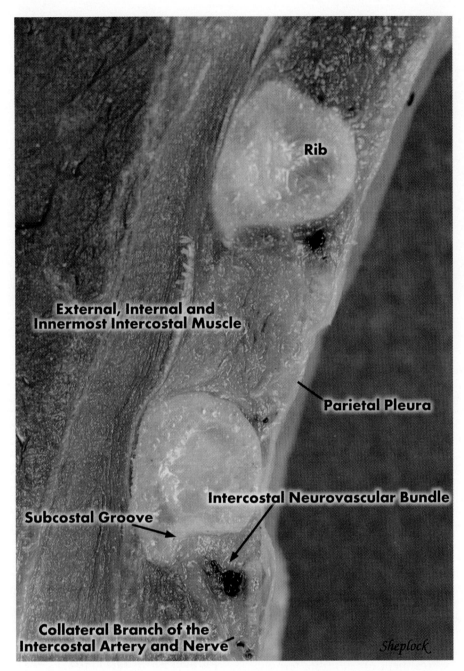

FIG. 34-2 *Corresponding computer-enhanced image of the anatomic section with annotation.*

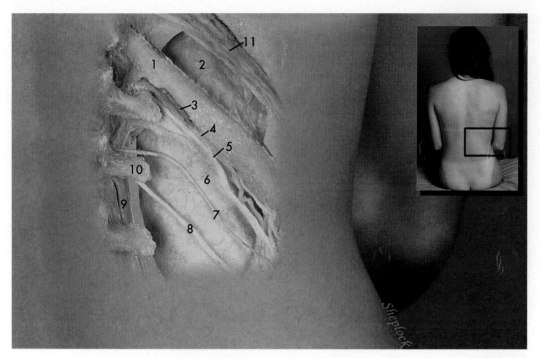

FIG. 34-3 *Dissection of the distribution for the branches of an intercostal nerve with most of the thoracic and abdominal muscles removed, superimposed over the surface anatomy. Key: 1, twelfth rib; 2, costophrenic recess of the pleura; 3, subcostal vein; 4, subcostal artery; 5, subcostal nerve; 6, kidney; 7, iliohypogastric nerve; 8, ilioinguinal nerve; 9, psoas major muscle; 10, transverse process of the second lumbar vertebra; 11, eleventh intercostal nerve.*

Minor surgical procedures of the chest or abdominal walls can be performed following blockade of the corresponding intercostal nerves. Postoperative and posttraumatic somatic pain can be adequately blocked with this technique. Intercostal nerve blocks may also be used in both diagnosis and treatment of various chronic pain states, such as intercostal neuralgias and metastatic lesions.

The use of neurolytic agents may be quite useful in the treatment of pain from terminal metastatic lesions.

REGIONAL ANESTHETIC TECHNIQUE
Lateral Technique
The patient is placed in a sitting or lateral position, with the involved side up. The ipsilateral arm is raised above the head to assist in abducting the scapula, thus exposing the angles of the ribs. The skin over the rib in the selected dermatome is retracted in a cephalad direction. A skin wheal with local anesthetic precedes the placement of a 3.75-cm, 22-gauge, short beveled block needle. The needle is advanced at a 45° angle toward the inferior border of the rib. After contact is made with the rib, the cephalad traction is slowly released, allowing the needle to be "walked" under the rib at the same angle and advanced 2 to 4 mm (Fig. 34-5). After careful aspiration for blood, 3 to 5 ml of local anesthetic is injected.

Paravertebral Technique
The patient is placed in a sitting, prone, or lateral position, with the involved side up. The thoracic spinous processes are palpated. They are at an acute angle and thus their tip lies adjacent to the transverse process of the vertebrae at one level inferior. The skin 3 cm lateral to the spinous process at the selected dermatome is retracted in a cephalad direction. A skin wheal with local anesthetic precedes the placement of a 8.75-cm, 22-gauge spinal needle. The needle is advanced at a 45° angle toward the junction of a transverse process and the adjoining rib, with a slight

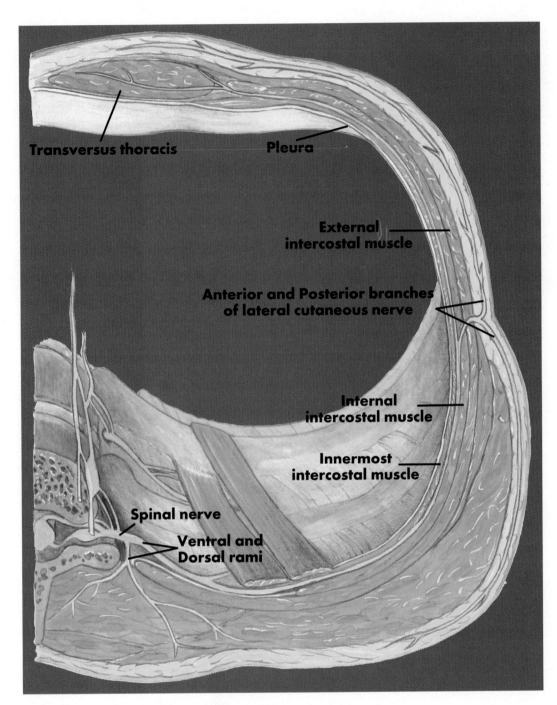

Fig. 34-4 *Line drawing demonstrating the distribution of an intercostal nerve.*

medial angle. After contact is made with the transverse process, the cephalad traction is slowly released, allowing the needle to be walked under the lateral processes at the same angle and advanced 2 mm (Fig. 34-6). After careful aspiration for blood and cerebrospinal fluid, 3 to 5 ml of local anesthetic is injected.

SIDE EFFECTS AND COMPLICATIONS

The primary concern following an intercostal nerve block is pneumothorax. However, this complication occurs infrequently. When it does occur, the pneumothoraces are usually small and the patient may be

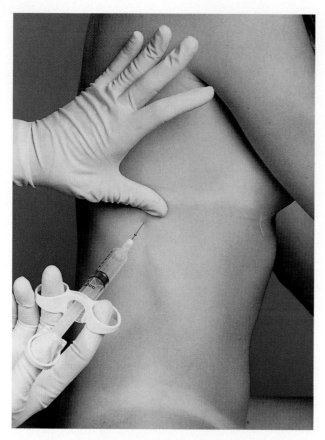

FIG. 34-5 *Intercostal nerve block at the angle of the rib.*

asymptomatic. Often treatment consists of oxygen therapy and needle aspiration; chest tubes are reserved for large or symptomatic pneumothoraces.

Local anesthetics are absorbed quite rapidly following an intercostal nerve block because of the increased vascularity of the intercostal space. Following multiple intercostal injections with large volumes of local anesthetic, the serum concentration may promptly reach toxic levels leading to neurologic or cardiovascular sequelae (see Chapter 2). Calculation of safe doses of local anesthetic is of paramount importance when performing multiple intercostal blocks.

Subarachnoid or epidural injection of local anesthetic may occur when using the paravertebral technique for intercostal blockade.

SUGGESTED READINGS

Carron H, Korbon GA, Rowlingson JC, editors: *Regional anesthesia*, Orlando, 1984, Grune and Stratton.
Netter F, Mitchell GAG: Nerve plexuses and peripheral nerves. In Brass, A, editor: *The CIBA collection of medical illustrations*, New Jersey, 1983, CIBA.
Snell RS, editor: *Clinical anatomy for medical students*, Boston, 1973, Little, Brown.

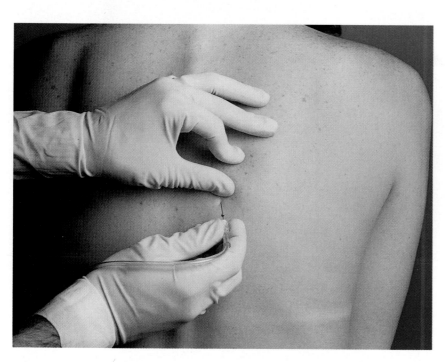

FIG. 34-6 *Intercostal nerve block via the paravertebral technique.*

CHAPTER 35

Ilioinguinal, Iliohypogastric, and Genitofemoral Nerves

Lynn Broadman

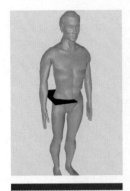

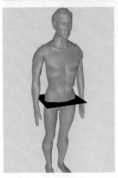

Introduction Blockade of ilioinguinal, iliohypogastric, and genitofemoral nerves produces anesthesia for unilateral surgical procedures of the groin. Blockade of these nerves may also be used to provide postoperative analgesia, as well as for the diagnosis and treatment of chronic pain syndromes.

ANATOMIC RELATIONSHIP

Innervation to the inguinal region is supplied by contributions from the lumbar plexus. More specifically, pain sensation to the inguinal region is transmitted by the ilioinguinal (L1), iliohypogastric (T12, L1) and the genitofemoral (L1, L2) nerves. The ilioinguinal and iliohypogastric nerves lie just medial to the anterior superior iliac spine and can be found between the fascial layers of the external oblique, internal oblique, and transversus abdominis muscle (Figs. 35-1 and 35-2). The iliohypogastric nerve provides skin sensation to the area above the inguinal liga-

ment. The ilioinguinal nerve travels in close proximity to the iliohypogastric nerve and, as previously mentioned, both lie about 2.5 cm medial to the anterior superior iliac crest. The ilioinguinal nerve then courses along the surface of the internal oblique muscle until it accompanies the spermatic cord and, finally, passes through the superficial inguinal ring. The ilioinguinal nerve then supplies skin sensation to the root of the penis and scrotum in men and the labia majora and mons pubis in women. The genitofemoral nerve passes through the psoas major muscle and divides into its two terminal branches, the femoral branch and the genital branch (Fig. 35-3).

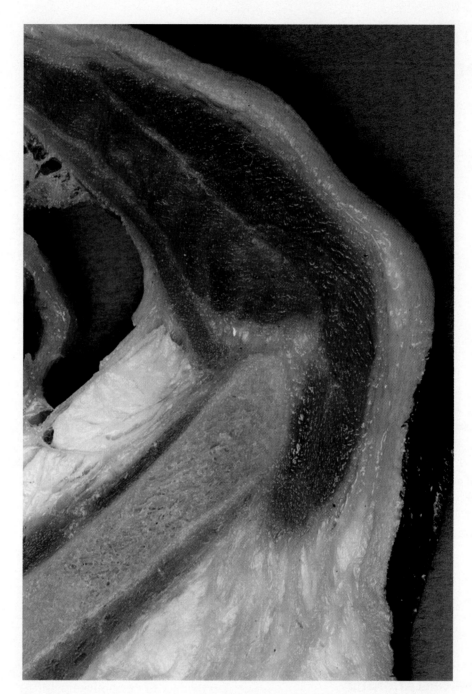

FIG. 35-1 *Transverse anatomic section through the pelvis at the level of the anterior superior iliac spine, revealing the relationship of the ilioinguinal and iliohypogastric nerves and related structures.*

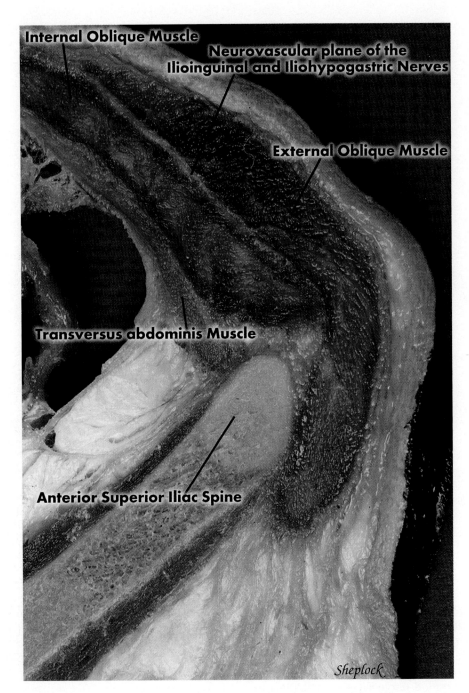

FIG. 35-2 *Corresponding computer-enhanced image of the anatomic section with annotation.*

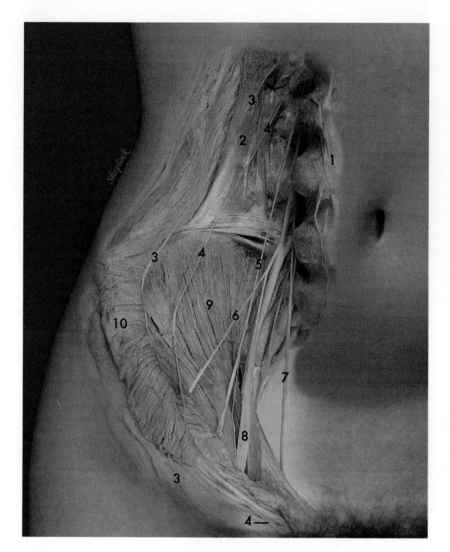

FIG. 35-3 *Dissection of the ilioinguinal, iliohypogastric, and genitofemoral nerves with the psoas muscle removed, superimposed over the surface anatomy. Key: 1, third lumbar vertebra and anterior longitudinal ligament; 2, quadratus lumborum muscle; 3, iliohypogastric nerve; 4, ilioinguinal nerve; 5, genitofemoral nerve; 6, lateral femoral cutaneous nerve; 7, obturator nerve; 8, femoral nerve; 9, iliacus muscle; 10, internal oblique muscle.*

This bifurcation takes place cephalad to the inguinal ligament. The femoral branch of the genitofemoral nerve joins the femoral artery and femoral nerve. The three structures then pass beneath the inguinal ligament and enter the femoral triangle. The femoral branch of the genitofemoral nerve supplies sensation to the skin just below the inguinal ligament. The genital branch of the genitofemoral nerve joins the spermatic cord and passes through the superficial inguinal ring (Figs. 35-4 and 35-5). Like the ilioinguinal nerve, it supplies sensation to the scrotum in men and labia in women (Fig. 35-6).

INDICATIONS

An ilioinguinal/iliohypogastric nerve block may be used in conjunction with a genitofemoral nerve block to provide operative anesthesia for inguinal herniorrhaphy, orchiopexy, or hydrocelectomy. The blocks may also be used to provide postoperative pain relief following these same surgical procedures and to assist in the diagnosis of postherniorrhaphy nerve entrapment pain syndromes.

REGIONAL ANESTHETIC TECHNIQUE
"Splash" Technique

If the blocks are being performed to provide postoperative pain relief following herniorrhaphy or orchiopexy surgery conducted under either general or spinal anesthesia, then splash bupivacaine is the easiest way to achieve this goal. The surgeon simply instills 5 to 10 ml of 0.25% bupivacaine into the inguinal herniorrhaphy wound at the completion of surgery just before skin closure (Fig. 35-7). No needle is used to perform this block;

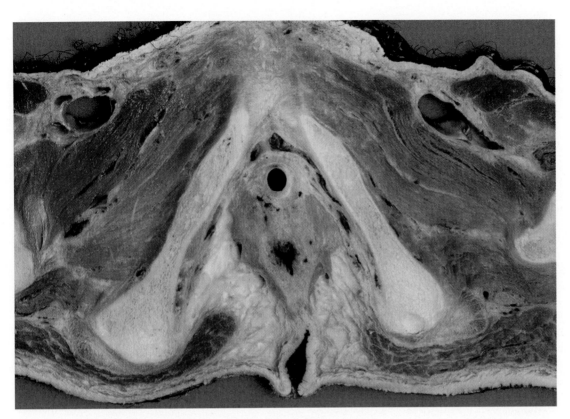

Fig. 35-4 *Transverse anatomic section through the pelvis at the level of the pubic tubercule, revealing the relationship of the genitofemoral nerve and related structures.*

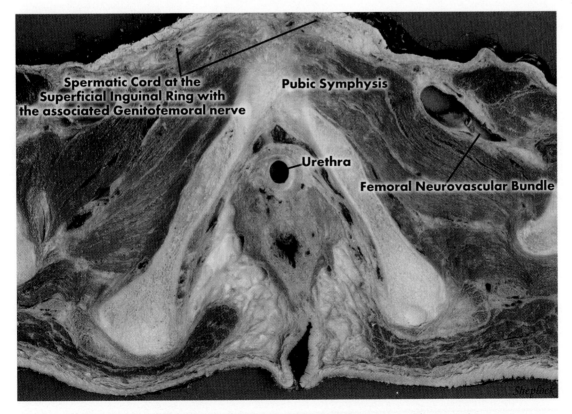

Fig. 35-5 *Corresponding computer-enhanced image of the anatomic section with annotation.*

therefore, little possibility exists of obtaining an intravascular injection. The surgeon "splashes" the local anesthetic solution into the wound and allows it to bathe the nerve endings and skin edges for about one minute. The iliohypogastric and ilioinguinal nerves are exposed to the local anesthetic solution as they cross the surface of the oblique muscles. Likewise, the ilioinguinal and genitofemoral nerves are bathed with local anesthetic solution, which passes down the exposed hernia sac and runs into the inguinal ring. Excess local anesthetic solution is removed with a sterile sponge before closure. Unfortunately the splash block cannot provide adjunct operative anesthesia, but it does provide excellent postoperative pain relief.

Percutaneous Technique

The percutaneous approach to blocking the ilioinguinal and iliohypogastric nerves can be used to provide operative anesthesia in addition to postoperative analgesia for herniorrhaphy and orchiopexy surgery. First the anesthetist raises a skin wheal over the needle puncture site with a 30-gauge needle using

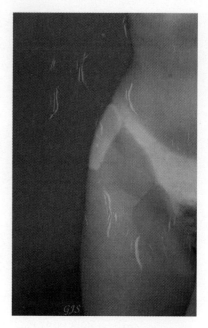

FIG. 35-6 *Sensory distribution of the genital (red) and femoral (blue) branches of the genitofemoral nerve and the iliohypogastric (lateral cutaneous branch) (yellow) nerve.*

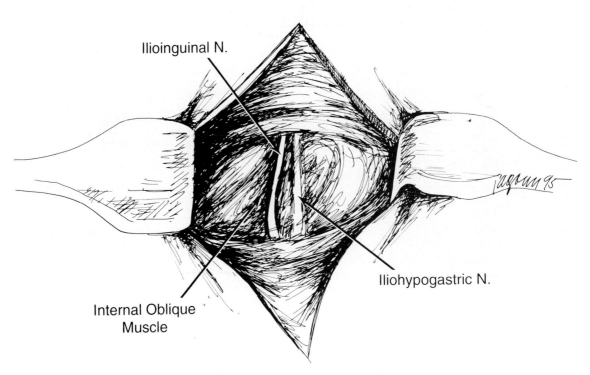

FIG. 35-7 *Blockade of the ilioinguinal, iliohypogastric, and genitofemoral nerves via the "splash technique." Local anesthetic is simply instilled into the herniorrhaphy site before skin closure.*

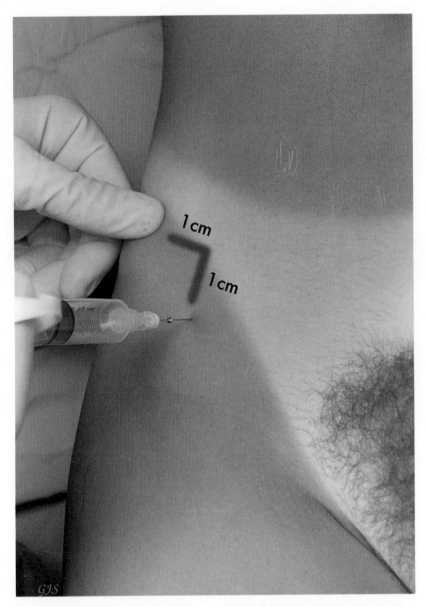

Fig. 35-8 *Blockade of the ilioinguinal and iliohypogastric nerves via the traditional percutaneous approach. Note the anesthetist's left thumb is palpating the patient's anterior superior iliac spine.*

local anesthetic. Then a 2.5 cm, 23-gauge needle is used to penetrate the skin about 2.5 cm medial and caudal to the anterosuperior iliac spine, and the oblique muscles are percutaneously infiltrated in a fanlike manner with 5 to 10 ml of local anesthetic (Fig. 35-8).

The genital branch of the genitofemoral nerve may be blocked percutaneously by injecting 3 to 5 ml of local anesthetic solution into the tissue that lies below the inguinal ligament just lateral to the pubic tubercle. This injection can be performed with a 2.5 cm, 23-

gauge needle (Fig. 35-9). Blockade of the genitofemoral nerve through percutaneous entry into the inguinal ring is discouraged because either the testicular artery or vein may be punctured, which may lead to the development of a sizable hematoma.

The blocks can also be performed at the completion of surgery by infiltrating the oblique muscles through the lateral edge of the herniorrhaphy incision in a fanlike manner with a 23- to 25-gauge needle and 5 to 10 ml of local anesthetic. Again, the genitofemoral

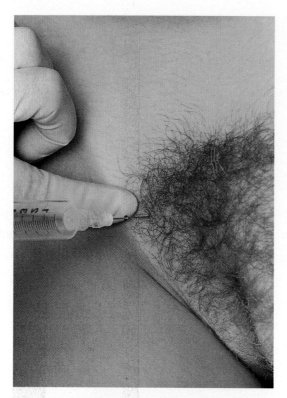

FIG. 35-9 *Blockade of the genitofemoral nerve via the percutaneous approach.*

nerve will be blocked when the excess local anesthetic solution runs down the hernia sac and enters the inguinal ring. If this block is performed early in the surgical procedure, it can be used to provide adjunct operative anesthesia; otherwise it will only provide postoperative pain relief. Performing this block at the completion of surgery has little advantage over the previously described "splash" technique.

SIDE EFFECTS AND COMPLICATIONS

Inadvertent blockade of the lateral femoral cutaneous nerve of the thigh is not uncommon when performing ilioinguinal and iliohypogastric nerve blocks.

SUGGESTED READINGS

Buleau Grant JC: *Grant's atlas of anatomy*, Baltimore, 1972, Williams and Wilkins.

Casey WF, Rice LJ, Hannallah RS et al: A comparison between bupivacaine instillation versus ilioinguinal/iliohypogastric nerve block for postoperative analgesia following inguinal herniorrhaphy in children, *Anesthesiology* 72:637-639, 1990.

Katz J: *Atlas of regional anesthesia*, Norwalk CT, 1993, Appleton and Lange.

CHAPTER 36

Suprascapular Nerve

Winston C. V. Parris

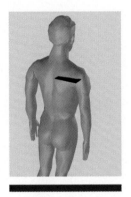

Introduction Many patients suffering from shoulder trauma or arthropathy may develop intractable pain syndromes that require aggressive management. A common approach for chronic shoulder pain is to perform a blockade of the suprascapular nerve with local anesthetics (with or without steroids) followed by appropriate physical therapy.

Suprascapular nerve blocks therefore have a major place in sports medicine and orthopedic shoulder manipulations. These blocks facilitate aggressive physical therapy and also serve to minimize pain after shoulder surgery.

ANATOMIC RELATIONSHIPS

The suprascapular nerve has both sensory and motor function. It is derived from the brachial plexus and is located in the posterior triangle of the neck. Its specific origin is the anterior primary rami of the fifth and sixth cervical nerve roots. It is located above the clavicle as it leaves the upper trunk of the brachial plexus, traversing posteriorly to disappear beneath the border of the trapezius. It then passes through the suprascapular foramen beneath the transverse scapular ligament and, at that level, supplies the supraspinatus muscle (Figs. 36-1 and 36-2). The suprascapular nerve then descends lateral to the spine of the scapula and, along with the suprascapular vessels, supplies the infraspinatus muscle. The suprascapular nerve also gives off sensory branches to the shoulder joint and to the tendinous portion of the rotator cuff (the subscapularis and teres major muscles) (Fig. 36-3). In patients in whom the transverse scapular ligament is not well developed, the suprascapular foramen is referred to as the suprascapular notch (fossa).

Paresthesias are often elicited at this point during the performance of the suprascapular nerve block.

INDICATIONS

Blockade of the suprascapular nerve is indicated for patients with shoulder pain secondary to rotator cuff lesions, osteoarthritis of the shoulder, or adhesive capsulitis ("frozen shoulder"). These lesions may follow trauma to the cervical or periscapular area, including the shoulder, or may be the result of degenerative disorders of musculoskeletal tissue in the shoulder region. This nerve block is usually followed by aggressive physical therapy to strengthen muscles and lyse adhesions. Suprascapular nerve blocks have been performed before shoulder arthroscopy and other orthopedic manipulations of the shoulder as a form of preemptive analgesia so as to minimize postoperative pain. Blockade of the suprascapular nerve alone may provide satisfactory relief in chronic pain syndromes but is usually most effective when given as a series of blocks followed by physical therapy.

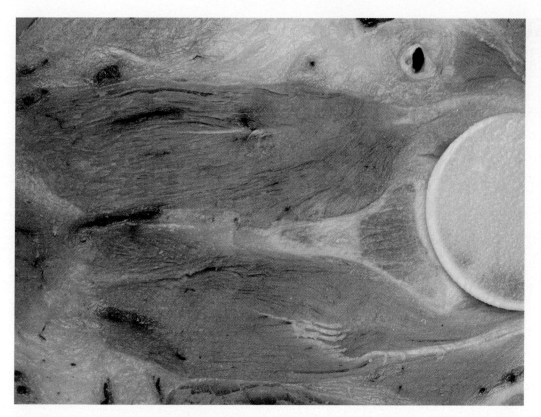

FIG. 36-1 *Transverse anatomic section through the scapula, revealing the suprascapular nerve in the suprascapular notch.*

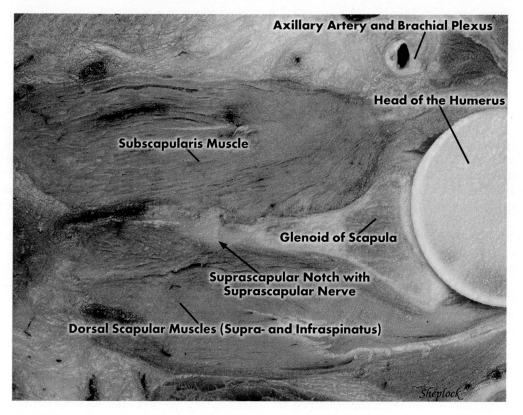

FIG. 36-2 *Corresponding computer-enhanced image of the anatomic section with annotation.*

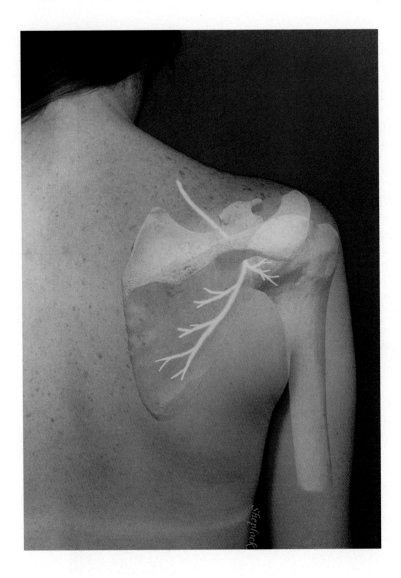

FIG. 36-3 *The scapula and the distributions of the suprascapular nerve superimposed over the surface anatomy.*

Suprascapular nerve block is also used to control severe pain produced by bursitis, tendinitis, and acute periarthritis of the shoulder. In patients with these conditions, the block is usually indicated when local trigger point injections, intraarticular and periarticular injection of steroids have failed to provide adequate pain relief. Suprascapular nerve block may be combined with cervicothoracic sympathetic block (stellate ganglion block) and other conservative measures to deal with resistant shoulder pain that may have a sympathetic nerve origin.

REGIONAL ANESTHETIC TECHNIQUES

Blockade of the suprascapular nerve is performed with the patient in the sitting position. After aseptic preparation of the supraspinous area of the scapula, a 22-gauge needle is inserted 1 to 2 cm superior to the midpoint of the spine of the scapula. The needle is advanced towards the suprascapular notch until a paresthesia is elicited in the affected shoulder. Approximately 10 ml of local anesthetic is usually injected for effective nerve block. Steroid medications may be added when indicated.

To reduce the risk of pneumothorax, the patient can be instructed to place the hand that is ipsilateral to the proposed suprascapular nerve block on the contralateral shoulder. After relocation of the hand, the needle is advanced in an inferior and slightly medial direction until a paresthesia to the shoulder tip is elicited (Fig. 36-4). This relocation of the hand from the anatomic position to the opposite shoulder causes rotation of the scapula away from the posterior chest wall, thus increasing the distance from the suprascapular notch to the chest wall (Figs. 36-5 and 36-6). This maneuver effectively eliminates or at least decreases the incidence of pneumothorax associated with suprascapular nerve blocks. The end point for successful needle placement is the perception of paresthesia to the tip of the shoulder on the side of the block.

SIDE EFFECTS AND COMPLICATIONS

The most serious, although rare, side effect of suprascapular nerve block is pneumothorax. The most common, though innocuous, complication of suprascapular nerve block is fail-

ure to achieve satisfactory postblock analgesia. This failure usually occurs if the local anesthetic is injected into the supraspinatus muscle mass and not in the region of the suprascapular foramen where the nerve emerges. Intravascular injections are also possible, with associated cardiovascular and neurologic complications including hypotension and seizure activity, respectively. These complications may be avoided by meticulous aspiration before injection of the local anesthetic. Muscle atrophy may occur, especially if bupivacaine or deposteroids are inadvertently injected into the muscle. Fortunately the muscle atrophy is not painful, and regeneration is complete after three months.

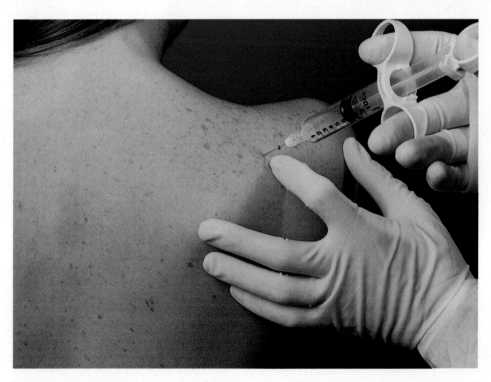

FIG. 36-4 *Blockade of the suprascapular nerve.*

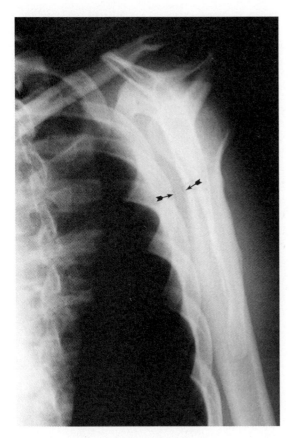

FIG. 36-5 *Oblique radiographic view of the chest with the patient's arm in the anatomic position. Note the close proximity of the scapula to the chest wall.*

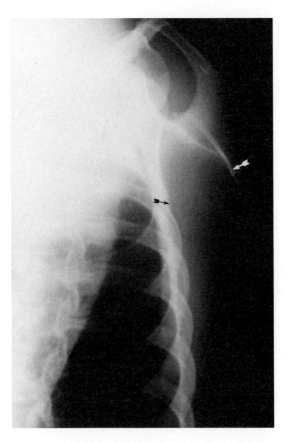

FIG. 36-6 *Oblique radiographic view of the chest, with the patient's arm flexed at the elbow and that hand on the contralateral shoulder. Note the markedly increased distance of the scapula from the chest wall.*

SUGGESTED READINGS

Breen TW, Haigh JD: Continuous suprascapular nerve block for analgesia of scapular fracture, *Can J Anaesth* 37(7):786-788, 1990.

Brown DE, James DC, Roy S: Pain relief by suprascapular nerve block in gleno-humeral arthritis, *Scand J Rheumatol* 17(5):411-415, 1988.

Emery P, Bowman S, Wedderburn L et al: Suprascapular nerve block for chronic shoulder pain in rheumatoid arthritis, *BMG* 299(6707):1079-1080, 1989.

Lee KH, Khunadorn F: Painful shoulder in hemiplegic patients: a study of the suprascapular nerve, *Arch Phys Med Rehab* 67(11):818-820, 1986.

Parris WCV: Suprascapular nerve block: a safer technique, *Anesthesiology* 72:580-581, 1990.

Vecchio PC, Adabajo AO, Hazleman BL: Suprascapular nerve block for persistent rotator cuff lesions, *J Rheumatol* 20(3):453-455, 1993.

CHAPTER 37

Penile Nerve

Linda Jo Rice

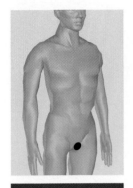

Introduction The penile block provides analgesia for surgical procedures of the glans and shaft of the penis, particularly the distal penis. This block has been found to be of particular use in newborns and children undergoing circumcision, although it is equally effective in older patients.

ANATOMIC RELATIONSHIPS

It is important to remember that the penile nerves are bilateral and adjacent to the midline, lateral to the paired dorsal arteries of the penis (Figs. 37-1 and 37-2). The dorsal nerves are terminal branches of the pudendal nerves (sacral 2, 3, 4). They arise in the pudendal canal, run forward along the ramus of the ischium, then along the margin of the inferior ramus of the pubis. The penile nerves then pass through the gap between the perineal membrane and the inferior pubic ligament, and emerge from under the pubis near the symphysis.

At the base of the penis the penile nerves divide into multiple filaments that encircle the shaft before reaching the glans. The suspensory ligament of the penis merges with the undersurface of the membranous layer of superficial fascia (Fig. 37-3). It then divides inferiorly to form two sides of a triangle fusing with Buck's fascia, which surrounds the penis. The dorsal nerves are covered by Buck's fascia and lie alongside the midline-paired dorsal arteries and vein of the penis, superficial to the corpora.

INDICATIONS

Penile blocks are safe, reliable, and easy to both perform and teach. They can be used as a complete anesthetic or as an adjunct to general anesthesia in pediatric, as well as adult, patients. These blocks are frequently used to provide anesthesia or postoperative analgesia for a variety of surgical procedures involving the glans and shaft of the penis, such as circumcision, laser fulguration of papilloma, or meatotomy.

REGIONAL ANESTHETIC TECHNIQUE

Several approaches exist to blockade of the penile nerves. The most popular are the techniques of dorsal penile nerve block. In the first technique, either a single injection or bilateral injections of local anesthetic are made deep to Buck's fascia, close to the paired nerves (Fig. 37-4). Both nerves may be blocked by one injection, although diffusion of local anesthetic is probably better if two injections are employed. Local anesthetic volumes of 0.5 ml in newborns to 5 ml in adults are employed. To provide adequate diffusion and a satisfactory block, adequate volumes of local anesthetics must be employed.

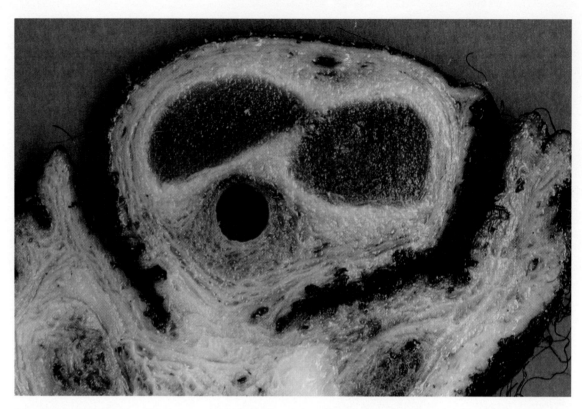

FIG. 37-1   *Cross-section of the penis near the base, revealing the dorsal penile nerves.*

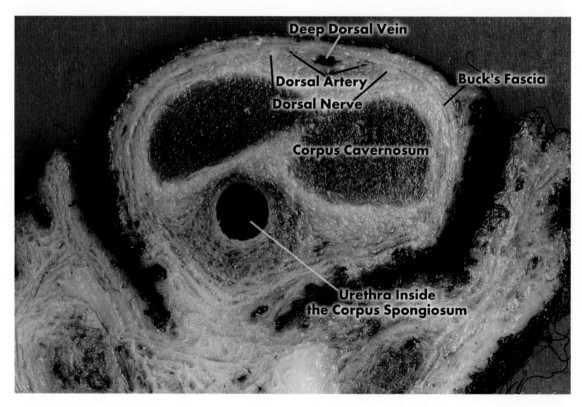

FIG. 37-2   *Corresponding computer-enhanced image of the anatomic section with annotation.*

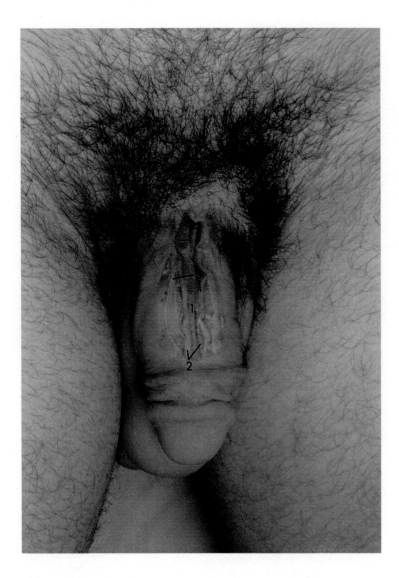

FIG. 37-3 *Dissection of the dorsal penis superimposed over the surface anatomy. Key: 1, deep dorsal vein; 2, dorsal arteries; 3, dorsal nerves.*

A second technique involves palpating the lower border of the symphysis pubis with the index and middle fingers, inserting the needle between them at right angles to the skin until the symphysis is felt (Fig. 37-5). At that point the needle is withdrawn and reinserted just below the symphysis until a "pop" is felt (1 to 5 mm, depending on the age of the patient). Local anesthetic is then injected, in a volume of 0.5 to 5 ml. Epinephrine-containing solutions must never be used to block the penis because vasoconstriction may seriously compromise its circulation.

A similar approach to neural blockade of the dorsal nerves of the penis is the subcutaneous ring block. This block consists of circumferential subcutaneous infiltration of the root of the penis with local anesthetic. It provides effective analgesia for circumcision (Fig. 37-6). A similar block with subcutaneous infiltration of the corona has also been reported.

Topical analgesia has been successfully used to provide analgesia following surgery of the glans penis. Of course, topical analgesia with lidocaine preparations must be performed following amputation of the foreskin, as lidocaine alone will not penetrate the intact skin. Application of lidocaine ointment, jelly, or spray to the exposed mucous membranes of the glans penis following circumcision provides excellent analgesia, equivalent to a more formal dorsal penile nerve block. Applications of topical lidocaine jelly every 6 hours provides significant analgesia during the first 48 hours following circumcision in both children and adults.

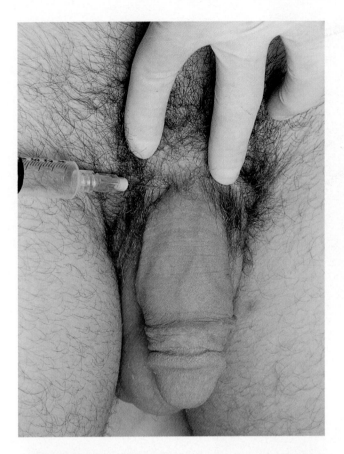

FIG. 37-4 *Blockade of the dorsal penile nerves at the base of the penis.*

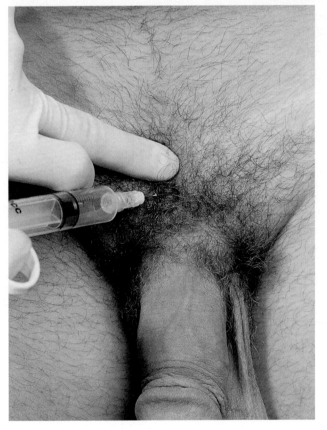

FIG. 37-5 *Blockade of the dorsal penile nerves at the symphysis pubis.*

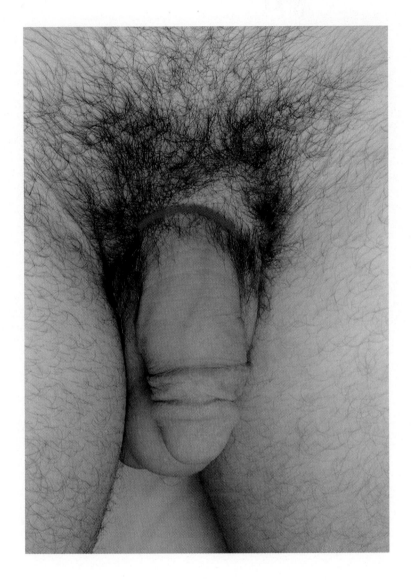

FIG. 37-6   *Ring block of the penis.*

SIDE EFFECTS AND COMPLICATIONS

Potential complications with blockade of the penile nerve include local anesthetic toxicity, although this is almost impossible as the dose of local anesthetic required is so small. However, injection directly into the corpora would provide blood levels of local anesthetic similar to intravascular injection.

Hematoma formation can also cause a problem. Several reports exist of problems with the dorsal penile nerve block technique. It may be technically challenging to place the local anesthetic just below Buck's fascia (not into the corpora) with no trauma to the dorsal vein or arteries. There is a case report of two occurrences of gangrene of the tip of the glans following blocks using this technique; it was postulated that trauma to the dorsal arteries, with ensuing hematoma, in addition to the local anesthetic volume compromised the circulation to the tip of the glans.

Finally, inadvertent use of epinephrine in the local anesthetic solution could be disastrous. A report exists of a 2-day-old who received a dorsal penile nerve block with an epinephrine-containing solution, resulting in profound vasoconstriction and ischemia of the genitalia. A caudal block was employed in this instance to provide a sympathectomy for successful treatment of this complication.

No complication have been reported with the ring block or with topical local anesthesia.

SUGGESTED READINGS

Andersen K: A new method of analgesia for relief of circumcision pain, *Anaesthesia* 44:118-120, 1989.

Benini F, Johnston C, Faucher D et al: Topical anesthesia during circumcision in newborn infants, *JAMA* 270:850-853, 1993.

Berens R, Pontus SP: A complication of circumcision and dorsal nerve of the penis block, *Reg Anesth* 15:309-310, 1990.

Broadman LM, Hannallah RS, Belman AB et al: Post-circumcision analgesia: a prospective evaluation of subcutaneous ring block of the penis, *Anesthesiology* 67:399-402, 1987.

Brown TCK, Weidner NJ, Bouwmeester J: Dorsal nerve of penis block: anatomical and radiological studies, *Anaesth Intens Care* 17:34-38, 1989.

Goulding FJ: Penile block for postoperative pain relief in penile surgery, *J Urol* 126:337, 1981.

Moldwin R, Valderrama E: Nerve distribution patterns within prepucial tissue: clinical applications in penile nerve blocks, *Anesth Analg* 70:S270, 1990.

Sara CS, Lowry CJ: A complication of circumcision and dorsal nerve block of the penis, *Anaesth Intens Care* 13:79-85, 1984.

Tree-Trackarn T, Pirayavaraporn S, Lertakyamanee J: Topical analgesia for relief of post-circumcision pain, *Anesthesiology* 67:95-399, 1987.

CHAPTER 38

Pudendal Nerve

Richard Sheppard

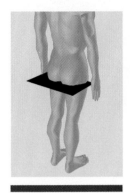

Introduction The pudendal nerve supplies sensation to the pelvic floor and perineum. As such, blockade with local anesthetic can provide pain relief and anesthesia for several therapeutic interventions, including obstetric and malignant syndromes.

ANATOMIC RELATIONSHIPS

The pudendal nerve is formed by the fusion of the second, third, and fourth sacral roots, and passes anterior to the sacral plexus. It then travels inferior to the piriformis muscle, between it and the coccygeus muscle whose gluteal surface is the sacrospinal ligament.

The nerve and the accompanying internal pudendal vessels pass out of the pelvis via the greater sciatic foramen, to pass around the ischial spine and reenter the pelvis through the lesser sciatic foramen by way of the pudendal canal (Figs. 38-1 and 38-2). At the ischial spine the vessels lie over the tip of the spinous process while the nerve lies more medially over the sacrospinal ligament. The nerve also lies more medially within the pudendal canal. The posterior cutaneous nerve of the thigh (S2, S3) lies lateral and posterior to the canal on its way to the buttock.

The pudendal canal is formed from the lateral prolongation of the perianal fascia, which splits and thickens to enclose the neurovascular bundle. It is bordered medially and superiorly by the ischiorectal fossa. Laterally it is boarded by the obturator internus and the ischium.

On entering the pudendal canal, the pudendal nerve is destined to branch into three major divisions: (1) the inferior rectal nerve, (2) the perineal nerve, and (3) the dorsal nerve of the penis or clitoris (Fig. 38-3).

Inferior Rectal Nerve

It is estimated that in nearly one half of individuals the inferior rectal nerve arises from the fusion of the third and fourth sacral roots alone to run anterior to the pudendal canal. In remaining individuals it branches off of the pudendal nerve from within the pudendal canal. Either having pierced the fascia of the canal or lying anterior to the canal, it travels obliquely over the lunate fascia (the cover of the ischiorectal fossa), together with the inferior rectal artery and vein. This neurovascular bundle then courses beneath the levator ani muscle, then downward and medial to its destination. It then divides to

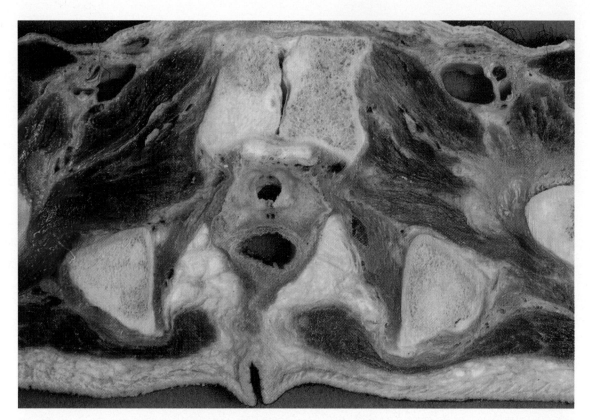

FIG. 38-1 *Transverse anatomic section through the pelvis at the level of the ischial tuberosity, revealing the relationship of the pudendal nerve and related structures.*

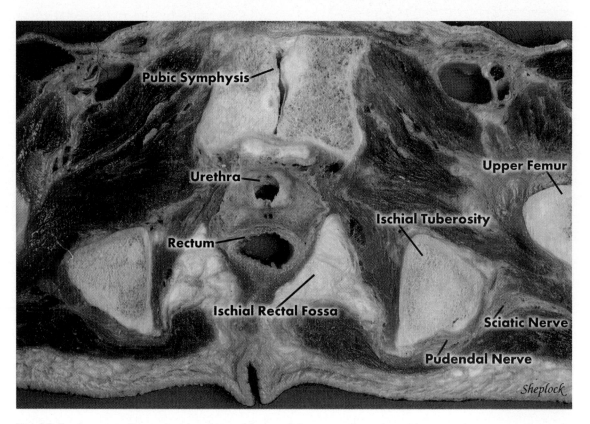

FIG. 38-2 *Corresponding computer-enhanced image of the anatomic section with annotation.*

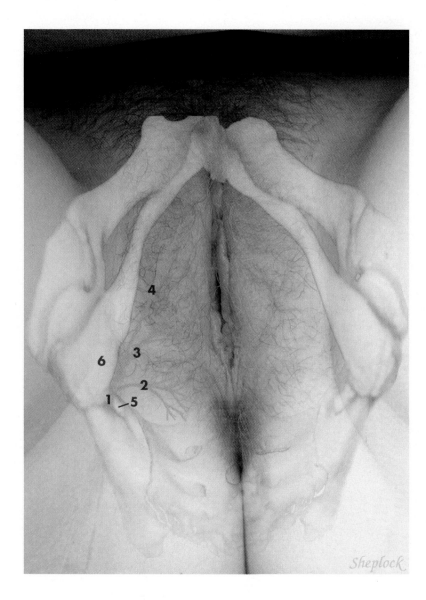

FIG. 38-3 *Distributions of the branches of the pudendal nerve and pelvis superimposed over the surface anatomy. Key: 1, pudendal nerve; 2, inferior rectal nerve; 3, perineal nerve; 4, dorsal nerve of the clitoris; 5, ischial spine; 6, ischial tuberosity.*

supply the profundus and subcutaneous part of the external anal sphincter and perianal skin. It also supplies the middle part of the levator ani muscle.

Perineal Nerve

The perineal nerve is the largest of the terminal branches of the parent nerve. It initially runs forward superficial to the perineal membrane, then pierces the membrane to supply the skin of the posterior two thirds of the scrotum or labia majora and the mucous membranes of the urethra or labia minora. It is the motor supply to the muscles of the urogenital triangle (i.e., ischiocavernosus, bulbospongiosus, superficial and deep trans-

verse perineal, and the sphincter urethrae). It also supplies the anterior part of the levator ani muscle.

Dorsal Nerve of the Penis or Clitoris

The dorsal nerve is the smallest terminal branch of the pudendal nerve, which passes superiorly over the perineal membrane to enter the deep perineal pouch. It pierces the perineal membrane just below the symphysis pubis to run forward to supply all of the skin on the dorsum of penis or clitoris, except for the root or base of the penis, which is supplied by the ilioinguinal nerve (L1). Another nerve that supplies many nearby structures is the perineal branch of S4.

This nerve arises on its own to supply the coccygeus and iliococcygeal muscles on the pelvic surfaces. It also supplies the intermediate (superficialis) part of the external anal sphincter, along with the skin at the anal margin. Sympathetic fibers travel with it to supply the dartos muscle.

INDICATIONS

The pudendal nerve block is usually considered in obstetric patients to provide pain relief during the second stage of labor or to assist in the performance of forceps deliveries.

The pudendal nerve or one of its branches can be affected by metastatic infiltration from local pelvic tumors.

The nerve can also undergo direct damage associated with trauma to the ischial spine due to its close proximity (e.g., straddle injury, horseback riding). Complete pain relief is provided in this instance by blockade of the pudendal nerve.

REGIONAL ANESTHETIC TECHNIQUE

Two techniques are employed to perform a pudendal nerve block: the transperineal and the transvaginal approaches.

Transperineal Approach

The patient is placed in the lithotomy position and the area to be manipulated is prepared in the usual sterile fashion.

A local anesthetic skin wheal is placed approximately 2.5 cm posterior and medial to the ischial tuberosity. Subcutaneous and deeper tissues are then infiltrated. A 22-gauge 8.75-cm needle is then inserted at right angles to the skin. The index finger of the free hand may be placed within the rectum to locate the ischial spine and the sacrospinal ligament to better direct the needle point just posterior to the junction of these two structures.

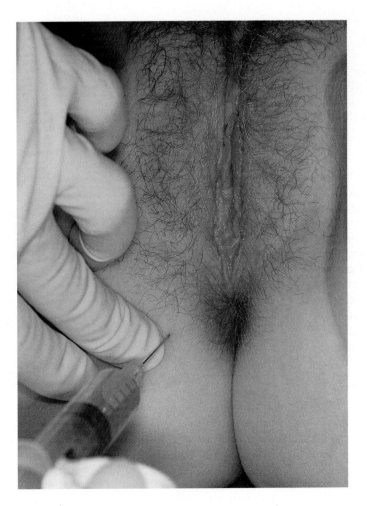

FIG. 38-4 *Blockade of the pudendal nerve via the transperineal approach.*

The needle will pass through the skin and ischiorectal fossa, behind the urogenital diaphragm and levator ani to the ischial spine. The rectal finger should assist in placing the needle posterior to the ischial spine. After careful aspiration to rule out intravascular placement, 5 to 20 ml of local anesthetic is injected just posterior to the ischial spine (Fig. 38-4).

Transvaginal Approach

The patient is again placed in the lithotomy position. The anesthetist's free hand is placed within the vagina to palpate the ischial spine and guide the needle to its correct placement just behind the ischial spine. In this instance the needle is passed to the spine within the vagina, and then through the vaginal wall to the sacrospinal ligament where significant resistance is met on the plunger. A loss of resistance occurs as the needle tip passes through the ligament and the area is then infiltrated after negative aspiration for blood. An Iowa Trumpet is often used as a needle guide within the vagina and also to limit the depth of needle penetration. This technique has a higher success rate, is less painful, and has a lower incidence of complications (Fig. 38-5).

Successful blockade of the pudendal nerve will provide analgesia to the posterior two thirds of the scrotum or labia and part of the buttock.

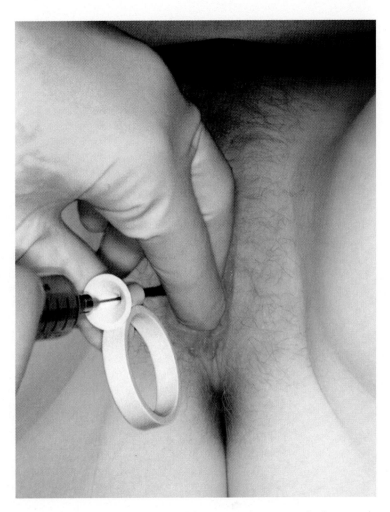

FIG. 38-5 *Blockade of the pudendal nerve via the transvaginal approach.*

SIDE EFFECTS AND COMPLICATIONS

Like any other regional anesthetic technique, the side effects and complications associated with pudendal nerve block are often associated with local anesthetic toxicity. The sciatic nerve may be blocked, but it is less likely if the dose is less than 5 to 10 ml of local anesthetic. The posterior cutaneous nerve of the thigh may be blocked due to its proximity to the pudendal canal. Intravascular injection can be minimized by careful aspiration to rule out intravascular placement of the needle.

SUGGESTED READINGS

Bonica JJ: *The management of pain*, ed 2, Malvern, PA, 1990, Lea and Febiger.

Cousins MJ, Bridenbaugh PO: Neural blockade. In Cousins MJ, Bridenbaugh PO, editors: *Clinical anesthesia and management of pain*, ed 2, Philadelphia, 1988, Lippincott.

Hoerster W, Kreuscher H, Niesel HC et al: *Regional Anesthesia*, ed 2, St. Louis, 1990, Mosby.

Last RJ: *Anatomy: regional and applied*, ed 6, New York, 1978, Churchill Livingstone.

Williams PL, Warwick R: *Gray's anatomy*, ed 36, Philadelphia, 1980, Saunders.

CHAPTER 39

Paracervical Nerve

Winston C. V. Parris

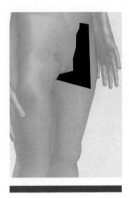

Introduction Before the established popularity of epidural anesthesia for labor and delivery, paracervical block was one of the more frequently used regional techniques administered for analgesia during the first stage of labor. Many reasons existed for this popularity. Paracervical block was a simple technique that was easy to administer both by obstetrician and anesthetist alike. It was successfully administered in approximately 80% of parturient patients, and was safe for the mother and relatively safe for the fetus.

Paracervical block is not usually administered now, mainly because epidural analgesia and natural childbirth methods are more acceptable to both patients and obstetricians. Nevertheless, a limited but distinct place for paracervical nerve blocks in obstetric anesthetic practice exists for patients in whom epidural analgesia is contraindicated or not acceptable by the patient, and also for patients who cannot tolerate natural childbirth techniques.

ANATOMIC RELATIONSHIPS

In order to appreciate the anatomic relationships associated with a paracervical block, it is important to review the anatomy of the female reproductive system. The sensory nerve supply to the uterus originates from T10, T11, T12, and L1, with the major contribution coming from T11 and T12. These afferent pain fibers accompany the sympathetic fibers to the uterus.

Thus pain arising from uterine contraction associated with the first stage of labor is referred to the dermatomes supplied by the same spinal cord segments that receive input from the body of the uterus and the cervix. As labor progresses, the dermatomal spread increases to involve T10 and L1, which are the two adjacent dermatomes. Thus the distribution of pain during the first stage of labor involves the lower three thoracic segments and the upper lumbar segment. Pain in the second and third stages of labor is mediated by the pudendal nerves (S2, S3, and S4) and a block of these nerves eliminates the pain associated with those stages of labor. The pain is essentially confined to structures in the pelvic cavity and includes the bladder, rectum, urethra, and adjacent structures in the perineal area.

Frankenhauser's ganglion, which contains all the visceral sensory nerve fibers from the uterus, cervix, and upper vagina, is located in the lateral fornix of the upper vaginal canal. It is that ganglion or plexus of nerves that is blocked by a paracervical block (Figs. 39-1 and 39-2). Thus a paracervical block essentially may relieve the pain of the first stage of labor but not the second and third stage (Fig. 39-3).

INDICATIONS

Paracervical block is indicated for analgesia associated with the first stage of labor. Repeated nerve blocks are usually required, especially in patients with a long labor, since paracervical block is associated with a limited duration (about 45 to 90 minutes). It is not indicated in second and third stage labor, which is more effectively relieved by either a caudal block or a pudendal nerve block.

Paracervical block should be avoided in prematurity, fetal distress, and uteroplacental insufficiency.

REGIONAL ANESTHETIC TECHNIQUE

Paracervical blockade is performed with the patient in the lithotomy position. Vaginal examination should be performed immediately before the block to determine the precise position of the presenting part. Maternal and fetal vital signs should be determined immediately before the block.

A 12- to 14-cm, 22-gauge needle is used to perform this block. The needle should be inserted with a guard (e.g., an Iowa Trumpet) so that the needle point cannot protrude beyond the guard for more than 5 to 7 mm. This maneuver prevents inadvertent intravascular injection and also prevents damage to the fetal presenting part. The needle is introduced through the submucosa into the lateral vaginal fornix, with the fingers of the examiner's nondominant hand being used to determine the precise location of the needle and to protect the vaginal tissues and the fetal presenting part from inadvertent puncture by the advancing needle. The point of injection of local anesthetic is at the 9 o'clock position and the 3 o'clock position in the lateral vaginal fornix, following negative aspiration (Fig. 39-4). Approximately 5 to 10 ml of the chosen local anesthetic should be used in each fornix for satisfactory paracervical block (Fig. 39-5).

The duration of the analgesia will vary with the local anesthetic, its concentration,

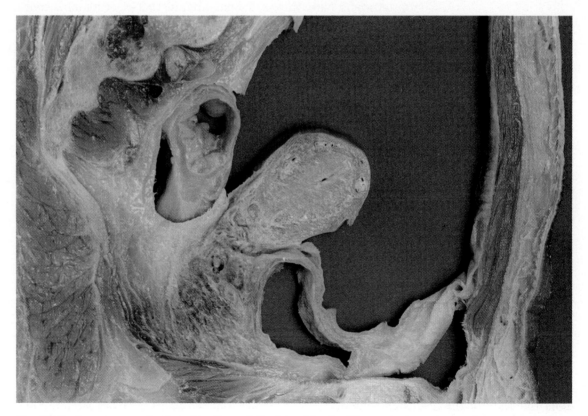

FIG. 39-1 *Transverse anatomic section through the lateral fornix of the vaginal canal, revealing Frankenhauser's ganglion.*

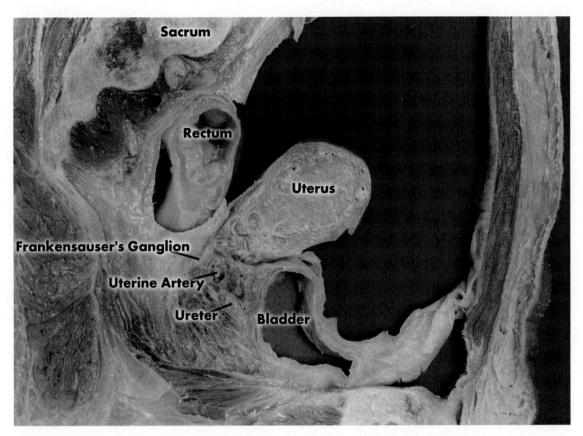

Sacrum

Rectum

Uterus

Frankensauser's Ganglion

Uterine Artery

Ureter   Bladder

FIG. 39-2 *Corresponding computer-enhanced image of the anatomic section with annotation.*

and the total dose used: 0.25% bupivacaine provides 90 to 150 minutes of analgesia; 1% mepivacaine provides 75 to 90 minutes of analgesia; whereas 1% procaine or 2% chloroprocaine provides 40 to 50 minutes of analgesia. The addition of epinephrine in 2.5 mcg/ml concentration may increase the duration of the analgesia by 25%, but may inhibit uterine contractions.

Continuous paracervical block techniques have been used but have not gained widespread acceptance mainly because it is difficult to adequately maintain the tip of the catheter in the correct position. Further, several cases of paracervical hematoma have been associated with continuous techniques, leading to major postdelivery perineal pain as a result of sacral plexus neuropathy.

When performing a paracervical block, fetal heart rate and maternal uterine contractions should be monitored immediately preceding and for some time following the block.

SIDE EFFECTS AND COMPLICATIONS

The major disadvantage associated with paracervical block is the unacceptably high incidence of fetal arrhythmia, the most common problem being bradycardia. Fetal bradycardia can occur within 10 minutes after the performance of the procedure, and its incidence occurs in up to 70% of the cases receiving paracervical block. Paracervical block is also associated with fetal acidosis and neonatal depression. Unexpected fetal death has also been associated with paracervical block when bupivacaine and mepivacaine have been used.

Possible mechanisms of fetal depression following paracervical block include direct depression of the fetal circulation by local anesthetics, uterine arterial vasoconstriction, increase in uterine tone, and mechanical distortion of the uterine vessels.

Paracervical block is associated with failure to produce satisfactory analgesia in

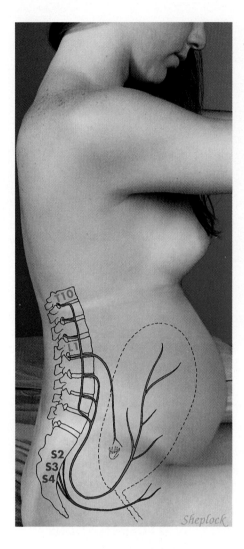

FIG. 39-3 *Sensory input from the uterus and cervix via nerves from the T10, T11, T12, and L1 spinal levels, versus sensory input from the perineum via nerves from the S2, S3, and S4 spinal levels. Distribution of these nerves is superimposed over the surface anatomy.*

FIG. 39-4 *The location of Frankenhauser's ganglion superimposed over the surface anatomy of the cervix and lateral fornix of the vagina.*

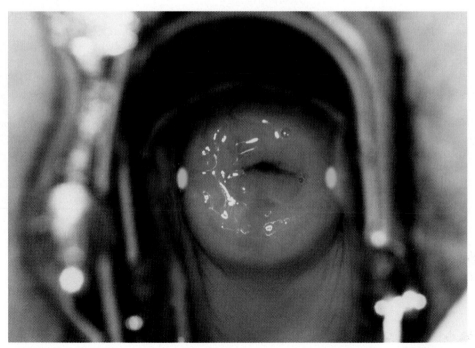

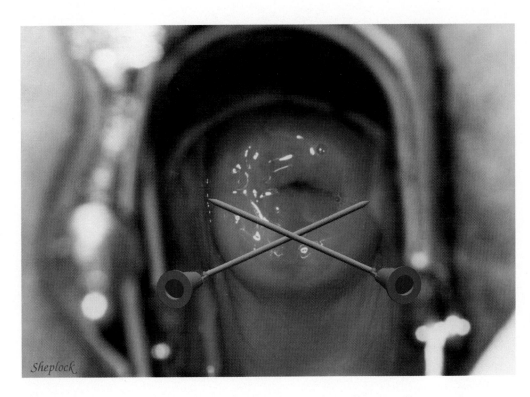

Fig. 39-5 *View of the cervix demonstrating needle placement for paracervical blockade.*

approximately 10% of patients. In the pregnant parturient, systemic toxic reactions including transient sensory disturbances in one or both limbs; damage to the uterine vessels, producing major hematoma, can occur. The hematoma may produce a severe chronic pain syndrome secondary to sacral plexus neuropathy. Postpartum paracervical abscess may occur on rare occasions.

A transient decrease in intensity and/or frequency of uterine contractions could be associated with the local anesthetic, especially when epinephrine is used to perform the block. Unlike epidural and subarachnoid block, paracervical block does not produce perineal anesthesia, which is necessary for the second and third stages of labor. Paracervical block may also inhibit the bearing-down reflex during the first stage of labor.

SUGGESTED READINGS

Goins JR: Experience with mepivacaine paracervical block in an obstetric private practice, *Am J Obstet Gynecol* 167(2):242-344, 1992.

Kangas-Saarela T, Jouppila R, Puolakka J et al: The effect of bupivacaine paracervical block on the neurobehavioural responses of newborn infants, *Acta Anaesthesiol Scand* 32(7):566-570, 1988.

LeFevre ML: Fetal heart rate pattern and postparacervical fetal bradycardia, *Obstet Gynecol* 64(3):343-346, 1984.

Mercado AO, Naz JF, Ataya KM: Postabortal paracervical abscess as a complication of paracervical block anesthesia: a case report, *J Reprod Med* 34(3):247-249, 1989.

Nesheim BI: Which local anesthetic is best suited for paracervical blocks? *Acta Obstet Gynecol Scand* 62(3):261-264, 1983.

Nielsen HK, Klunder K, Moller JT et al: Midazolam combined with paracervical blockade compared to general anaesthesia for curettage of the uterus, *Acta Anaesthesiol Scand* 33(8):643-646, 1988.

Williamson JG: The use of paracervical nerve block anaesthesia in labor, *Ir J Med Sci* 3(12):581-586, 1970.

CHAPTER 40

Transsacral Nerve Root

Jon W. Blank
Cynthia H. Kahn
Carol A. Warfield

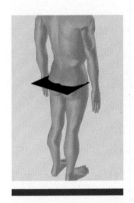

Introduction Transsacral nerve root blockade can play an important role in the diagnosis and treatment of sacral nerve root lesions. The utility of sacral nerve root block is demonstrated in patients with lumbosacral radiculopathy, perineal pain, or bladder dysfunction.

Transsacral nerve root blockade is not commonly used for surgical or obstetrical analgesia, due to the technical difficulty required of the blockade of bilateral multiple nerve roots in those settings.

ANATOMIC RELATIONSHIPS

The sacrum is a triangular wedge of bone composed of five fused sacral vertebrae. The normal S-curve of the vertebral column has its greatest obliquity at the sacrum (see Fig. 40-1). The sacrum is at approximately 40° to 45° from the horizontal plan during upright stance. This obliquity is more pronounced in females than males.

The intervertebral foramen in the sacrum contains the cauda equina, with the filum terminale extending to the base of the coccyx. The anterior and posterior primary rami of the sacral nerve roots exit through the anterior and posterior sacral foramina, respectively (Figs. 40-1 and 40-2). There are three sacral crests, each of which represent the fusion of elements of the sacral vertebrae. The median sacral crest is the fusion of the spinous processes of the first four sacral vertebrae and is a midline, unpaired structure. The dorsal sacral foramina, through which the posterior sacral roots exit the sacrum, are just lateral to a paired series of tubercles, the intermediate sacral crests. These intermediate processes represent the fused articular processes of sacral vertebrae. Lateral to the posterior sacral foramina are the lateral sacral crests, which correspond to the fused transverse processes of the sacral bodies. Thus the depression between the intermediate and lateral sacral crests is the location of the sacral foramina. This depression is often palpable in thin individuals, and can be used as a surface landmark. Overlying the median and intermediate sacral crests are the deep and superficial posterior sacrococcygeal ligaments, which blend laterally with the medial portions of the posterior sacroiliac ligaments.

The sacral canal contains the five paired sacral nerves as they extend caudad to exit through the sacral foramina. The sacral plexus consists of the anterior divisions of the fourth and fifth lumbar and first through third sacral nerves. These nerves course medial to the piriformis muscle and converge toward the lower part of the greater sciatic foramen, where they unite to form the sciatic nerve (Fig. 40-3). The inferior gluteal nerve exists the pelvis through the infrapiriform space to supply the gluteal muscles.

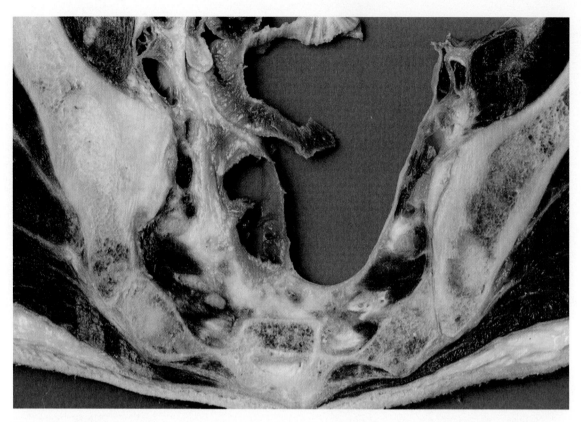

FIG. 40-1   *Transverse anatomic section through the sacrum, revealing the sacral nerves, foramen, and related structures.*

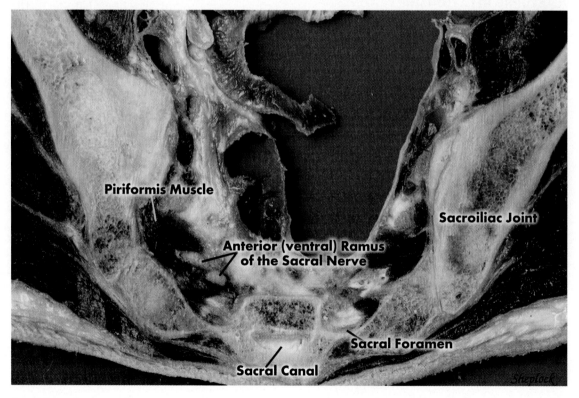

FIG. 40-2   *Corresponding computer-enhanced image of the anatomic section with annotation.*

The pudendal plexus, composed usually of branches of the anterior divisions of second through fifth sacral nerves and the coccygeal nerve, gives rise to the pudendal nerve (see Chapter 38). The third and fourth sacral nerves give sensory innervation to the anorectal region and motor supply to the external anal sphincter, levator ani, and coccygeus muscles through the inferior hemorrhoidal branch of the pudendal nerve. The S2-S4 nerves are the principal sources of visceral innervation to the bladder, urethra, and external genitalia.

The usual articulations of the bony sacrum are to the fifth lumbar vertebra cephalad and to the coccyx caudad. Approximately 10% of patients have "transitional" bony anatomy at the lumbosacral junction. Four to five percent of anatomic specimens have unilateral fusion between the fifth lumbar and first sacral vertebra, with 1% of specimens demonstrating complete fusion of the fifth lumbar vertebral body to the sacrum ("sacralization of L5"). Five to six percent of lumbosacral spines demonstrate an unfused first sacral vertebra, often described as "lumbarization of S1." In these patients the thoracolumbar segment is effectively lengthened, with corresponding increase in mechanical stress on the lower lumbar segments.

It should be noted that marked variability exists in the dorsal anatomy of the sacrum. However, the posterosuperior iliac spine and sacral cornua are helpful surface landmarks. The inferior portion of the posterosuperior iliac spine (PSIS) is at the level between first and second sacral foramina, and indicates the level of the termination of the subarachnoid space. The sacral canal is open at its inferiormost extent as the sacral

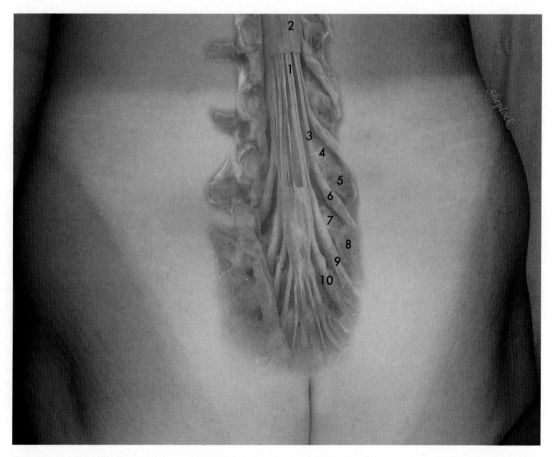

Fig. 40-3 *Dissection of the sacrum and nerve roots with parts of the vertebral arches and meninges removed, superimposed over the surface anatomy. Key: 1, cauda equina; 2, dura mater; 3, roots of fifth lumbar nerve; 4, fourth lumbar intervertebral disk; 5, pedicle of fifth lumbar vertebra; 6, dorsal root ganglion of fifth lumbar nerve; 7, fifth lumbar intervertebral disk; 8, lateral part of the sacrum; 9, root of first sacral nerve; 10, root of second sacral nerve.*

hiatus, and this structure is invariably in line with the median sacral crest. The sacral hiatus represents the incomplete fusion of the laminae of the lowest 1 to 2 sacral segments. Bridged only by ligaments, the bilateral sacral cornua correspond to pedicles and articular processes of the S4 and/or S5 vertebrae. The fourth dorsal foramen, through which the S4 root emerges posteriorly, is lateral to the sacral hiatus.

INDICATIONS

The use of transsacral nerve root blocks can aid in the localization of symptomatic nerve root(s) for patients with lumbosacral radiculopathy. For those patients with back pain and multilevel lumbosacral pathology, transsacral nerve root blocks can aid in diagnosis of the specific nerve roots causing symptoms. By preoperative localization of the specific symptomatic nerve root, successful surgical outcome may be more likely. In addition, antiinflammatory therapy with injected steroids at the site of the involved root may alleviate the pain and obviate the need for invasive surgery.

Transsacral nerve root block may be of benefit in management of intractable perineal or suprapubic pain. As an alternative to intrathecal neurolysis, transsacral nerve root block is associated with a lower incidence of prolonged incontinence and loss of motor function.

Urinary bladder dysfunction is another clinical scenario where transsacral nerve root block can play an important role. The spinal centers of micturition are subserved by sacral nerves 2 to 4. Usually, the S3 or S4 root is most responsible for control of the muscles of micturition. Selective transsacral nerve root blockade can identify the dominant nerve root. After diagnosis, treatment with local anesthetic may provide relief of bladder dysfunction caused by detrusor instability or severe urge incontinence not remedied by other means. If local anesthetic alone is insufficient for prolonged relief, transsacral nerve root block with neuroablative agents such as phenol or cryoneurolysis can be performed.

In the obstetric suite or for surgical analgesia, transsacral nerve root block is seldom the regional technique of choice. Since few surgical procedures are performed in a single dermatomal region, multiple blocks would be required for appropriate anesthesia. Furthermore, successful blockade may be difficult without the use of radiographic imaging. Thus time and equipment constraints mitigate against the use of transsacral blockade in the surgical or obstetric environment.

REGIONAL ANESTHETIC TECHNIQUE

Due to the variability of sacral anatomy, use of radiographic correlation is recommended. The anatomic landmarks of note are the PSIS superiorly and the paired sacral cornu inferiorly. In thin individuals it is often possible to palpate the sacral foramina as a depression in the sacrum approximately 10 to 15 mm lateral to the midline (Fig. 40-4).

The patient is placed prone, with the hips slightly rotated internally to relax the gluteal muscles. A pillow placed under the iliac crests facilitates exposure. The PSIS and sacral cornu are identified. The S1 foramen is located approximately 1 cm medial to the PSIS, while the S2 foramen is 1 cm medial and 1 cm inferior to the PSIS. The S4 foramen is immediately lateral and just superior to the sacral cornu. The S3 foramen is located midway between S2 and S4 foramina. The S5 root is 1 to 2 cm caudad to the S4 foramen, below the level of the sacral cornu. It is important to confirm landmarks and foramen location radiographically.

A skin wheal using local anesthetic is made with a 25-gauge needle before placement of a 8.75 cm, 22-gauge spinal needle. The needle is inserted perpendicular to the skin until it contacts periosteum. The angle of the needle is the adjusted slightly medial and cephalad until the posterior sacral foramen is entered. Because of the wedge-shaped sacral anatomy, the distance between anterior and posterior sacral foramina decreases from S1 to S4 foramina. There is approximately 2.5 cm distance at S1, decreasing to approximately 0.5 cm interforaminal distance at S4. The depth of needle insertion as it passes from posterior to anterior sacral foramen should reflect this distance (Fig. 40-5). Radiographic correlation should confirm placement of the needle tip at the anterior border of the sacrum, in the anterior sacral foramen.

If paresthesia is elicited, adjust the needle placement slightly. If aspiration of the needle for blood or CSF is negative, a total of 1 to 2 ml of local anesthetic agent (1% lidocaine or 0.5% bupivicaine) is instilled. The local anes-

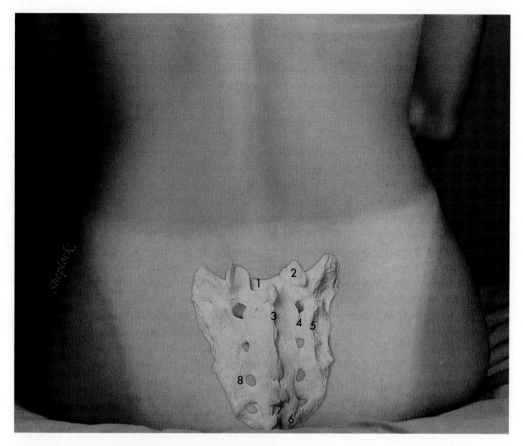

FIG. 40-4 *Image of the sacrum superimposed over the surface anatomy. Key: 1, sacral canal; 2, superior articular process; 3, median sacral crest; 4, intermediate sacral crest; 5, lateral sacral crest; 6, sacral cornu; 7, sacral hiatus; 8, third dorsal sacral foramen.*

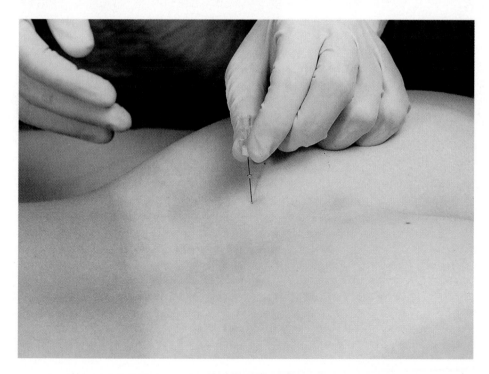

FIG. 40-5 *Blockade of the second sacral nerve with the patient in the prone position and the needle redirected into the sacral foramen.*

thetic may be mixed with steroid (25 to 40 mg of triamcinolone or 25 mg of methylprednisolone). For radiographic correlation, 1 ml of radiocontrast agent may be injected as well. Radiographic evidence of appropriate needle position is especially important for neurolytic block (1 to 2 ml 6% phenol) (Fig. 40-6).

SIDE EFFECTS AND COMPLICATIONS

Injection into false passages or improper sites is possible because of the variable anatomy of the sacrum. Because of the close approximation of the sacral hiatus to the fourth dorsal foramen, inadvertent caudal block is sometimes performed when attempting an S4 root block. Transient pain due to needle placement or sensory disturbance due to block of the posterior primary ramus of the sacral root may occur, as may block of the perineal branches within the anterior division. Theoretic risks include bowel or bladder incontinence, impotence, and subarachnoid injection. As with other needle techniques, needle fracture, local infection, and hematoma are also potential risks.

SUGGESTED READINGS

Awad SA, Flood HD, Acker KL: Selective sacral cryoneurolysis in the treatment of patients with detrusor instability/hyperreflexia and hypersensitive bladder, *Neurol Urodynamics* 6:307, 1987.

Clark AJ, Awas SA: Selective transsacral nerve root blocks, *Reg Anesth* 15:125, 1990.

Cousins MJ, Bridenbaugh PO: *Neural blockade in clinical anesthesia and management of pain*, Philadelphia, 1988, Lippincott.

Hollinshead WH and Rosse C: *Textbook of anatomy*, Philadelphia, 1985, Harper & Row.

Robertson DH: Transsacral neurolytic nerve block: an alternative approach to intractable perineal pain, *Br J Anesth*.

Simon DL, Carron H, Rowlingson J: Treatment of bladder pain with transsacral nerve block, *Anesth Analg* 61:46, 1982.

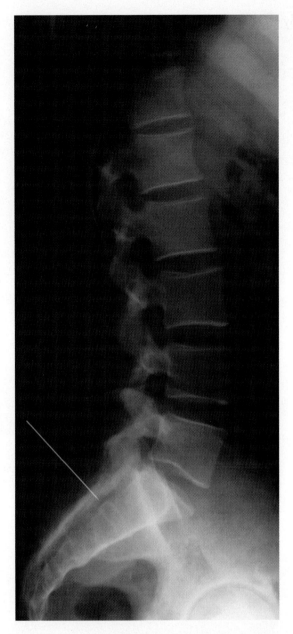

FIG. 40-6 *Lateral radiograph demonstrating proper needle placement for blockade of a sacral nerve root at the S2 foramen.*

CHAPTER 41

Lumbar Spinal Nerve Root

Cynthia H. Kahn
Jon W. Blank
Carol A. Warfield

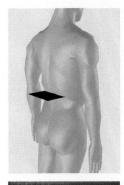

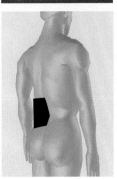

Introduction Lumbar somatic nerve root blocks can be used in conjunction with intercostal nerve blocks to provide anesthesia for surgery of the lower abdomen and upper portion of the lower extremity. The blocks can also serve as important diagnostic and therapeutic aids in the evaluation and treatment of low back pain syndromes.

ANATOMIC RELATIONSHIPS

At each of the five lumbar levels, the ventral motor and dorsal sensory roots combine to form a mixed nerve. These mixed nerves exit their respective intervertebral foramina and diverge as ventral and dorsal rami (Figs. 41-1, 41-2, 41-3, and 41-4). The dorsal ramus innervates the paraspinous muscles and zygapophyseal (facet) joint of each intervertebral level. The lumbar nerve also carries fibers of the lumbar sympathetic system, via the gray and white rami communicantes, at the anterolateral aspect of the lumbar vertebral bodies (Fig. 41-5). The ventral lumbar nerve roots traverse the psoas muscle and continue in the fascial plane between psoas and quadratus lumborum. It is at this juncture that a neural plexus is formed (see Fig. 19-3). This plexus consists of the ventral divisions of L1-L4 (and frequently receives contributions from T12 and occasionally L5). The peripheral nerves derived from the lumbar plexus provide sensory and motor innervation to the lower abdomen and legs. The iliohypogastric and ilioinguinal nerves (L1) supply the lower abdominal wall. Inferomedial sensory information is conveyed by the genitofemoral nerve (L1-L2). The lower extremity is supplied by the lateral femoral cutaneous (L2, L3), femoral (L2-L4), and obturator (L2-L4) nerves (Fig. 41-6).

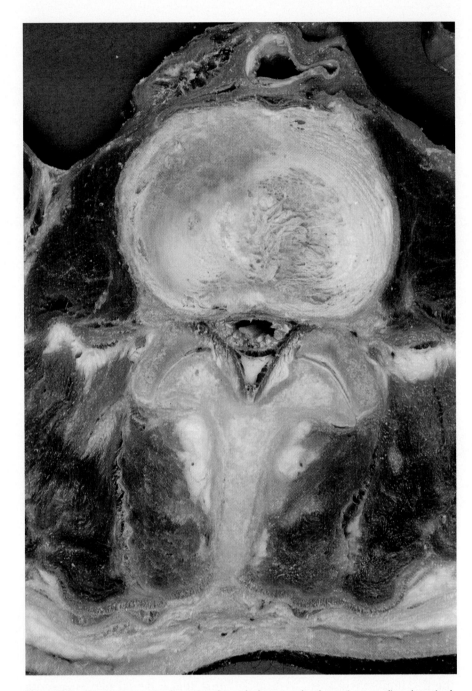

FIG. 41-1 *Transverse anatomic section through the upper lumbar spine revealing the spinal cord, lumbar nerve, and related structures.*

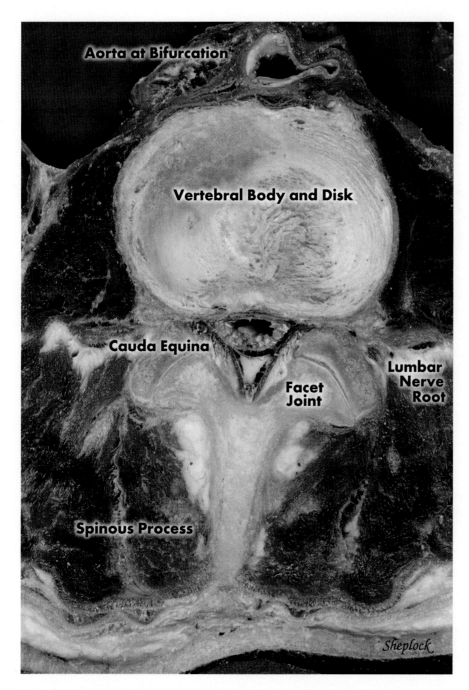

Fig. 41-2 *Corresponding computer-enhanced image of the anatomic section with annotation.*

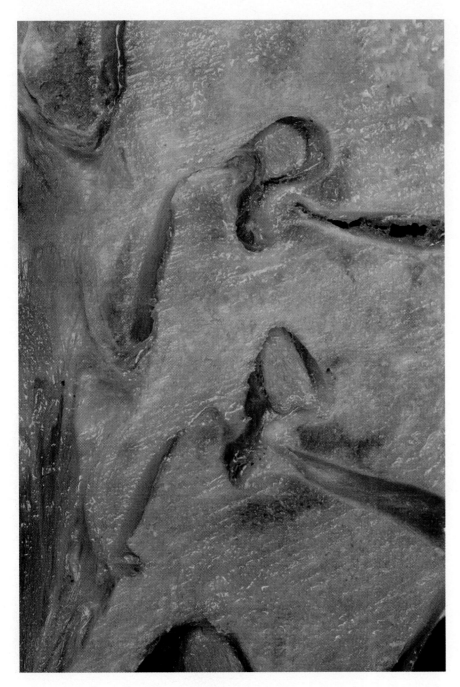

FIG. 41-3 *Parasagittal anatomic section through the lumbar spine, revealing the facet joints, lumbar nerve roots, and related structures.*

Effective blockade of selective lumbar nerve roots is facilitated by understanding the anatomic relationships of the root as it exits the intervertebral foramen. The lumbar nerve root angles caudad and immediately passes anterior to the lateral border of the transverse process of the vertebral body below (Fig. 41-7). The spinous process of each lumbar vertebra is at the midline in patients without spinal deformity. The transverse process of each vertebral body extends 3 to 4 cm lateral to the most cephalad portion of the corresponding vertebral body. The iliac crests usually lie at the level of the L4 spinous process (see Fig. 30-2). Orientation based on these landmarks assists positioning in preparation for neural blockade. Confirmation can be achieved radiographically.

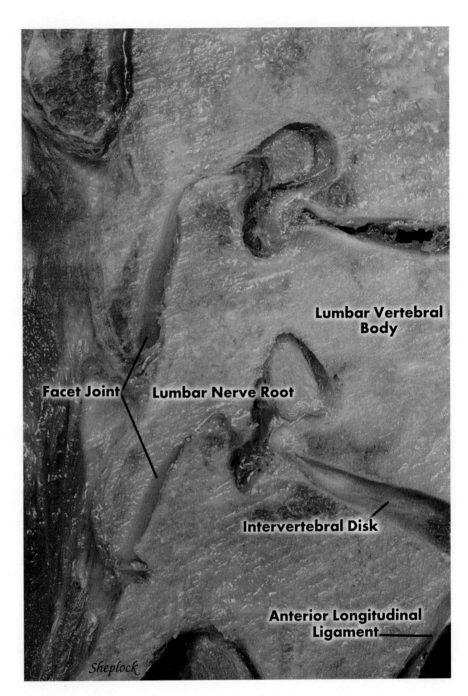

Lumbar Vertebral Body

Facet Joint   **Lumbar Nerve Root**

Intervertebral Disk

Anterior Longitudinal Ligament

Sheplock

FIG. 41-4 *Corresponding computer-enhanced image of the anatomic section with annotation.*

INDICATIONS

Surgical indications for lumbar somatic blocks include procedures performed on the upper leg or lower abdomen when used in conjunction with intercostal nerve blocks. For example, inguinal herniorrhaphy has been successfully undertaken after blockade of the T12-L2 nerve roots. Use of lumbar somatic nerve blockade, accompanied by lower intercostal blockade, has also been used in patients undergoing lithotripsy.

Lumbar somatic blocks are of particular benefit in the diagnosis of low back pain syndromes. The blocks can aid in localization of the pathologic lesion and thus confirm the desired operative level for the surgeon. Their utility is especially noteworthy for patients with multilevel disk pathology, spondylolisthesis and/or spondylolysis, "hip-spine syndrome," spinal stenosis, and for diagnosis in those patients who have undergone previous spine surgery.

In some cases surgery can be avoided altogether. Some patients obtain significant symptomatic relief after selective lumbar nerve root blockade with local anesthetic, steroids, or a combination of the two agents. In these cases, the selective lumbar nerve root blockade provides both diagnostic and therapeutic benefit.

REGIONAL ANESTHETIC TECHNIQUE

Two commonly used approaches to lumbar somatic nerve root blockade have been described. One is performed with the patient in the prone position, the other with the patient in the lateral position.

For the prone patient, it is helpful to place a pillow under the patient's abdomen to increase the lumbar intervertebral space.

After sterile preparation of the skin, the lumbar spinous processes are identified. Using the spinous processes as a landmark, a line is drawn from the most cephalad portion of the process laterally. The transverse process is located 3 to 4 cm lateral to the midline along this line.

To determine the lumbar vertebral level, it is helpful to draw a line connecting the superior aspect of each iliac crest. This line is at the L4-L5 interspace or the L4 spinous process. Using the L4 spinous process, the cephalad and caudad lumbar spinous processes may then be counted and marked. Confirmation of the desired lumbar level can be achieved by placing a radiopaque marker at the expected level and obtaining radiographic correlation.

The skin and subcutaneous tissues are anesthetized with 1 to 3 ml of local anesthetic via a 25- or smaller gauge needle. A 8- to 10-cm, 22-gauge needle is then introduced perpendicular to the skin, 3 to 4 cm ipsilater-

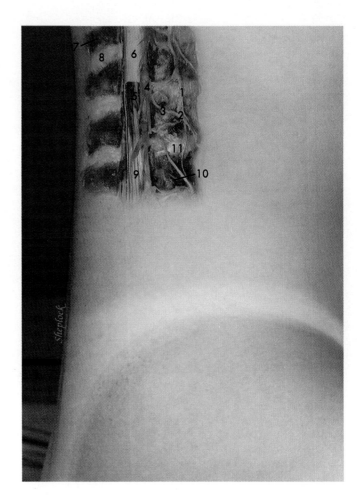

FIG. 41-5 *Dissection of the spine viewed from the right with parts of the vertebral arches and meninges removed to reveal the rami communicantes and related structures, superimposed over the surface anatomy. Key: 1, sympathetic trunk; 2, sympathetic ganglion; 3, rami communicantes; 4, dorsal root ganglia of the first lumbar nerve; 5, spinal cord; 6, dura mater; 7, spinous process of the twelfth thoracic vertebra; 8, interspinous ligament; 9, cauda equina; 10, body of the third lumbar vertebra; 11, intervertebral disk.*

al to the spinous processes at the desired nerve root level. At a depth of 3 to 5 cm, the transverse process should be identified. Once the transverse process is contacted by the tip of the needle, the needle is retracted and redirected slightly caudad. The needle is then "walked off" the transverse process (Fig. 41-8). The nerve root is 1 to 2 cm anterior to the lateral aspect of the transverse process. The patient may note pain in the nerve root distribution (Fig. 41-6).

An alternate method is to place the patient either prone or with the affected side uppermost. A small pillow placed under the patient's flank, extending from iliac crest to costal margin, increases the lumbar intervertebral spaces and facilitates needle placement. The spinous process of the desired level is identified as previously described for the prone position block, and a skin wheal of local anesthetic is made 10 cm ipsilaterally and just cephalad to the transverse process. One to three ml of local anesthetic is infiltrated into the subcutaneous tissues. A 8- to 10-cm, 22-gauge needle is introduced under fluoroscopic guidance at a 45° angle to the sagittal plane, and advanced to the intervertebral foramen (Fig. 41-9). Paresthesia in the lumbar nerve root distribution may result (Fig. 41-6).

For both techniques, confirmation of proper needle placement may be undertaken using 1 ml of radiocontrast dye to visualize the nerve root (Fig. 41-10). Before injection of the dye, it is necessary to aspirate through the needle to ensure absence of blood or CSF. If severe pain is elicited and injection of the agent is difficult, intraneural injection must be suspected and the needle repositioned. After injection of radiocontrast agent through a properly placed needle, radiographic imaging will demonstrate a clear outline of the nerve root. If radiographic imaging reveals only a localized collection of dye, the needle must be repositioned before performance of the block.

Once satisfactory needle position has been achieved by either technique, 1 to 2 ml of local anesthetic with our without steroid may be injected in those patients undergoing diagnostic or therapeutic block for low back pain. Patient response to blockade should be assessed by provocative testing. A good test is to have the patient undertake a motion or series of actions that had previously resulted in pain or discomfort.

When the selective nerve root block is used for the provision of surgical anesthesia, the volume of local anesthetic agent injected should be 5 to 7 ml at each level. As with any block, the anesthetist must ensure that the volume of local anesthetic injected does not exceed the recommended dosage limit for the patient.

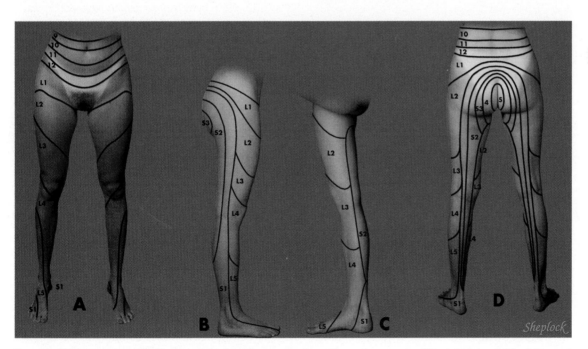

FIG. 41-6 *Dermatome distribution of the lumbar nerves viewed from the anterior (**A**), right lateral (**B**), right medial (**C**), posterior (**D**) aspects.*

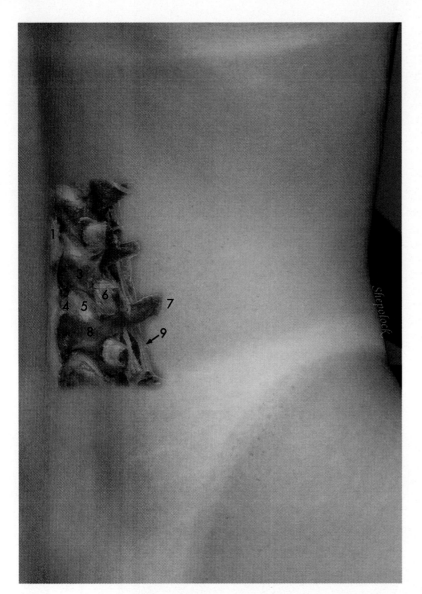

FIG. 41-7 *Dissection of the lumbar spine, demonstrating the relationship of the transverse processes and nerve roots superimposed over the surface anatomy from a posterior oblique view. Key: 1, supraspinous ligament; 2, spinous process of the fourth lumbar vertebra; 3, lamina of the fourth lumbar vertebra; 4, interspinous ligament; 5, ligamentum flavum; 6, facet (zygapophysial) joint; 7, transverse process of the fifth lumbar vertebra; 8, lamina of the fifth lumbar vertebra; 9, fifth lumbar nerve root.*

SIDE EFFECTS AND COMPLICATIONS

Radiographic confirmation of appropriate needle placement is recommended before performing lumbar somatic nerve root blockade. For those patients with an allergy to radiocontrast dye, it is still advisable to use radiography (without dye) to visualize needle position in relation to the bony structures. Improper positioning of the needle can result in subarachnoid, epidural, or intraneural injection. Severe pain in the distribution of the nerve root that increases with injection will occur with intraneural injection. If the needle is advanced beyond the transverse process, it is possible to induce sympathetic ganglion blockade. This is more likely if a larger volume of local anesthetic was used for the attempted lumbar nerve root block. Symptoms of sympathetic blockade include flushing or increased surface temperature of the ipsilateral lower extremity and a subjective sensation of warmth in the limb. Other theoretic risks include infection, CSF leak, nerve root laceration, hematoma formation, and damage to intraperitoneal hollow or solid viscus. With the use of radiographic imaging, such complications are unlikely to occur.

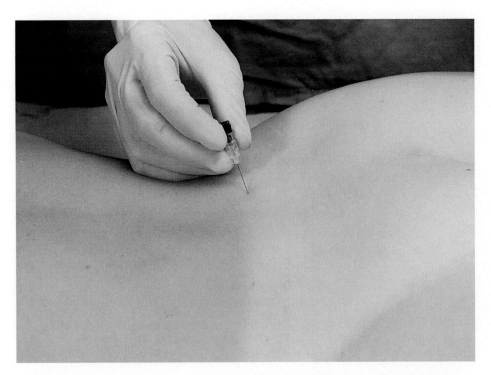

FIG. 41-8 *Blockade of the fourth lumbar nerve root with the patient in the prone position and the needle "walked off" the corresponding transverse process.*

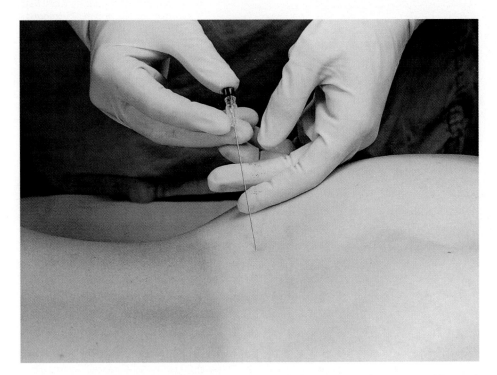

FIG. 41-9 *Blockade of the fifth lumbar nerve root with the patient in the prone position and the needle advanced toward the intervertebral foramen.*

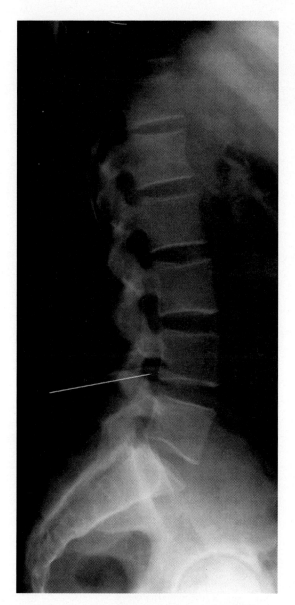

FIG. 41-10 *Lateral radiograph demonstrating proper needle placement for lumbar nerve root blockade at the L4 foramen.*

SUGGESTED READINGS

Cousins MJ, Bridenbaugh PO: *Neural blockade in clinical anesthesia and management of pain,* ed 2, Philadelphia, 1988, JB Lippincott.

Dooley JF, McBroom RJ, Taguchi T et al: Nerve root infiltration in the diagnosis of radicular pain, *Spine* 13:79, 1988.

Haueisen DC, Smith BS, Myers SR et al: Diagnostic accuracy of spinal nerve injection studies, *Clin Orthop* 198:179, 1985.

Herron LD: Selective nerve root block in patient selection for lumbar surgery: surgical results, *J Spinal Disord* 2:75, 1989.

Jonsson B, Stromqvist B, Annertz M et al: Diagnostic lumbar nerve root block, *J Spinal Disord* 1:232, 1988.

Krempen JF, Smith BS: Nerve root injection, *J Bone Joint Surg* 56:1435, 1974.

Stanley D, MacLaren MI, Euinton HA et al: A prospective study of nerve root infiltration in the diagnosis of sciatica: a comparison with radiculopathy, computed tomography, and operative findings, *Spine* 15:546, 1990.

Quinn SF, Murtagh, Chatfield R et al: CT-guided nerve root block and ablation, *Am J Radiol* 151:1213, 1988.

Tajima T, Furukawa K, Kuramochi E: Selective lumbosacral radiculography and block, *Spine* 5:68, 1980.

van Akkerveeken PF: Diagnostic value of nerve root sheath infiltration, *Acta Orthopaed Scand* Suppl 251(64):61, 1993.

INDEX

Page numbers followed by i *indicate illustrations;* t *indicates tables.*